Most phenomena, physical problems, mental problems, and social problems

and how to solve them

Talent
Outliers
Belief system
Natural learning
Autism - ADHD

***

Stress
Meditation
Depression
Fibromyalgia
Pain management

***

Mindfulness
Natural healing
Self-healing
Metabolic disorders
Autoimmune disease

AWAKEN YOU WONDERFUL WE

How do we create heaven on earth?
The secret of the one - page table reveals the real causes of most phenomena and problems

VAN DUY DAO

Awaken parents – the conversation of the old

Is autism, depression, obesity, mastery, outliers, talent, ADHD, poor learning, stress, chronic illnesses, abilities, seizures, diabetes, cancer, hypertension, autoimmune diseases, violence or PTSD born or created by a continuous and stoppable process? What is the role of the environment? And how can we master it?

Facts about health and natural healing:

"It is the deep breathing, not the smoke, makes people lose weight. It is the diaphragm breath, not the smoke, to reduce the rate of getting Parkinson's disease. The obvious fact is the deep breathing by the mouth of the smokers can reduce the rate of getting Parkinson's disease."

"Why laughing has good effects on health? Happiness and moving all organs in the stomach. It is like to make all the organs in the stomach upsidedown. If we make the fake laugh, we do not get the result as the real laugh. If we just feel joy but not laughing, we do not get a good impact on health as a real laugh."

The key for most chronic illnesses, stress and flu may lie in the "Keto flu". Keto flu used to describe the side effects of having a keto diet to reduce weight, the diet has limited Glucid. The fat man may have keto flu in the first week of having a keto diet, he may have all symptoms like flu symptoms but he does not have flu. The symptoms of the flu that the man on the keto diet has are the results of the hunger cells and hunger organs of the whole body. These hunger cells do not have enough glucose for the energy source. The hunger of the billion cells in the body make the man have the signs live the flu-signs. All of these flu-like signs will be removed by just several cups of sugar juice!

The common advice for all health problems is having suitable exercise and having the right diet. Baking soda, papaya, fruits, vitamins, minerals, alternative therapies, and traditional medicine also play an important role in dealing with these diseases. If there are a lot of trigger points or blocking points around the vessels, it will make the distribution of the glucose and oxygen in the body disorder. On the other hand, there are many sensors of the autonomic nervous system that lie along the vessels in the head, liver, legs, hands and all other organs to have the autonomic responses to maintain balanced homeostasis. The chronic trigger points will create longterm changes in the homeostasis and make the autonomic nervous system out of balance. To some extent, traditional therapies, suitable diets, and alternative therapies seem to be effective for treating some chronic diseases because these therapies help to remove trigger points. There are some Vietnamese Qigong exercises to remove trigger points and remove many chronic symptoms in just 10 to 30 minutes of practicing.

We all know that millions of other healthy kids:

• "You do not need to teach healthy kids to learn any of these languages: English, Japanese, Chinese, and Vietnamese... but kids can make it become their native language with the language of the land they grow. That is the nature of learning without learning, Kid under three years old never have to sit at the table to learn, but they learn naturally every time with joy"

• "Nature of learning is learning without stress, learn just with joy, enthusiasm, love, curiosity, endless energy, and participate in all senses. The environment just supplies Unconditioned Love, Connection – Understanding, Encouraging Environment, and Chances of Building Abilities."

• "Walking, thinking, speaking native languages, studying countless skills, one-year-old kids, two-year-old kids, three-year-old kids never have to sit at a table to learn. But these kids can learn more than anybody can imagine. Think about that before any blind intervention."

- "Playing is learning, watching is learning, sleeping is learning, and doing is learning… Kids may experience "Flow" from the early stage of life. Kids' most powerful tools are the weakness, beloved, cute, enthusiasm, attention, curiosity, asking, imagining, and learn, try, fail, think, learn, try, fail, think, learn, try, fail, think with Joy and safety. Think about that before each time of intervention."

- "Best for kids: accept we may wrong to create more chances for kids to grow naturally. Socrates was smart because he said he did not know anything. I feel cramp of gut feelings when seeing the parents of kids with lots of problems said they know all things and start to blame all things except themselves for their problems."

But why many of our angels: "They live in stress, eating in fear, sleeping in anxiety, playing in the boring safe side, wearing luxury clothes in discontentment, studying with pressure, getting lifesaving vaccination with hysterical doubt, and sexing with contempt. They never find real joy and happiness. Stress chemical: Adrenalin, noradrenalin, and cortisone can create countless side effects on patients, which listed in all medical books."

Value of character, the adjective used to describe the character and the adverb form use to describe the pattern of the behaviors that people have: Discontented men react to good unwanted things discontentedly.

"Contented man has conditioned responses to response contentedly to any unwanted things, problems and challenges. He has ADJECTIVE character means he has conditioned his responses to things ADJECTIVELY."

- "Contented men are happy, joyful and hopeful when seeing a rose in the bushes of thorns"

- "Discontented men maybe angry or upset when seeing bushes of roses have a thorn."

- "Worst of all, he is intelligent but corrupted. It means, in spite of countless regulations, he finishes well the corrupted works so intelligently that no one can realize until a hundred years later."

Then:

- "The ignorant stressed world: The world is spending half of it money: $ thousand billion on buying the weapon for finding safety, certainty, and peace; and they spend $ thousand billion on fashion, luxury products, cars, villas for find the feeling of significance, recognition, importance. Then they spend other $ trillions on drugs and healthcare with the hope of sleeping well, relaxing, relieving, and enjoying the temporary comfort, and artificial happiness?"

Reminding of Zen masters:

- "Just remember the moment of doing good to each other, the acts of kindness, respectfulness and trust, which are described by positive adjectives or positive adverbs, all will going to sleep easily, happily, and peacefully."

I love you

I am sorry

Please forgive me

Thank you!

ALL IN ONE, ONE IN ALL:

Dear Neurologist, psychiatrist, sociologist, gastroenterologist, urologist, educators, sleep therapists, cardiologist, language therapists, educators, trainers and teachers: there is no separation in the health of heart, stomach, muscle, cognitive thinking, sleeping, hormones system: all are interdependent in the interdependent world and all are under the state of mind.

PARETO IN HEALTHCARE

Remember when working with the mind: irrational mind, the giant brain evolved for millions of years, illogical mind and Placebo effects, Neuro-plasticity, Mirror neurons, affirmation, self-talk, nocebo effects, T1/2 or half-life of all substances, taboos, rituals, religious belief, compound effects, conditioned responses, and magical adaptability, illusive mind, self-healing or self-destroying, irrational thinking, Subliminal message, marketing of luxury brand, benefit of expensive products, and Hysteria. Remember the question of the old: "What do we feed our mind every day?" And what if all of foods of mind lead to negativity or positivity? Maybe Outliers or Failures!

This book is dedicated to

My mother, Muot T. Nguyen, my fathers: Dung D. Dao and Thinh N. Duc, my wife, Hoa N. T. Kieu, and my children: Khang, Khai, whom I learn the most and motivate me the most to write the book.

I want to say thank all the authors, speakers, teachers who give me invaluable materials, proofs, citations, references, and instructions to write this book directly and indirectly. I really appreciate and want to say thank them all. I thank the authors listed on the references in this book. Their works, teachings, and findings have shaped my mind.

I also want to say thank all my teachers, friends, colleagues, brothers, and sisters because of their work, their supports have shaped my mind.

I want to thank the Vietnamese government has to support invaluable chances for me to work, study, and access to advanced knowledge with an incredibly cheap price.

Best of all, I want to thank you :_____
(Your name)

You are the readers chose to participate with me on the way to help the needed people. You are my greatest inspiration for me to finish the work. And I know that together we can help more, because:

Awaken you, wonderful we
Awaken you, wonderful world.

You are approved for fair use of any part which less than 1000 words.

If you make profits from the material, I am grateful if you donate any part of it to one of these sites with the subject: "Awaken You Wonderful We"

- Charitable organizations in countries around the world.

- Charitable organizations in Vietnam to help the needed students advised by Professor Ngo Bao Chau.

- Vietnam Association for Victims of Agent Orange/dioxin – VAVA from http://vava.org.vn

Hanoi, 26/09/2017
Van Duy Dao

Thank you, these are some of the feedbacks:

Thank you Van, your words are true. We need healing now. True love is expressed in action and how we live. True love is unconditional. Without expectation or desire, or craving.

You are an amazing healer and have such deth of knowledge in naturel medicine and understanding of the human body and energy systems. More than anyone I know. I appreciate you and all of your work and for helping to kee everything on the right path.

Alex Valdes

Interesting information from a Vietnamese health practitioner. You may already know that hospital personnel will "pound" the chest in specific ways to assist in removing phlegm and other toxins from the lungs?

Well, it seems that in Vietnam this is performed as part of very important "self-care" to relieve lungs of toxins for example... tobacco resin, residue from a viral infection, inhales smoke, etc... The instructions need to be read carefully before self-treatment. One example of this is the warning not to go near the heart area... Good luck with your self-care friends!!!

p.s I've tried it and it leaves one with a lovely warmth in the lung area, and a sense of general well-being.

Ellen Steadman

Oh, I have just farted. Thanks for triggering the point. Big relief. Lots of air. - **Mok Malvin**

Very informative and beneficial. Thank you. - **Arnab Kumar DE**

Thank you, I thought your take on health and some of these methods sounded great (I had heard of some) and you explain so well. And of course, people have access to these methods they can employ as they choose. Thanks again. – **Maz Aspen**

Thank you for sharing! Yes, this technique is very helpful, and can clear stagnant energy in many areas of body. Much Love and Light. - **Denise**

I see you online and read everything I can find that is posted in English. Thank you. I show a lot of people how you helped me too. Thank you again.

My CT scans are perfect now cause beat on my back and front pretty regularly the last couple of years.I Could see progress using your instructions. I have had ZERO asthma this summer. Amazing and no allergy symptoms either. I attribute that directly to the tapping. Thank u Dao

Jeanette Lindow

Thank You, Duy.

I am happy there are more people who know we are all humans and we can all heal.

As you might have read, I already healed part of my 'autism'

And still integrating more towards oneness with all of myself and with all that is. I am so thankful for this experience and happy to share this with the world. Because iII have been there I can show the world it is possible!!

And yes, I'm into meditation, healing, energy work. Many experiences of Oneness/Dao /Source. We all are one.

Thank you for your offer, and your message,

You also are doing great work for humankind!

Love, Els

Van Duy Dao well read the article, I agree with it, some on here are assuming Autism is a disease or caused by pesticides, I have limited social skills as well as my boys, only downfall. assumptions like these are what keeps people looking at us like we are freaks, there is no cure and never will be, hate to say it but my parents had mental disorders my mom bipolar my dad OCD, maybe the cause all it is I am unique therefore blessed, I can go through life wishing or I can go through life accepting and coping, I wish I could do a lot others can like socialize, I wish my kids were like everyone else, then I realize that all 3 of us are truly blessed with health, family and love, love for ourselves and others even those who judge us, you are a very intelligent individual and reading your comments has enlightened me.

T.y

AWAKEN TO THE WORDS OF OUR BLESSED LORD AND SAVOR, VAN DUI DAO. HIS WORDS HAVE GRACED US WITH UNDERSTANDING OF COSMOS, LOVE PAPER PLANES, AND MATTERS OF LIFE YET UNDISCOVERED.

I LEARN PERSONAL DEVELOPMENT, FORGOTTEN THINGS, AIDS, TALKING WELL, AND SUCH OTHER GREAT ENDEAVORS YOU WANT NOT TO NOT LEARN. ENGLISH, WORDS.. YES. VERY MUCH YES. AUTISM EXSITS! DO NOT LET ROBOTS WHO SAY OTHERWISE GET INTO YOUR MIND BOX AND SPEAK SLANDEROUS AUTISMIC LIES. AS OUR CREATOR SAYS, "Life is not paradoxical, life is art. Life is not calculated by the autistic robot, life is must felt and created" <----- THIS!!! (p.s. I love you)

Nathan THE AWAKENED

We will discuss in this book:

We will discuss the surrounding phenomena: Autism, depression, obesity, mastery, outliers, talent, ADHD, poor learning, stress, abilities, seizures, drugs, violence, gut feeling, PTSD and how to deal with other chronic diseases, how to self-healing chronic diseases and how to have good health just by simply eating and deep breathing and doing Vietnamese Qi Gong exercises. I want to start with a series of questions to trigger our mind and old paradigm.

A. Self-healing and natural healing

The stomach, a place where digestion, absorption, and elimination has taken place, should be in a good state.

- In Vietnam, we are told to put a small blanket across the stomach of the kids during the sleep to make them sleep well and not ill.
- In traditional, when people have cold stomach pain, we are told to rub the topical hot medical ointments, drink sweet ginger juice or massage the stomach.

• These facts and the experience make the author think of the vital role of blood circulation in health and chronic illness. Poor blood circulation may come from the blocking points in the vessels or from low blood pressure or low blood glucose. In the body, all the billions of cells of all body systems need the energy to have normal functions; which is mainly generated from metabolizing glucose. When the cells hunger for glucose, it can start to use structure stored glucose or stored lipids or polysaccharides or structure lipid or structure protein. To take stored glucose, the body needs good blood circulation and right body temperature. The people with chronic illness often have hormonal imbalanced – which need glucose as the main source of energy also, and poor blood circulation and disorder of thermoregulation. If we do not stop these disorders, these people may have metabolic disorders or metabolic diseases. The main energy source for the cells is from the catabolism of glucose. So any problem for glycemia and oxygen saturation will make the billions of cells of the body are out of balance.

A metabolic disorder can generate free oxygen and free radicals. On the other hand, the immune system is not in a good state because of the hunger for energy may fail in repairing the damage caused by metabolic disorders.

In traditional medicine, the pain mainly caused by trigger points, so all alternative therapies like acupressure, dry needle, massage aim to remove trigger points. In the metabolic view, the author saw that the trigger points mainly in the muscle which presses the surrounding vessels of blood circulation. The signs of trigger point are pain, numbness, coldness, or rigidity. Poor blood circulation may make the target cells and target organs hunger for the glucose and poison by the metabolic wastes which are not carried out well by the poor blood circulation.

Glycemia, oxygen saturation and blood pressure are mainly control by heart, vessels, liver, pancreatic, intestine, lungs and kidneys. Any problems that happen to the heart, vessels, liver, pancreatic, intestine, lungs or kidneys will make the whole body have the various problems described by syndromes or metabolic diseases. Only oxygen can not create energy, the body does not have stored oxygen we do need breath continuously. To have a good metabolism, the blood needs to supply glucose or substrates for the cells at the optimum levels. Supplying substrate for metabolic reactions depend on the blood circulation to carried stored glucose and stored lipid in the abdominal area

B. Effortless teaching the kids and how to have effortless self-help

Is there any relation between autism, ADHD, poor learning, stress, depression & mental health? Some by genes, some are not by genes but they are comorbid!

What if we can have the diagnostic since the kids 2, 3, 4, 5, 6, 7, or 8 months old? What if we can have the diagnostic long before they can officially be diagnosed? then what these kids will be if we can give them effective intervention since that time 24/7 for kids with love, compassion, and patience?

What if autism is just viewed as having substantially poor social skills? According to the definition of autism, will kids recover from autism if they have full communication skills, emotional skills, and social skills?

The big question for autism is which causes make kids poor at these skills? This cause is also the cause of autism. And in the changing world, all are changing with different speed, genes, and brain change also. The changing of the brain is described well by neuroplasticity.

If the defect in genes and brain is by nature, scientists can test and detect it to predict autism since the time of pregnancy, infant, but the facts is no, they cannot see any warning until the behaviors, poor skills are obvious! This makes me think problems in genes and the brain is just the symptoms in the rainbow of autism.

Sorry, I am not satisfied with the explanation for if the kids get autism or not as the random chances or luck. I will work to find out why!

At least Autism: obvious facts are boys vs girls; city vs countryside; past vs present. In facts, the rate of autism is soaring in the U.S.A. and the rate of poor state: Alabama is 1 per 175 while the rate of rich state: New Jersy 1 per 45; boys are 5 times higher than girls.

Why are girls Outliers? Kids in my rural areas are outliers also with the rate is less 1/1000 kids while in U.S.A is 1/60?

After all, when we know the whole process, have a big view of opposite directions, we can understand and master it. We can become the outliers with the awakened mind so that we can master the art of living wealth, health, joy, inner peace and happiness.

14A

Part I: The cause and possible cure for cancer and chronic diseases from applying Papaya, baking soda, aspirin, sugar, Vietnamese Qi Gong breathing and traditional medicine.

In practice, the author has seen many cases that have been successfully recovered from cancer by alternative therapies without using the medicine. On the one hand, Some of them are recovered by Papaya leaf juice, some of them are by baking soda, some of them are by Qi Gong breathing or other therapies. On the other hand, the scientists also found that baking soda and raising body temperature also have a positive impact on cancer treatment so that physicians using baking soda and raising body temperature when applying chemotherapy for cancer. The question is how and why these cases are successful? The answer will give us an overall view of most diseases that we are dealing with. This is just part of my view and I have seen it had positive impacts on many cases. During studying the functions of the cells and organs, the author thought: "All of these functions will poorly execute or do not happens at all if we give its poor fuels or cut important parts of the metabolic reactions. The cells and organs are in an ecosystem. All fuels or ingredients should at the precise biological amounts. Nothing more, nothing less. Too many sugars can be seen as too much fuel, it can destroy the body, most are described well with hyperglycemia, hypoglycemia, hypotension, and hypertension.

Trigger points of the diseases in the body are the points that can prevent and have negative impacts on the body functions, blood circulation, fluids circulations. Overtime, the trigger points not removed may create a lots of unwanted signs, negative feelings, weakness, chronic symptoms, chronic illneses and systemic diseases.

The trigger points in the body and organs may have abnormal sensations when we create normal force on the areas like pressing, scratching, pounding, massaging or claping on it. The abnormal sensations, the feelings that healthy people usually do not have when receiving these forces, are relieved, comfortable, percing, pain, numbness, itching.

Self-checking the health and trigger points in the body, the hands, the feet.

Self-checking the health and trigger points	
It is not good if it is higher or lower than normal. It indicates that there are some forgotten health problems.	Checking the blood pressure on both hands several times a day to see if it is normal, low or high
	Checking glycemia when you hungry, tired, and after eating, drinking sweet juice to see if it is normal.
Check the state of the important organs in the stomach.	Just press the thumb on the stomach of people: right upper stomach (liver), Left upper stomach (gastric), and middle-lower stomach (intestine, ovule or prostate), if it pain, there may be block for fluidity
Forgotten trigger points along the way will make	Quick and slight clap on the shoulder, neck, back, lumbar, head, and forehead

people have abnormal sensations.	to see if there are the sensations of pain, piercing, burning, or comfortable.
Checking blood circulation to the feet, hands	Check the hands, feet to feel if it warm, and scratch on the feet to feel if there are abnormal feelings
Check the blood circulation to the head well or not	Bend and the neck and the back to see if it feels uncomfortable. Close the eyes than sit down and stand up 10 times to see you have the feeling of dizziness or vertigo. Turning the head to the left and to the right to see if it have uncomfortable
Check the blood circulation to the eyes	Pressing along the eyebrows to see if there is pain or piercing.
Check the health of the lungs	Clapping or quick punching on the chest to see if it is pain, piercing or comfortable feelings.
Self-finding any trigger points on the body	Clapping and pressing many points in the body to see if there are abnormal feelings.
Reflexology points on hand and foot	Pressing every area of the hand and the foot on the edge of the table, chairs or any hard objects: spoon, conner of the phone, a rock, piece of wood, if there are abnormal feelings, these are the

	trigger points and the body may not in good health.

The main reflexology points in the foot are said to be as follows:

    Spine – instep

    Liver – outside of right foot

    Spleen – outside of left foot

    The head and face – toes

    Lower back, lower limbs, genitals – heel

    Kidneys – sole of the feet

Chapter 1: Cells with metabolic reactions are the basic structure of all tissues and organs

Table 1: Catabolic reactions

Substrate + Oxy = Product + H2O + Energy (ATP/heat)

These are the factors that the author withdraw from inorganic reactions, organic reactions, and intercellular metabolic reactions catalyzed by enzymes.

Table 2: The factors that impact the catabolic reactions in the body

The factors that impact the catabolic reactions in the body: the cell, the reactions, the environment, and the whole body.
Factor 1: Concentration of Enzyme
Factor 2: Concentration of Substrate from digested foods
Factor 3: Concentration of Oxy
Factor 4: Concentration of products
Factor 5: Mobility of blood circulation or the mobility of fluid in the cells and around the tissues.
Factor 6: The state of the solution: homogeneous or inhomogeneous

Factor 7: Temperature: When two reactants are in the same fluid phase, their particles collide to have a reaction. If the reactants are uniformly dispersed in a single homogeneous, then the number of collisions per unit time depends on concentration and temperature.
Factor 8: PH of the environment.
Factor 9: Effect of Activators or cofactors. Some of the enzymes require certain inorganic metallic cations, like Mg^{2+}, Mn^{2+}, Zn^{2+}, Ca^{2+}, Co^{2+}, Cu^{2+}, Na^+, K^+, etc., for their optimum activity.
Factor 10: Some of the properties in this category are the state of matter, molecular size, bond type, and bond strength. - State of Matter - Bond Type - Bond Strength - Number of Bonds/Molecular Size

If we do not feed right ingredients, forget biology, forget biogenetics, forget biochemistry, forget immune system, forget the metabolism when there are the problems that reduce normal circulation: Glycemia and blood pressure.

What is oxygen in the blood circulation for? When we talk about the vital role of oxygen, we forget that the vital role of oxygen is to interact with glucose in the cells catalyzed by many enzymes to generate energy. The main source to generate energy in cells is from glucose, enough glucose is as vital as enough oxygen.

The circulatory, or the vascular system, is an organ system that permits blood to circulate and transport nutrients (such as amino acids and electrolytes), oxygen, carbon dioxide, hormones, glucose and blood cells to and from the cells in the body to provide nourishment and help in fighting diseases, stabilize temperature and pH, and maintain homeostasis.

> Globally, the average blood pressure, age-standardized, has remained about the same since 1975 to the present, at approx. 127/79 mmHg in men and 122/77 mmHg in women.

Blood pressure is influenced by cardiac output, total peripheral resistance, and arterial stiffness and varies depending on the situation, emotional state, activity, and relative health/disease states. In the short term, blood pressure is regulated by baroreceptors which act via the brain to influence the nervous and endocrine systems. The main purpose is to give the cells enough energy to function well which varies depending on the site, situation, emotional state, activity, and relative health/disease states

Blood pressure that is too low is called hypotension, and pressure that is consistently high is hypertension.

We do know that Blood the pressure is the vital signs, but we are taught that hypotension is so dangerous that we forget the danger of lower blood pressure. So that most of the therapists only afraid of hypertension and skip the dangerous of hypotension. Blood pressure is the vital signs of a healthy body. Blood pressure tell us the state of the circulatory system, also called the cardiovascular system, an organ system that permits blood to circulate and transport nutrients (such as amino acids and electrolytes), oxygen, carbon dioxide, hormones, glucose and blood cells to and from the cells in the body to provide nourishment and help in fighting diseases, stabilize temperature and pH, and maintain homeostasis.

In practicing, the author recorded: healthy people only have the feeling of dizziness or vertigo when they have hypotension or hypoglycemia.

Interruptions of coronary circulation quickly cause heart attacks, in which the heart muscle is damaged by oxygen starvation and glucose starvation. Such interruptions are usually caused by ischemic heart disease (coronary artery disease) and sometimes by embolism from other causes like obstruction in blood flow through vessels. Cardiologists are taught well about the vital role of blood circulation to the heart so they pay attention very closely the to the healthy of the coronary arteries. Coronary artery disease causes the blood flow to the heart below the optimum level. but the facts are all the living cells of the body need an optimum level of the blood circulation. Many tissues and organs are not as important as the heart, so we do not see immediately the signs of localizedizing ischemic of these tissues. Poor localized circulation will make the localized disordered metabolism which will lead to abnormal functions of the organs, and the cells may die quicker than normal, withdraw to an inactive state or speed up the degeneration of the tissues. If too many tissues and organs have poor circulation for a long time, we may soon have systemic diseases or severe syndromes. This is why the hypotension should be paid more attention than normal. Any number of blood pressure below the normal number will cause the cells and organs to work below the normal level. The author has seen many practitioners who said they feel more tired, dizziness, fatigue or weakness since recent years, but when they went for a check-up, doctors could not find any diseases and problems. After checking their blood pressure, the author usually got the number below the normal number, the systolic pressure may be around 110 mmHg or 100 mmHg. This made the author think that, if these people have these low blood pressure for years or decades, they will get specific diseases. It is just the blood flow to all organs and tissues are below the optimum level.

Table 3: The signs and the effects of hypotension.

The signs and the effects of hypotension	The possible mechanism
· Lightheadedness or dizziness.	Not enough glucose and oxygen
· If the blood pressure is sufficiently low, fainting may occur.	Severe lacking glucose and oxygen
· Chest pain	Not enough glucose and oxygen make the heart and lung have to work more, this causes the pain
· Shortness of breath	The brain stimulate to take more breath to get oxygen
· Irregular heartbeat	Not enough glucose and oxygen
· Fever higher than 38.3 °C (101 °F)	Impaired thermoregulation
· Headache	Not enough glucose and oxygen
· Stiff neck	Not enough glucose and oxygen make the muscle

	cells become inactive. These are muscle we use most of the time.
· Severe upper back pain	Not enough glucose and oxygen make the muscle cells become inactive. These are muscle we use most of the time.
· Cough with sputum	
· Prolonged diarrhea or vomiting	Not enough glucose and oxygen make the muscle cells become inactive or semi-paralyzed mixed with overactive
· Dyspepsia (indigestion)	Not enough glucose and oxygen for the cells act well.
· Dysuria (painful urination)	
· Acute, life-threatening allergic reaction	The reduction of the immune system
· Seizures	Severe lacking glucose and oxygen make the brain cells overactive disharmony mixing with inactive.
· Loss of consciousness	Not enough glucose and oxygen
· Profound fatigue	Hypotension is the vital

	signs
· Temporary blurring or loss of vision	Not enough glucose and oxygen
· Black tarry stools	Not enough glucose and oxygen for the intestine cells.

In practice, the author did see that when the glycemia below the normal level, most practitioners feel dizziness, vertigo, weakness, these signs can be deal well with just glass of sugar juice. This makes the author realized that glycemia, blood pressure and physical health is interdependent. People have good health when they have these indicators in the normal range. It is also the aim that most traditional aim to deal with. The traditional medicine aims to solve the cause and make the whole body is balanced. Modern medicine merely treats the symptoms which are the results metabolism disordered.

Chapter 2: Hypoglycemia and hypothermia

Glycemia and temperature of specific tissues are crucial for the functions of the tissues, in practice, traditional therapist always feel the cold or low temperature in the pain legs, pain arm or irritational stomach. It is the signs that abnormal areas temperature links to physical pain. If they check the blood glucose in the finger of healthy hand and the finger of the tingling hand, they can see that there is a variation of these two numbers. These numbers are not the same even we do at the same time and to the same people. It is because of localized knots can prevent blood circulation.

When the body's ability to thermoregulate becomes hindered and is left untreated, organ failure is imminent. Blood flow will be reduced, leading to ischemia, and, ultimately, multiple organ failures.

Table 4: The signs and the effects of hypoglycemia

The signs and the effects of hypoglycemia		
Sympathetic nervous system	Central nervous system	
• Produced by the counterregulatory hormones	• Abnormal thinking, impaired judgment	• Difficulty speaking, slurred speech
• Shakiness, anxiety, nervousness	• Nonspecific dysphoria, moodiness, depression, crying, exaggerated	• Ataxia, incoordination, sometimes mistaken for drunkenness

	concerns	
• Palpitations, tachycardia	• Feeling of numbness, pins and needles (paresthesia)	• Focal or general motor deficit, paralysis, hemiparesis
• Sweating	• Negativism, irritability, belligerence, combativeness, rage	• Headache
• Pallor, coldness, clamminess	• Personality change, emotional lability	• Stupor, coma, abnormal breathing
• Dilated pupils (mydriasis)	• Fatigue, weakness, apathy, lethargy, daydreaming, sleep	• Generalized or focal seizures
• Hunger, borborygmus	• Confusion, memory loss, lightheadedness or dizziness, delirium	• Abnormal thinking, impaired judgment
• Nausea, vomiting, abdominal discomfort	• Staring, glassy look, blurred vision, double vision	• Nonspecific dysphoria, moodiness, depression, crying, exaggerated concerns

• Headache	• Flashes of light in the field of vision	• Feeling of numbness, pins, and needles (paresthesia)
Shakiness, dysphoria. Significant hypoglycemia appears to increase the risk of cardiovascular disease	•Automatic behavior, also known as automatism	• Negativism, irritability, belligerence, combativeness, rage

Hypoglycemic symptoms can also occur when one is sleeping. Examples of symptoms during sleep can include damp bed sheets or clothes from perspiration. Having nightmares or the act of crying out can be a sign of hypoglycemia. Once the individual is awake they may feel tired, irritable, or confused and these may be signs of hypoglycemia as well. What if localizedized hypoglycemia, localized hypotension appears in the brain, and other tissues of the body for years or even the decades? The author did record glycemia, temperature, and stiffness of the pain, numbness areas, the recorded results are much different from the normal areas of the same body. And when practitioners take sugar juice with suitable exercise, the author did see when the localized glycemia, localized temperature back to normal, most of the pain and numbness disappeared.

Long-term effects of hypoglycemia may lead to permanent brain damage. The longterm effects of diabetes show the results that cells, organs, and tissues are under severe degeneration for years. It has been frequently found that those type 1 diabetics found "dead in bed" in the morning after suspected severe hypoglycemia had some underlying coronary pathology that led to an induced fatal heart attack.

Hypothermia

Hypoglycemia is also found in many people with hypothermia, as hypothermia, may be a result of hypoglycemia. The distribution of temperature in the body will lead us to know where the cells may suffer hypoglycemia and low temperature. The level of sugar in the blood is like the level of supplying energy for the billions of cells and organs function normally. Body temperature is also maintained by the function of the body cells. The whole body is a big biologic machine that all of the activities of the cells in the body are belong to the energy supplied by the reaction that control by enzymes and these enzymes are very sensitive to the changing of the temperature.

Table 5: The signs and the effects of hypothermia

The signs and the effects of hypothermia		
Mild	**Moderate**	**Severe**
With sympathetic nervous system excitation.	Mental status changes such as amnesia.	Cold
Shivering	Confusion	No shivering
High blood pressure	Slurred speech	Hallucinations
Fast heart rate	Decreased reflexes	Inflamed skin
Fast respiratory	Loss of fine	Pulmonary edema

rate	motor skills.	
Contraction of blood vessels	Mental status changes such as amnesia	Lack of reflexes
Increased urine production due to cold		Fixed dilated pupils
Mental confusion		Low blood pressure
Liver dysfunction may also be present		Physiological systems falter and heart rate, respiratory rate, and blood pressure all decrease.
		Pulse and respiration rates decrease
		Fast heart rates: ventricular tachycardia, atrial fibrillation

Chapter 3: Possible results of metabolic disorders proves that metabolic disorders are the real cause.

These are the possible results of metabolic disorders that are proven by scientists. All of these problems do not have medicine but adequate diets and regular physical exercise, vitamins can help.

The metabolic disorder creates reactive factors like hydrogen peroxide (H_2O_2) hypochlorous acid (HClO), and free radicals such as the hydroxyl radical (•OH) and the superoxide anion (O_2-). In traditional therapies, when to apply silver rings or silver spoons, we can see that the silver spoons have to change the color to darken. It is the results of reactions between silver and products of metabolic disorders. The facts are when the ill people usually have silver bracelet change the color into darker colors. These products of metabolic disorder will damage to DNA can cause mutations and possibly cancer, if not reversed by DNA repair mechanisms, while damage to proteins causes enzyme inhibition, denaturation and protein degradation.

A. Oxidative stress

Oxidative stress is thought to contribute to the development of a wide range of diseases including Alzheimer's disease, Parkinson's disease, the pathologies caused by diabetes, rheumatoid arthritis, and neurodegeneration in motor neuron diseases. Oxidative damage in DNA can cause cancer.

Radicals are only under controlled in a balanced state – Parkinson diseases

Radicals may also be involved in Parkinson's disease, senile and drug-induced deafness, schizophrenia, and Alzheimer's. The classic free-radical syndrome, the iron-storage disease hemochromatosis, is typically associated with a constellation of free-radical-related symptoms including movement disorder, psychosis, skin pigmentary melanin abnormalities, deafness, arthritis, and diabetes mellitus

B. Neuritis is the general inflammation of the peripheral nervous system may link to Parkinson diseases, Leprosy, and diabetic complications.

Nerve injury is an injury to nervous tissue. Neurapraxia is a disorder of the peripheral nervous system in which there is a temporary loss of motor and sensory function due to blockage of nerve conduction, usually lasting an average of six to eight weeks before full recovery. Symptoms depend on the nerves involved but may include pain, paresthesia (pins-and-needles), paresis (weakness), hypoesthesia (numbness), anesthesia, paralysis, wasting, . and the disappearance of the reflexes.

C. Carcinogen

Carcinogen is any substance, radionuclide, or radiation that promotes carcinogenesis, the formation of cancer, these also may be the byproduct of metabolic disorder. When there is poor circulation, the repairing for the DNA damage also reduced.

Is it genes or accumulation? We do see that genes are attacked by many factors and under continuous repairing. When the repairing is too weak, we may have damaged genes and a genetic disorder. Inside the cells, gene expression needs ATP and a series of anabolic reactions; these reactions also depend on the nature of substrates and nature of the environment, like PH, temperature, enzymes, and homeostasis. Carcinogen: this may be due to the ability to damage the genome or to the disruption of cellular metabolic processes.

After the carcinogen enters the body, the body makes an attempt to eliminate it through a process called biotransformation. The purpose of these reactions is to make the carcinogen more water-soluble so that it can be removed from the body, how can the body gain well this purpose when there is systemic or localizedized blood circulation

D. Pain in many illnesses and in fibromyalgia

"Far away from the optimum level, all things may out of balanced."

Lacking nutrients, and oxygens: cells go into inactive state, cold or stiffness as the bacteria or the cancerous cells in the research of Dr. Dang Chi Van did to test the role of baking soda and cancerous cells. When in this state, the cell does not help the vessels in carrying blood, and it may press on the nearby vessels so that it reduces the supplying blood of the vessels to the targets organs. On the other hand, these cells can press on the nerve tissue that causes pain or irritable sensations. The stiffness of the muscle cells in the back, neck and lumbar may impact the neurons and vessels in the back. The compression makes the related cells, related vessels and related tissues function below the optimum level. In these areas, the rate of dying may exceed the rate of reproducing. This may be the reason why in many alternative therapies, we use heat to pain areas or using back therapies on the back may help many painful conditions.

These disordered metabolic reactions create poisonous products, in traditional medicine, therapists called these organs to have negative Qi or negative energy. The oxidative stress, oxidative factors, and free radicals may change the color of the silver bracelet.

E. Other medical conditions that share similar symptoms as systemic metabolic disorders that need to have deeper research.

- AIDS: acquired immune deficiency syndrome maybe a kind of degenerative the immune system.

- Parkinson disease may be view as degeneration of peripheral neurons and mild degeneration of central nervous neurons. Scientists found that Parkinson has similarity to leprosy in genes. The reason maybe it has relation to the degenerative of peripheral neuron cells.

- More research in ulcer prevention and treatment in leprosy is needed to better guide management of skin changes caused by leprosy-induced nerve damage. In many people who are exposed, the immune the system is able to eliminate the leprosy bacteria during the early infection the stage before severe symptoms develop a genetic defect in cell-mediated immunity may cause a person to be susceptible to develop leprosy symptoms after exposure to the bacteria. The region of DNA responsible for this variability is also involved in Parkinson's disease, may be linked at the biochemical level.

- Alzheimer may be viewed as the degeneration neurons in the brain. This is about Alzheimer's disease (AD), also referred to simply as Alzheimer's, is a chronic neurodegenerative disease that usually starts slowly and gradually worsens over time.

- May Alzheimer is the combination of severe brain nerve injury and mild peripheral nerve injury

- HIV makes immune injury? What is the role of nutrients and physical exercise to speed up the repairing of the injury?

- May the problems of diabetes: part of Parkinson, part of leprosy, and part of Alzheimer and all other degenerative of relating cells?

- Diabetic is a group of metabolic disorders characterized by high blood sugar levels over a prolonged period. Symptoms of high blood sugar include frequent urination, increased thirst, and increased hunger. If left untreated, diabetes can cause many complications. Acute complications can include diabetic ketoacidosis, hyperosmolar hyperglycemic state, or death. Serious long-term complications include cardiovascular disease, stroke, chronic kidney disease, foot ulcers, and damage to the eyes. Diabetic is simply seen as the high glucose in the blood and low glucose in all cells. When the problems are unsolved, the long-term complications are the results of severe degeneration of the cells and tissues because of the lacking glucose – an important material for metabolic reactions. Balanced diets and regular exercise play an important role in preventing the diabetic complications mainly because it increases the blood circulation which increases the chances for the cells to catch glucose.

PH acidity is also the by-product of disordered metabolism, PH acidity is not good for the cells and metabolic reactions, this is why baking soda may help many illnesses.

Chapter 4: Science of the Qi

Combining the factors that affect metabolism, the cause of most diseases and health problems with the Chinese traditional medicine, mechanism of alternative therapies, the author assume that these are the factor to create balancing or the optimum of Qi.

Table 6: Balancing Qi

Balancing of the body can be measured by Qi. Balancing Qi may equal to all vital signs are in balanced. We can feel the Qi by the energy radiating from the cell, organs, and body by asking, seeing, examining and touching. Balancing Qi means there is no localized abnormal signs and systemic abnormal signs.
All these vital signs are interdependent to the changing of the intracellular and extracellular environment.
Localized or systemic vital signs become imbalanced for a long time can lead to metabolic diseases.

Blood pressure	Glycemia	Oxygen saturation	Body temperature

We usually use the general medical indicators to tell whether or not these vital signs are in balanced. The measured indicators tell us about the whole body still in balancing
For so long, we forget these vital signs of the specific areas, specific organs. Because of the vasodilation, contraction, blocking factors, the vital signs of the specific areas may be

varied. Therapists of traditional medicine use all localized signs of the body, combine it to find the root of diseases.

Localized hypertension	Localized hyperglycemia	Localized good oxygen saturation	Localized hyperthermia
Localized hypotension	Localized hypoglycemia	Localized low oxygen saturation	Localized hypothermia

Then we will have the specific signs of lacking nutrition, lacking oxygens, lacking glucose, poor circulation. Just see the signs of hypotension, hypoglycemia, low oxygen saturation, hypothermia, hypertension, and hyperglycemia. The organs' functions may fluctuate with the fluctuation of these vital signs.

Result of right Qi or balancing of all vital signs: warm areas, the right temperature, the right skin color, healthy cells, and healthy organs, all function well.

The places that have abnormal metabolic can be seen as trigger points or knots. Trigger points, blood clots or knots cause a lot of symptoms in the tissues and organs.

All these localized vital signs can go up and down according to the physical needs of the body and cells. Increasing and decreasing state alternative replace each other.

If not balancing, we can have acute localized or systemic hypotension and localized or systemic hypotension. The imbalance makes the metabolism of the cells become disorder, this may make the process of degeneration or aging may

> become faster.

When traditional therapists touch the patients' shoulders. They feel bumps with the fingers that they call 'knots' or trigger points.

Fibromyalgia – a mild systemic disorder of metabolism that makes many muscles in the inactive state. Inactive muscle will make us feel pain, numbness, irritation. I remember the image of the cancerous cells light up when the mice were fed with baking soda by Dr. Dang Chi Van. I see that with suitable impact, we can make these inactive cells will light up again, so the pain and irritation will diminish.

Myofascial trigger point: Activation of trigger points may be caused by a number of factors, including acute or chronic muscle overload, activation by other trigger points (key/satellite, primary/secondary), disease, psychological distress via the hormonal the system, homeostatic imbalances, direct trauma to the region, collision trauma such as a car crash which stresses many muscles and causes instant trigger points, infections. These are the factors that directly or indirectly impact on metabolism. The combination of some technique in the next witing will show you how to remove the trigger points in just 10 minutes.

Chapter 5: Effect of deep breathing, Vietnamse Qi Gong exercise and smoking on the glycemia.

"It is the deep breathing, not the smoke, makes people lose weight. It is the diaphragm breath, not the smoke, reduce the rate of getting Parkinson disease. Obvious fact is the deep breathing by the mouth of the smokers can reduce the rate of getting Parkinson disease."

"Why laughing has good effects on health? Happiness and moving all organs in the stomach. It is like to make all the organs in the stomach upsidedown. If we make the fake laugh, we do not get the result as the real laugh. If we just feel joy but not laughing, we do not get a good impact on health as real laugh."

Respiration therapy in Khi Cong Y Dao Vietnam, an alternative form of health exercise founded by Master Do Duc Ngoc in 1980, Master Do is widely respected by many people for his expert knowledge of the ancient Eastern concept "Qi" or "Chi" energy. At its core, Khi Cong Y Dao Vietnam combines the idea of Chi energy with simple, specific physical exercises, which is able to stimulate the body to repair damage and regenerate itself. The nutritions, herbs, sugar intake and suitable physical exercises of Vietnamese Qi Gong can make us gain most of the results of most alternative therapies.

Inner exercise: best of all is the exercise for the stomach. We do know the good effect of deep breathing in yoga, Qi gong, and meditation. We do know the negative effect of shallow, quick breathing. During my practice, I discover that this relationship to the metabolism of the billions of cells in the abdomen areas which can be a trigger to increase multifold just by practicing. The deep breathing and normal breathing do not change much in the volume of the lungs, but it is relating to the voluntary movement of the stomach muscle and diaphragm muscle during the deep breathing, this leads to the activation of billons cells of many organs in the stomach accidentally. This process increase the blood flow to the stomach, increase the glycemia to the stomach cells, this makes the semi-rigid cells in the stomach activate again. Just a little of practicing the deep breathing by mouth, practitioners may feel the stomach more soften and warmer than before. This is the signs that the cells activate again, the inactivate cells or semi inactive cells activate fully again. The full activation of the billions of cells in the organs still continue after stop practicing the breath, because I can still see the glycemia of practitioners still reducing when they take the rest, some practitioners still feel tired after practicing so that they have to take glasses of sugar juice to feel well again. The activated cells may uptake the sugar in the blood too much to compensate for the hunger of the cells for too long. It is like the cells may bright up with the practicing of deep breathing like the experiment of the dr Dang Chi Van found in the cancerous cells in mice brighten up when let the mice drink the juice have baking soda. In other words, all the cells in the stomach may have full metabolism as normal cells. Why deep breathing is so effective: firstly, it is synergy with the breath to continuously activate the cells in the abdomen so that practitioners do not feel tired. Secondly, is not the breath, but the activation of the billions of cells in the stomach and increase the blood flow to stomach areas gradually, leading to the metabolism of the billions of cells activated then the functions of repairing the damage and removing the temporary blockages in the vessels and organs are at a peak. Metabolism, blood flow, balanced glycemia, and the heat will make all enzymes in the stomach at peak of actions, these enzymes are vital for repairing, removing, controlling and active transporting functions of the cells in the stomach. Just by placing an object in the lower abdomen in lying posture, then slowly breath by mouth can make people feel warm in the abdomen, hands, and feet – even the ones who always have cold hand and cold feet.

To make the stomach, a place where digestion, absorption, and elimination has taken place, in a good state

> In Vietnam, we are told to put a small blanket across the stomach of the kids during the sleep to make them sleep well and not ill.
>
> In traditional, when people have cold stomach pain, we are told to rub the topical hot medical ointments, drink sweet ginger juice or massage the stomach

Due to the lung expansion being lower (inferior) on the body as opposed to higher up (superior), it is referred to as 'deep' and the higher lung expansion of the rib cage breathing is referred to as 'shallow'. The actual volume of air taken into the lungs with either means vary.

Several conditions are marked by or are symptomatic of, shallow breathing. The more common of these conditions include various anxiety
disorders, asthma, hyperventilation, pneumonia, pulmonary
edema, and shock. Anxiety, stress, and panic attacks often accompany shallow breathing.

Before the test, we check the blood pressure: systolic pressure/diastolic pressure. Then during the breathing, we check the blood pressure regularly and when the participants said they have some strange feeling that they do not have before taking the breathing test. You can do for yourself to compare the signs of the table below. Note that you should have a glass of sugar juice next to you to drink when you have strange signs because it is the signs caused by hypoglycemia when you blow out:

- Blow out quickly, strongly and deeply by mouth

- Blow out slowly, gently and deeply by mouth

Table 7: Experiments of quick, strong and deep breathing in respiration therapy

Experiments of quick, strong and deep breathing in respiration therapy				
Breathings by mouth	Changes inside the body	Glycemia during the breathing	Blood pressure during breathing	Hypoglycemia
Group one: blow out quickly, strongly and deeply by mouth	Burn out glucose quickly so that people started to yawn and the feeling of vertigo, dizziness, and the	Glucose in the blood reduce quickly	Systolic pressure reduced substantially and diastolic pressure reduced substantially	Most of the signs in the body were clear by a glass of sugar juice.

pain, stiffness, and numbness, in the face and the body's parts after five or ten minutes of practicing. If they have back pain and neck pain before, their pain will become severer when taking deep and fast breathing in and out		.	The more severe of the symptoms, the more sugar juice they need to take to clear it out

Awaken you wonderful we

Table 8: Experiments of slow, gentle and deep breathing in respiration therapy

Experiments of quick, strong and deep breathing in respiration therapy				
Breathings by mouth	Changes inside the body	Glycemia during the breathing	Blood pressure during breathing	Hypoglycemia
Group two: blow out slowly, gently and deeply by mouth	Burn out glucose slowly so that after five or ten minutes, they do not have as many signs as group one. These people only started to yawn and the feeling of vertigo, dizziness, and the pain, stiffness, and	Glucose in the blood reduce slowly, and it was reduced substantially when participants start to have a strange feeling	systolic pressure and diastolic pressure reduce slowly, and it was reduced substantially when participants start to have a strange feeling	Only some participants need to take sugar juice to clear out the strange signs.

	numbness, in the face and the body's parts after ten or twenty minutes of practicing.			

By practicing and recording the signs, I see that blowing out will reduce the glycemia. If we blow out quickly and strongly, we will reduce the level of glucose in the bloodstream quickly and we will soon have the signs of hypoglycemia after 5 minutes of practicing. Our participants who had high blood pressure just blowing out strongly by mouth in five minutes had systolic pressure reduced 10 mmHg.

If we blow out slowly and deeply, we will not have signs of hypoglycemia after 5 minutes of practicing. This kind of breathing is similar to breathing in smoking. During smoking time: people start to breathe in deeply and slowly by mouth. Breath The participants taking a breath by mouth slowly and deeply for 20 minutes can reduce both systolic pressure and diastolic pressure substantially, and their glycemia also reduced. Some participants had a feeling of reducing glucose level in the blood like yawning and the feeling of vertigo, dizziness, and the pain, stiffness, and numbness, in the face and body's parts. I confirm these feelings appeared caused by reducing glucose level in the bloodstream because all of these feelings had been cleared out immediately just by taking a glass of sugar juice. These are the simple experiments that you can do by yourself. The deep breath of smoking may be the answer for why people who smoke tend to have

These kinds of breathing can be done by you and all other participants so that you can self prove the signs, symptoms, and applications? As a pharmacist and a trainer of respiration therapy in Qi Cong Y Dao Viet Nam, I see the immense application of the breathing in controlling glucose level and many metabolic diseases that we are facing.

Any higher amount or lower amount of ingredients than balanced level will lead to metabolic disorder of the cells and dysfunctioning of the organs. Most of the techniques of Vietnamese Qi Gong is to aim at balancing the circulation system to the important organs and on the whole body. To have healthy circulation, therapists aim at the exercise that increases the mobility of the blood to the five important organs, nutritions, sugar intake, herbs and the techniques removing the blocking points or trigger points. The poor circulation and the blocking points are the main cause of most symptoms like pain, numbness, irritation, stiffness. When the blocking points are near the blood circulation to the head, it can cause a lot of hypotension and hypoglycemia on the central nervous system. These points may around the neck, shoulder and upper back. During the practicing, just within ten minutes, the author could remove these trigger points and these central nervous system disappeared immediately.

These are the exercise for Kungfu Master, who has a lot of experience in controlling the body, so if we want to follow this exercise, one crucial thing is that we have to drink sugar juice or eat sugar after five minutes of taking exercise or when we feel any abnormal senses during the exercise, these are the senses of hypoglycemia. To the people who have hypoglycemia or hypotension, they should drink sweet juice as soon as possible: sugar juice, coke, sweet juice.

Always place these juice nearby when start to take the exercise, and drink it immediately whenever you feel strange feelings: pain, numbness, tingling, vertigo, dizziness, short of breath, cold hand, cold sweating... it is the signs of hypoglycemia, all of these signs will be clear when you drink sugar juice. If these signs do not disappear after taking sweat juice, it means that the amount of juice is not enough.

To know more detail of the changing in the body, you should have the blood pressure machine and glucose blood machine to measure before, during and after the exercise, especially whenever you have strange symptoms. Do not do this exercise when feeling hunger. Eat some things before taking exercise.

Note that the glycemia still reducing after 20 minutes when you stop taking the exercise because when you remove the knots, increase the circulation, the hungry, inactive cells start to act and take up much more glucose.

Table 9: Vietnamese Qi Gong instructed by master Do Duc Ngoc

Vietnamese Qi Gong instructed by master Do Duc Ngoc		
The exercise	**The steps**	**Benefits**
1. Tie the feet then walk on a step or stair for 10 minutes	Slightly rolls the elastic crepe around the calves, tighten a little more around gastrocnemius muscle because of this muscle have a lot of	Activate the blood circulation

		arteries: it will have a strong impact on the arteries and blood circulation when we walk the step.	
2. Loading energy for the middle body – the stomach			Activate the organs in the stomach
		With hypertension: 2 hands placed on the lower abdomen	Men: put a left hand under the right hand
			Women: Put right hand under the left hand
		Normal blood pressure	Men: left hand on the upper abdomen
			Right hand on the lower abdomen
			Women: right hand on the upper abdomen left hand on the lower abdomen
		Hypotension: 2 hands	Men: put the

	placed on the upper abdomen	left hand under the right hand
		Women: Put right hand under the left hand
3. Loading energy for 5 organs	Places 2 plates together on the floor. Stand with your feet slightly broader than shoulder-width, then twist the feet to make the toes move closer together, the toes make a V shape. Then bend the knees to make the 2 knees against each other, lower the body part, still keep the back upright, Stretch the arms in front keeping the fingers together then the palms up. Look at both the thumb alternatively in slow succession	Stand like this for 5 to 10 minutes to make the body and the back warm or sweating. Activate the flow of energy in the body.
4. Exercise for the lower abdomen: breathing lower abdomen	Place a little heavy object like a stone, can of Coca-Cola on the lower abdomen, then breath via the mouth, When breath in, pay attention to the object, then breath out via	

		the mouth slowly and deeply.	
5. Pull the knee to the chest and blow the air deeply and slowly		Just press the thumb on the stomach of people: right upper stomach (liver), Left upper stomach (gastric), and middle-lower stomach (intestine, ovule or prostate), if it pain, there may be block for fluidity	Lie on the floor, place the hand to pull the knee to the chest, during the pulling, blow out slowly and deeply when stopping the breath, loosen the hands for a while then move straight the foot to the floor, when moving the foot, just breath in quickly via the mouth, then repeat with another foot, do this for 5 to 10 minutes.
6. Blow 3-5 minutes: to reduce blood pressure and glycemia, to prevent		To hypertension: blow strongly and deeply	Reduce blood pressure by 10 to 20 mmHg after 5 to 10 minutes of

vertigo because of reducing glycemia		blowing.

Clapping, massaging, pressing on pain areas when having heat and enough sugar in the blood.

Clap on the pain area, on the shoulder, neck, back, lumbar until have the sensations of form and roughness, pain, burning. When you feel the warmth on the back or warm sweating know the sensation of blocking, just clap on the ribs, it is the normal sensation, then clap on the pain areas: it is the different sensation: maybe numbnessClap on the areas of pain, it will make the numbness sensation, clap until they feel roughness or burning, it means that the areas are getting clear the small blocking. To that time, the person will not feel the pain when they bend the neck or the back.

Chater 6: Applying self-healing techniques, the natural healing for pain, hypertension, hypotension, fibromyalgia, cancer, ulcer, respiratory diseases, and metabolic disorders

The simple techniques that give the healing for most illnesses. It is so simple that most people can do it. And this can give us a new view of most illnesses.

> - The first, eat more, drink more, have more intake to have normal body weight. If overweight, no need to have more intake, just do the exercises, when feel tired, take a rest, and continue later.
> - The second: cover the tower and clap the lungs, and back if you feel pain, piercing, or comfortable, continue to do it until you feel normal. When you feel normal, all trigger points will be removed.
> - The third: place object weigh 0.5 kg - 1kg on lower stomach, 30 minutes each time, 2 to 3 times a day. During waking time, you can use an object to press on the lower stomach, this can be seen as a passive Qigong exercise.
> - The fourth, tie the leg with elastic crepe during running, jogging, or walking on stairs.
> - The fifth, use the bottle to press on the stomach, when slowly blow via the mouth, press the bottle, at the end of blowing, stop pressing, then loosen the bottle to breathe in via the mouth. Repeating for 10 minutes.

> The sixth, clapping all along the back, neck, and head, forehead 10 minutes each time, do with suitable force, several times a day until you feel roughness. Roughness feelings mean all trigger points in these areas are gone.

> The seventh, hand and foot massage: using stick, or top of the bottle or any tool to press on hands, all areas of hands, until you feel no pain, ni piercing. Or press the hands on the corner of the hard object. Any abnormal sensations when you pressing mean that all trigger points in your hands are gone.

> The eighth, have gently deep breath all the time you can. To do it easily, breathe in via the mouth, and during the blow out make the gently, long O, or U sound as long as possible. This exercise will make your body warm and feel healthier.

> The ninth, slightly and quickly clapping table, chair, or any objects to warm up the body, boosting blood circulation. It should be 5 - 10 minutes each time.

Do these exercises and self-healing tips, feel the changes of the body during and after, you can find out the best suitable exercises for you. The best healing techniques will make you healthier, not take much time because you can do it passively with other activities and not taking much effort.

If it is good and understandable do it gradually, the destination of health is at hand.

When you do this, if you feel healthier, you are on the right track of healing, if you feel tired, your glycemia may drop below the normal level, stop and, take a glass off sweet, or take the rest and do the exercises another time, you will feel healthier.

Do this continually, when you do this, your body will become

> healthier than before, the body can digest and absorb nutrients needed for the body to function better. Exercises not only can remove trigger points, but also can make the body absorb better you will feel more appetite.
>
> Do this gradually exercise, eating, drinking,… until you have normal health and normal body weight.
>
> The body needs about 2000 kcal or 3000kcal/a day for daily functions. The nutrients and energy of the foods and drink will not only supply for the body to work well, but also it uses to heal all impaired organs which work below normal functions.
>
> So that the more energy you intake during self-healing with these exercises, the better and faster the body is healed.
>
> A weak body means many organs have been hungry for a long time, we need to feed more to compensate the hungry cells, organs to make them back to a normal/healthy state. In a healthy state, all indicators will normal, you have normal functions, and your and hands, feet warm all the time.

A. Ten minutes to remove trigger points cause pain in the back, neck, head and shoulder.

Ten minutes removing these trigger points reduces most of the central nervous symptoms: dizziness, vertigo, headache, balanced disorders, and vestibular disorders. Trigger points or stiffness areas: clap on it, there will no normal sensual, it is just the sensual of numbness.

When we know the mechanism is to loosen the stiffness, there are better and natural ways: by increasing body temperature with exercise Tie the feet then walk on a step or stair for 10 minutes or Load energy for 5 organs, then clap on the stiffness

Doing exercise one for 5 minutes to warm the body, then clap on the pain areas: shoulder, neck and the back. Just by touching on the back or seeing the pattern of sweat, you will know the sensation of blocking. Just clap on the ribs, it is the normal sensation, then clap on the pain areas: it is the different sensation, maybe numbness. Clap on these areas of pain, it will make the numbness sensation, clap until they feel roughness or burning, it means that the areas are getting clear the small blocking. When having the feeling of roughness, the person will not feel the pain when they bend the neck or the back. People who have back pain only feel the roughness when they have enough warmth and glucose in the body. If clap around 30 seconds to 1 minute on pain areas, the patients do not feel burning, it means that they do not practice enough to have enough warm or do not drink sugar juice enough to have enough glycemia. Let they drink more sugar juice then.

B. 10 minutes to reduce irritation bowel, irritation on the stomach or pain in the liver.

Pulling the leg on the stomach, or using bottle or objects to press the stomach along with the breathe . This makes to clear the gas in the stomach and make the organs in the stomach work harmoniously.

C. 10 minutes to make warm the hand and feet and the whole body

When it warm, most of the irritation in hands and legs reduce substantially.

With the people with hypotension, they usually have cold hands, cold feet, after removing the pain areas, they can lie down and start exercise 4, after five or ten minutes, they will feel warm in the hands, then in the feet.

To the skinny people or weak people, if after 10 minutes they do not feel warm in the feet, it means that the glucose level in the body has reduced to the below normal level, ask them to drink sugar juice as much as possible before starting the exercise.

During the exercise, if they feel the hands or feet start to warm, but then stop warming after that, it means that they are in hypoglycemia, stop the exercise and start to drink as much as sugar juice as possible before taking the exercise.

D. 30 minutes to have a natural sleep for the people with insomnia.

- First, remove the pain areas

- Then start taking some of the exercises below about 5 minutes

- Then start exercise placing an object on the lower abdominal for 30 minutes before sleep.

E. Control glucose in the blood, blood pressure, metabolism of the body

To control glucose in the blood, blood pressure, metabolism of the body, to lose weight or gain weight: do these exercises regularly 5 – 10 minutes a day with suitable nutrition to help increase blood circulation, metabolism and make the organs in the bodywork harmoniously.

F. Remove trigger point and balance metabolic reactions simply in three steps

The facts about laughing and the experience make the author think of the vital role of blood circulation to health and chronic illness. Poor blood circulation may come from the blocking points in the vessels or from low blood pressure or low blood glucose. In the body, all the billions of cells of all body systems need the energy to have normal functions; which is mainly generated from metabolizing glucose. When the cells hunger for glucose, it can start to use structure stored glucose or stored lipids or polysaccharides or structure lipid or structure protein. To take stored glucose, the body needs good blood circulation and right body temperature. The people with chronic illness often have hormonal imbalanced – which need glucose as the main source of energy also, and poor blood circulation and disorder of thermoregulation. If we do not stop these disorders, these people may have metabolic disorders or metabolic diseases. The main energy source for the cells is from the catabolism of glucose. So any problem for glycemia and oxygen saturation will make the billions of cells of the body are out of balance.

A metabolic disorder can generate free oxygen and free radicals. On the other hand, the immune system is not in a good state because of the hunger for energy may fail in repairing the damage caused by metabolic disorders.

In traditional medicine, the pain mainly caused by trigger points, so all alternative therapies like acupressure, dry needle, massage aim to remove trigger points. In the metabolic view, the author saw that the trigger points mainly in the muscle which presses the surrounding vessels of blood circulation. The signs of trigger point are pain, numbness, cold, or rigid. Poor blood circulation may make the target cells and target organs hunger for the glucose and poison by the metabolic wastes which are not carried out well by the poor blood circulation.

Glycemia, oxygen saturation and blood pressure are mainly control by heart, vessels, liver, pancreatic, intestine, lungs and kidneys. Any problems that happen to the heart, vessels, liver, pancreatic, intestine, lungs or kidneys will make the whole body have the various problems described by syndromes or metabolic diseases. Only oxygen can not create energy, the body does not have stored oxygen we do need breath continuously. To have a good metabolism, the blood needs to supply glucose or substrates for the cells at the optimum levels. Supplying substrate for metabolic reactions depend on the blood circulation to carried stored glucose and stored lipid in the abdominal area.

The common advice for all people who have any diseases is the right laboring exercise like gym, exercise, yoga, qigong; and right diets.

Eating too much can make the body have too much stored-nutritions, this stored nutrition will create a lot of poisons for the body and have a burden for blood circulation and important organs. So the right advice to the people who have overweight is reducing eating and exercise more.But the skinny and the weak people, the right advice for them are eating more and the right exercise. During practice, the author saw that weak people have the cells are hunger and out of balanced; they all experience symptoms of weakness, dizziness, trouble in eating, trouble in sleeping and trouble in studying.

The symptoms of the hungry cells are easily found in transient hypoglycemia in diabetic patients, when they late for meals or when they skip meals. The most common cause of death in these extreme cases of starvation is myocardial infarction or organ failure. To healthy people, can easily feel hypoglycemia, hypotension and the hungry cells of the body when they have hard labor work and skipping meals. The more they skip meals the more obvious they have the symptoms of hypoglycemia and hypotensions. If the chronic patients skipping meals too much, they may have cold sweating, cold hand, trembling, vertigo, headache, dizziness or fainting which are described well in Vestibular disorder. All of these symptoms can be easily eradicated by sweat juice, sweet candies, food or intravenous glucose transfusion.

During practice, the author sees that with right eating or drinking sweet juice, and right exercise to increase blood circulation to all organs and cells in the body, and removing trigger points by clapping on it, most of the chronic symptoms disappear immediately in 10 minutes to 30 minutes of practicing.

Self-healing with right eating, right drinking sugar juice and doing the exercises below.

- **The first step: eat and drink first**

The heat comes from metabolic reactions. To remove the trigger points more heat the better. Just touching on the skins of the forehead, the back, the shoulder to feel whether or not the body has normal body temperature. To the weak, skinny or chronically ill people, they need to take a lot of sugar juice to supply enough glucose for the cells. During practice, there are some learners had chronic illnesses taken nearly 400 mg of sugar to have enough glucose for the cells. After two - hours practicing some qigong exercise, checking their glycemia, we got the number ranged from 6.0 mmol/l to 8 mmol/l. The author was surprised that how the cells of their bodies were undergone. [97]

To the people who have the right body weight or overweight and have a warm back and warm forehead, do not need to drink sugar juice.

- **The second step: lie down and place an object on the lower abdomen**

Lie down and place an object weight about 1 kg to 2 kg on the lower abdomen. The object the author usually uses was the bottle of water, a rock, a brick or a handy bag. Place from 10 minutes to 30 minutes until they have warm hands and warm feet. During practice, the author usually saw that the hand will warm first, then the stomach, and the foot.

- If the hands and the foot warm, then do the third step

- If the hands warm and the foot are not warm, these people can take more sugar juice then continue to lie down and put an object on the lower abdomen.

- If the hands and the foot are not warm, even worse, the hand become colder and have cold sweating, stop immediately to start the first step to eat more and drink more sugar juice

- The warm of the skin is from the heat of the metabolic reactions of the cells under the skin. When the cells under the skin hunger for glucose for the metabolic reactions, the skin is cold or dry. During practice, the author saw that there were some practitioners have the temperature in the hands increased just a little then it started to decreased immediately; this can explain that that glucose level in the blood starts to reduce substantially. The author asked the practitioners to start to take more sugar juice if they want to continue.

All the physical exercises will increase the blood circulation to the muscle, organs, and cells in the whole body. The disadvantage of physical exercise make many people do not persist to follow because to gain good health from physical exercise, some people have to take hard physical exercise. There are a lot of soft tissues, soft organs and large vessels in the lower stomach so changing the vibration or movement of the lower stomach can make a great impact on blood circulation. This is the reason why deep breathing and abdominal breathing in yoga or qigong have many benefits on health. After many times of practicing, the author realized that by placing an object in the lower stomach, lying down and breathing normally, we put a rhythmic force directly on the blood circulation to boost the blood circulation.

- **Third step: clapping on trigger point until having the sensation of roughness.**

Clap on the muscle of the back, the shoulder, the neck, the nape, and the head

When the practitioners have warm hand and/or foot, start to clap on the muscle on the back, the muscle on the lumber, the muscle on the neck, the muscle on the nape and the muscle on the head; these are the areas have many trigger points. Clapping on trigger points, people only feel numbness, continue clap on it until people have the sensation of roughness or burning. The trigger point will be removed when people have the sensation of roughness or burning. Clap on those areas until all have a sensation of roughness.

- The stiffness of the muscle in the lumbar may make the lumbar pain and prevent blood circulation to the foot which causes pain, irritation, tingling and weakness in the legs, hips, knees, and feet.

- The stiffness of the muscle on the shoulder may press the vessels to the arms and hands, which causes the hands' pain, weakness, numbness, and tingling.

- The stiffness of the muscle on the neck and the nape will prevent the blood circulation to the neck, spine, and head, which cause Degenerative spine, headache, dizziness, tingling, vertigo, Alzheimer's & Neurodegenerative Diseases and Vestibular disorder.

- The cold and abnormal function of the muscle in the vessels, intestine muscle, stomach muscle will also prevent the blood circulation and substances exchanging between the heart, lungs, intestine, liver, kidneys and soft tissues, which will make these organs function poorly. We do know that we will have heart ischemia when the blood to the heart is poorly. These trigger points in the muscles in the abdominal if not being removed will prevent blood circulation in the abdominal. The chronic poor blood circulation in the abdominal may create heart diseases, lung diseases, liver diseases, kidneys diseases, and organs failure. The kind of diseases and the severity of the diseases depends on the degree and the sites of poor blood circulation.

- Poor blood circulation to the soft tissues may make people feel pain. Most of these symptoms and the symptoms of fibromyalgia will be removed or reduced substantially by practicing these three steps. Furthermore, during practicing, the author saw that increasing the heat of the body and removing the trigger point, we can deal with a lot of health symptoms and diseases.

Chapter 7: The cold, flu A, cough, asthma, bronchitis, pneumonitis, and Covid-19.

These can also applying for chronic obstructive pulmonary disease, chest pain, difficulty breathing, tonsillitis, rhinitis and flu complication will be relieved well by removing the trigger points in the lungs.

Herbal oils for health, cold, flu, sinusitis and systemic body

Inhale herbal oils can treat sinusitis, cold, kill viruses, and boost the resiratory system. It creates great benefit for the health of the body so that the body can heal faster and prevent the cold, flu better.

To inhale the herbal oil, we can rub the oil on the face mask. Or we can use plastic tubes 2 feet in length, placing tissues paper or cotton on the one top of the tube, rub the oil on the tissues paper/cotton, then placing the other top the tube in the nose. The oil will be inhale little by little. The plastic tube not only prevents the oil do not have direct contact to the skin of the nose but also it can store the oil for inhaling gradually for 10 to 30 minutes.

The herbal oil maybe eucalyptol oil, cinnamo oil, mint oil or many herbal oil sell in drug stores.

By finding and removing trigger points in the lungs we can help to treat the diseases. On the other hand, removing trigger points in the lungs can boost the health of the lungs, supply well oxygens for all important organs and the whole body in critical situations. Quickly and slightly punch on the back under which there are the lungs, if there are places that the patients feel hurt, pain, breathlessness, causing the coughing or feel comfortable these are the trigger points which can make the lungs ill or pneumonitis. The trigger points I usually find are on the bottom of the lungs. We can remove these trigger points in the lungs by continuous punching on the lungs and the bottom of the lungs, which are the site of trigger points, for about 10 to 30 minutes each time. By asking the feeling of the patients and the sound during punching on the back we can know whether or not the trigger points have been removed? Continous doing these several days can remove all the forgotten trigger points in the lungs. During the time of practicing, I always find these trigger points in the lungs of the practitioners even they are healthy by quick and slight punching on the back, and I make them feel better and healthier by continuous punching. The video in this writing also illustrates the way that I usually do. The health of the lungs also impacts the health of the heart, intestine, liver, kidneys, blood vessels and the billion cells in the body, so removing the forgotten trigger points in the lungs we can make all the body in a good shape. Epidemiology of SARS may reveal that it is not the condition of the treatment but the health of the patients or the health of the lungs decides the results of recovery or complication. Especially living in the polluted environment, people inhale a lot of contaminations that may deposit in the whole lungs and on the bottom of the lungs. By quick and slight punching on the back, we can make the whole lungs, bronchitis and blood vessels in the lungs vibrate with a rhythm. The virus spread quickly in a large community, the virus is not dangerous to the people, but its complications on the lungs and the whole body are life-threatening. We do not have medicine for virus flu but we do know that by boosting the immune system, have good health can prevent and stop the flu. The complication of the SARS mainly on the lungs. Reading the epidemiology of the SARS, the author sees that by making the lungs in good health, we can stop the epidemic of flu.

> *We can use hands or rubber hammer to punch or clap on the back.*

"Keto flu", the key for the flu and the most chronic illnesses.

Keto flu used to describe the side effects of having a keto diet to reduce weight, the diet has limited Glucid. The fat man may have keto flu in the first week of having a keto diet, he may have all symptoms like flu symptoms but he does not have flu. The symptoms of the flu that the man on the keto diet has are the results of the hunger cells and hunger organs of the whole body. These hunger cells do not have enough glucose for the energy source. The hunger of the billion cells in the body make the man have the signs live the flu-signs. All of these flu-like signs will be removed by just several cups of sugar juice!

> So to the patients of flu, patients of chronic diseases, or any patients feel tired or exhausted, we should give them more sugar juice or add more sugar in their drinking juice to make them feel better, to remove all flu symptoms, to make all other cells have enough energy to beat with diseases and to prevent the dangerous complications.
>
> After having the sugar juice, patients can do simple Qigong exercises like slow deep breathing

> via the mouth for 30 minutes each time of practicing to mobilize the sugar into the cells. Or they can do any of the Vietnamese Qigong described in this chapter. People should pay attention to the symptoms before and after having sugar juice to know the role of sugar. If anyone has a doubt of drinking sugar juice, you should have check blood glucose levels every day.

Tips to help self treating COVID-19, cold, asthma, coughing, difficult breathing, COPD, chest pain, Shortness of breath, cough with sputum.

Herbal oils for health, cold, flu, sinusitis and systemic body: head, heart, hormones, circulations..

> Inhale herbal oils can treat sinusitis, cold, kill viruses, and boost the resiratory system. It creates great benefit for the health of the body so that the body can heal faster and prevent the cold, flu better.
>
> To inhale the herbal oil, we can rub the oil on the face mask. Or we can use plastic tubes 2 feet in length, placing tissues paper or cotton on the one top of the tube, rub the oil on the tissues paper/cotton, then placing the other top the tube in the nose. The oil will be inhale little by little. The plastic tube not only prevents the oil do not have direct contact to the skin of the nose but also it can store the oil for inhaling gradually for 10 to 30 minutes.
>
> **The herbal oil maybe eucalyptol oil, cinnamo oil, mint**

> oil or many suitable herbal oils sell in drug stores.

Preventing and treating for Coronavirus, Covid-19 or Corona outbreaks lie in the finding and removing trigger points in the lungs and the whole body.

From statistics, the same condition of treatment, how can the young, the healthy men, and the females can self-prevent, self-heal flu caused by Coronavirus or COVID19. Not yet medicine cure viruses, asthma, COPD, chronic bronchitis, difficult breathing, but the health of the patients makes a great difference. Most death cases had other diseases.

A. First step: eat and drink first to warm up the body

The heat comes from metabolic reactions. To the weak, skinny, or chronically ill people, they need to take a lot of sugar juice to supply enough glucose for the cells. During practice, there are some learners who had chronic illnesses taken nearly 400 mg of sugar to have enough glucose for the cells. The glycemia should be maintained ranged from 6.0 mmol/l to 8 mmol/l.

B. Second step: boosting the blood circulation, warm up the body and cut the fever by one or some of these exercises.

- Lie down and place an object on the lower abdomen, this will make the blood circulate well to the whole body
- Clapping the objects or flapping the hands for 10 minutes.
- Tying the legs with plastic rubber string or elastic crepe then go for walk or walking up and down a step.
- Practicing relaxed deep breathing

Lie down and place an object weigh about 1 kg to 2 kg on the lower abdomen. The object the author usually uses was the bottle of water, a rock, a brick, or a handy bag. Place from 10 minutes to 30 minutes until they have warm hands and warm feet. During practice, the author usually saw that the hand will warm first, then the stomach, and the foot.

- If the hands and the foot warm, then do the third step
- If the hands warm and the feet are not warm, these people can take more sugar juice then continue to lie down and put an object on the lower abdomen.
- If the hands and the feet are not warm, even worse, the hand become colder and have cold sweating, stop immediately to start the first step to eat more and drink more sugar juice

There are a lot of soft tissues, soft organs and large vessels in the lower stomach so changing the vibration or movement of the lower the stomach can make a great impact on blood circulation. This is the reason why deep breathing and abdominal breathing in yoga or qigong have many benefits on health.

Do COVID-19, coronavirus, flu virus reveal that too many people have forgotten, untreated problems in systemic cardiovascular? Some of its drugs caused coughing because the lungs contain lots of veins! Test by slightly punching/clapping on the back.

Virus, fear, and worry makes people self-reduce from greed to basic needs. The earth becomes much cleaner. Needs: just small space, quiet, simple eating, enjoy!!!

Benefits of relaxed deep breathing which is proven by science.

How can we know if someone has deep breathing: just count that in one minute, how many breaths that they take.

One a simple way to have relaxed deep breathing is:

1. Just try to breathe out via mouth or nose gently and slowly and as long as possible, when breathing out, we can pronounce a small voice of OOOO or UUU or hahahahaha. By having this

small sound, practitioners can have the breathing out longer 2-5 seconds than the breath without small sound. This can make the breath longer, deeper but the practitioners are not tired and do not have to try hard.

2. Do not try to breathe in, just breathe in normally.

During practicing, when practitioners have relaxed, long deep breaths, they can have the hand warm, feel much healthier, and soothes the pain in the muscle and the lungs. By practicing this, practitioners can have only 6 to 12 breaths in a minute. While the patients of asthma usually have 20 - 40 breaths per minute. The shorter the breath, the weaker they are. The shorter of the breath can make patients have more chest pain.

Practice for 10 to 20 minutes, practitioners will have warmer hands and feel healthier than not practicing this.

C. Third step: Removing trigger points in the lungs

We can use hands or rubber hammer to punch or clap on the back.

You may feel like this is similar to postural drainage, No, this is better. The postural drainage technique makes patients feel lots of roughness on the back but do not make the lungs vibrate much. Punching on the back makes the whole lungs vibrate, this will make patients breathe easier. Do this in the right degree can be seen as a massage for the lungs to boost the health of the lungs.

· Quickly and slightly punch/clap on the upper back, if there are places that the patients feel hurt, pain, breathlessness, causing the coughing or feel comfortable these are the trigger points that can make the lungs ill or pneumonitis. The trigger points I usually find are on the bottom of the lungs. We can remove these trigger points in the lungs by continuous punching on the site of trigger points for about 10 to 30 minutes each time. By asking the feeling of the patients and the sound during punching on the back we can know whether or not the trigger points have been removed?

- Continous doing these several days can remove all the forgotten trigger points in the lungs.

D. Fourth step: finding and removing the trigger points on the whole body.

Clap on the muscle of the back, the shoulder, the neck, the nape, and the head.

When the practitioners have warm hand and/or foot, start to clap on the muscle on the back, the muscle on the lumber, the muscle on the neck, the muscle on the nape, and the muscle on the head; these are the areas that have many trigger points. Clapping on trigger points, people only feel numbness, continue clapping on it until people have the sensation of roughness or burning. The trigger points will be removed when people have the sensation of roughness or burning. Clap on those areas until all have a sensation of roughness.

Some of traditional alternative healing techniques that help for pain, fever and systemic illnesses:

- ✓ Using stick, or top of the bottle or any tool to press on hands, all areas of hands, neck and the head gradually until you feel no pain, ni piercing. Or press the hands on the corner of the hard object. Any abnormal sensations when you pressing mean that all trigger points in your hands are gone.
- ✓ Using herbal oils rub on the palm of hands a feet before sleep.
- ✓ Soaking feet with herbal warm water. To simply have herbal warm water, using salt and ginger, cinnamo or any herbal at hands.

> ✓ Using the papaya leaves soaking the alcohol to rub a long the back for 10 minutes.
>
> ✓ Using hairdryer to warm up the back, hands, feet, palm of the hands and the pain areas for 10 minites each times.

E. FACTS: Covid-19 mortality rate, profoundly disturbing. It is not by the virus, but it may reveal the weakness of the modern medical system.

1. The forgotten health problems

Covid-19 mortality rate, profoundly disturbing. It is not by the virus, but it may reveal the weakness of the modern medical system. It does not heal people, it just makes them feel temporary relief. It creates a term like chronic illness and asks them to take medication for blood pressure, glycemia, itchy, pain, irritation for years, decades, or lifetime. Many patients of chronic diseases have to take 4 - 5 pills for diabetes, cholesterol, hypertension, and impotent at the same time.

They may wrong, they may create their own conflict, paradoxes in even one branch of medicine. Worst of all, they are come from the wrong belief on lifestyle, on the heath. When having problems with lipidemia, glycemia, blood pressure, nutrition in blood, they all taught to think of medication. Poor physical lifestyle caused a lot of health problems in developed countries, just google or Wikipedia. This is a fact.

Many religious leaders infected and dying, even the high position in their religions, they even die when they are praying. It makes me doubt God. Just a kind of belief and power of belief. If Darwin was right, then we have roots from animals, we do not need too much clean and isolating lifestyle. Look at the lives of 2300 years ago, 2000 years ago, 1400 years ago, 1000 years ago, 400 years ago, 100 years ago, if based on the modern standard of hygiene, the modern theory of diseases, theory in eating, drinking, all these people of these time should be dead because of a lot of diseases.

We may forget that the condition of living can have an impact on overall health and the immune system. I can only describe the paradoxes of living, paradoxes of David and Goliath, the advantages and disadvantages of having, pr of richness, of leisure/lazy lifestyle. Modern men may lazy caused they have too much and not think much of right giving, right taking. They may have a shallow view on physical and material life, tangible and intangible life, of giving or taking are the two faces of a coin/act/phenomenon.

> Do COVID-19 and flu viruses reveal that too many people have forgotten, untreated problems in systemic cardiovascular? Some of these drugs caused Coughing because the lungs contain lots of veins! Test by slightly punching/clapping on the back.

2. Facts of drugs for chronic health problems

Drugs: just simply make the statistic that a drug can reduce a kind of symptom, it can be approved by FDA and mass prescriptions. No need for total healing or recovered, just proves that it can reduce a kind of symptom in a cluster of symptoms call disease or syndrome. That is why patients may take a bag of prescription medication months. And they may take for years, decade, until they die. Or until they stumble to Flu, flu A, cold, or stroke (overreact/too many changes of the body to the changing environment).

3. Removing trigger points by comfortable clapping or punching.

Blood vessels are the reason why some kind of medicine to treat high blood pressure that effect of contraction and expending of blood vessel cause the side effect of coughing – try this: just punching or clapping on the back and the chest to remove the trigger points, we can clean the airway and stop the chronic cough immediately. Any kind of coughing, even the coughing caused by the side effects of hypertension medications.

Right clapping or right punching that does not make patients feel pain or roughness but has an impact on the vibrations of inner organs, vibrations of the cells, vessels,... can clear the ways, tubes, vessels that are inside the organs or connecting organs. This will make a great impact on health if we do it on the right degree. That is why the right nutrition and regular physical exercises are the best advice for patients of all kinds of diseases. Nutrition just gives energy to the body. The exercises just to mobilize the cells, expansion of the vessels, and make the whole body more.

The movement of the muscles helps the vessels and the heart in circulating the blood. The facts are if we spleen the normal right arm for a month, we will have a weak right arm and a little atrophy on this arm. It is proved that the physical movements have great impacts on the blood circulation and the health of cells and organs.

4. Forgotten chronic diseases that make profoundly disturbing the Covid-19 mortality rate.

Nutrition, mineral, vitamins, and physical exercises are good advice for all diseases, but a single factor of these does not create meaningful therapeutical effects. I just combine and make it better. Right calories from nutrition, combine to 3 to 5 Qigong exercises that have a strong impact on blood circulation, and right clapping/physical impact that makes rhythmic pressure on trigger points will make meaningful therapeutic effects. Up to 90% patients of many symptoms like tiredness, weakness, pain, stomach pain, back pain, headache, dizziness, insomnia, vertigo, hyperglycemia, hypoglycemia, hypotension, coughing, difficult breathing, cold hands, cold feet, cold the stomach will be recovered after a day or a week. On helping people on heath, I do not take the fee if I do not help them feel better/recovered/totally healed.

The Qigong exercises describe the writings. All can try it. I just combine and explain general knowledge, simple exercises, nutrition, and alternative therapies on the eye of medical science. It is so simple that all can try or test it. It is so obvious that the

Ph.D., doctors and scientists have to admit it. Best of all, in treating the chronic symptoms, the experienced patients can treat as well as modern doctors. Learning more, they can do better. The results have not come from they are smarter, but they are awakened to the basic, simple knowledge. Experiences make them awake to the core of healing, mechanism of illness, of chronic illnesses.

Forgotten chronic diseases make patients tend to overreact to the changing of the environment. Like the kind of health problems change with time of the day, time of the month, time of the years. Seasonal diseases. The profound disturbing mortality rate of Covid-19, a kind of flu, a kind of cold, mainly come from complication in the lungs. They have too weak lungs, or lungs with the blood vessels have a lot of problems. Cardiovascular disease is the disease with the vessels have a lot of problems. It has a link to the health of the lungs. Of the tiny vessels in the lungs. The giant square of blood vessels surfaces that magically exchange the air will be impaired in patients of cardiovascular diseases.

5. Systemic effects, the organs are interdependent

If the body has hundreds of Km blood vessels, the main part of the body's vessels are in the lungs, then the stomach. The medication causes systemic effects, on the whole, body, describe in effects, and side effects in the drug leaflets.

NOTE: side effects are the effects that we do not want, but it really exists. We want some effects on other organs, but also we have to bear the effects on other organs that we may not welcome.

The lungs take oxygen for the body, but the health of the lungs are interdependent to the health of other important organs and the whole body. Relaxed deep breathing makes the lungs healthier and equipped well oxygen for the whole body. Scientists and researchers do find out the great benefit of deep breathing - a kind of exercise in Yoga, meditation, and Qigong.

Source of the oxygen in in the lungs, all health problems should check the health of the lungs

> The Nobel Assembly at Karolinska Institutet has today decided to award the 2019 Nobel Prize in Physiology or Medicine jointly to William G. Kaelin Jr., Sir Peter J. Ratcliffe, and Gregg L. Semenza:
>
> "for their discoveries of how cells sense and adapt to oxygen availability"

For self treating fever, pain, cough, phlegm, difficult breathing and many other chronic diseases: finding and removing the trigger points.

- ❖ Inhale herbal oils
- ❖ Practicing Qigong, and right eating, exercises to have good health
- ❖ Clapping on the chest and back.
- ❖ Massaging or pressing on the hands and feets
- ❖ Placing the object on the lower abdominal

Chapter 8: Changing lifestyle, adequate diet is the advice for most diseases

We do know the vital role of exercise, but what mechanism we have not yet fully know, the author just want to sum up some questions and facts of health relating to physical activity. Hope that the right answer will soon be found by the scientists.

Preventive therapies and alternative therapies are to aim to make the metabolic rate at the optimum level.

1) Why exercise?

2) Why a healthy diet, with good nutritions and rich fruits?

3) How does lifestyle help?

4) Why Do Women Live Longer Than Men?

It is maybe because of the combination:

- Women eat and drink less than men. Most pubs in Vietnam only have male guests.

- Women have less intense physical exercise than men, so it makes them have more rate of fibromyalgia.

- Women have more moderate laboring work then men, especially in developing countries, these laboring activities may help to increase the mobility of the blood circulation, reduce the free oxidants and make metabolic reactions more balanced than men have. This may be the reason why women do live longer than men. Especially in Eastern countries, where there is the domination of Confucianism, Men have more rights, more benefits, and more delicious food than women. And the women still have to do moderate laboring work than men like housework, kitchen work, taking care of children, taking care of grandchildren. Eating less and working more maybe the answer for why do women live longer than men.

Table 10: Mechanism of alternative therapies that help to prevent and heal chronic illness

Mechanism of most application on preventing and healing chronic illness
To make the metabolic reactions have optimum rate, blood circulation, PH, nature of the substrate, temperature, enzymes, the concentration of substrate, the concentration of products, repairing damages, immune cells, homeostatic, motility of surrounding fluid should be at the optimum levels.
1. Aspirin, papaya, baking soda, acupressure, massage, statin drugs, and NSAIDs help to prevent and remove the blood clots, trigger points in the vessels and tissues.
2. Exercise, suitable physical laboring work increases the blood circulation, fluid mobility and exchanging particles between blood and cells.
3. Vitamins, minerals in fruits and balanced diets play an important role in contributing substrates and activating enzymes. Enzymes are important for all metabolic reactions.
4. Vitamines also play important roles as the antioxidants.
5. Mindfulness, meditation, and positive affirmation help the body relaxed and in balanced which facilitates the process of healing and preventing blood clots, free oxidants and free

radical.
6. Baking soda reduces PH acid from disorder metabolism. PH acid is not good for the cells, tissues, and metabolism.
7. Deep breathing and diaphragm breathing help to mobilize all cells, tissues, and organs of important systems in the abdominal, which increases the temperature of the abdomen, make the abdomen softer more flexible than before. This breathing also increases the blood circulations between organs, increase rate and efficiency of the metabolic and catabolic in the abdomens. This leads to increasing the metabolic rate of the whole body.
8. Balanced diets may make all participants of metabolism at an optimum level: macrobiotic, balanced diets or rich fruits diet

These are the review that needs deeper researches, some of the techniques carried by the author can be easily tested by the readers and researchers and we can gain the results immediately. Master Do Duc Ngoc is profound in teaching and combining these techniques to get the best results. This writing hope that scientists can do more research to find evidence and prooves to combine all advantages of modern medicine, traditional medicine, traditional techniques and alternative therapies to get effective treatments for all patients.

The illnesses and diseases can be benefit from these exercises:

The common advice for all these health problems is having suitable exercise and having the right diet. Baking soda, papaya, fruits, vitamins, minerals, alternative therapies, and traditional

Table 11: Top ten causes of death in high income/affluent countries – lifestyle diseases

Top ten causes of death in high income/affluent countries
1. Ischemic heart diseases
2. Stroke
3. Alzheimer disease and other dementia
4. Trachea, bronchus and lung cancer
5. Chronic obstructive pulmonary disease
6. Lower respiratory infections
7. Colon and rectum cancers
8. Diabetes
9. Kidney diseases
1. Breast cancer

[58] [83] [45] [46] [47] [55] [59] [81]

medicine also play an important role in dealing with these diseases. If there are a lot of trigger points or blocking points around the vessels, it will make the distribution of the glucose and oxygen in the body disorder. On the other hand, there are many sensors of the autonomic nervous system that lie along the vessels in the head, liver, legs, hands and all other organs to have the autonomic responses to maintain balanced homeostasis. The chronic trigger points will create longterm changes in the homeostasis and make the autonomic nervous system out of balance. to some extent, traditional therapies, suitable diets, and alternative therapies seem to be effective for treating some chronic diseases because these therapies help to remove trigger points:

- To make the hand warm, reduce irritation in the patients who have Raynaud

- Removing backache, pain in the neck and headache.

- Removing Vestibular disorder hay vestibular trouble

- To remove the headache, dizziness, vertigo and floating and most of the symptoms of Alzheimer's and neurodegenerative diseases.

- Preventing Alzheimer's & neurodegenerative diseases

- Removing numbness and tingling in hands and feet.

- Removing the weakness and hands and legs

- Removing lumbar pain

- Making balancing for diabetes patients

- Reducing blood pressure by removing the trigger points, the resistance of the vessels will back to normal.

- Preventing heart failure, renal failure by increase blood circulation

- Liver inflammation relating to the poor blood circulation into the liver

- Heart pain relating to the poor blood circulation to the heart

- Intestine problems relating to the poor blood circulation to the intestine systems: irritation bowel movement, chronic diarrhea, chronic constipation

- Removing nerve pain and nerve inflammation

- Removing chronic fatigue.

- Treating insomnia because it increases the blood circulation to the brain and by placing a small object on the lower stomach will make people pay attention to it during breathing, which can make their head is empty from unwanted thinking.

- Stress makes the blood circulation and the whole body imbalanced.

Chronic poor blood circulation can make people suffer hypoglycemia, hypotension. These symptoms make be found in localize organs or localized tissue or the whole body.

For self treating fever, pain, cough, phlegm, difficult breathing and many other chronic diseases: finding and removing the trigger points.
❖ Inhale herbal oils   ❖ Practicing Qigong, right eating, exercises to have good health   ❖ Clapping on the chest and back.   ❖ Massaging or pressing on the hands and feets   ❖ Placing the object on the lower abdominal.

Some of traditional alternative healing techniques that help for pain, fever and systemic illnesses:

- ✓ Using stick, or top of the bottle or any tool to press on hands, all areas of hands, neck and the head gradually until you feel no pain, ni piercing. Or press the hands on the corner of the hard object. Any abnormal sensations when you pressing mean that all trigger points in your hands are gone.

- ✓ Using herbal oils rub on the palm of hands a feet before sleep.

- ✓ Soaking feet with herbal warm water. To simply have herbal warm water, using salt and ginger, cinnamo or any herbal at hands.

- ✓ Using the papaya leaves soaking the alcohol to rub a long the back for 10 minutes.

- ✓ Using hairdryer to warm up the back, hands, feet, palm of the hands and the pain areas for 10 minites each times.

❖ Always bear in mind the exercises that make the hands and feet warm and a little moistured.

> During and after practice, to remain the results, always make the body have enough nutrition by eating and drinking and make the veins clear. To gain this state you can maintain these interdependent signs:
>
> 1. Achieved the hands and feet warm
>
> 2. Maintain the palm of the hands warm and moistured
>
> 3. Keep glycemia at least 6.0 mmol/l when hungr, and at normal level when full.

When we maintain the hands warm, soft and a little moisture for a long time, we can achieve the optimal level of blood pressure, which is around 120/80.

Ho'oponopono techniques and the combination to calm the mind – forget it , all are rubbishes, we can only accept the terms, definitions and diseases put on us only when they give us the solutions also.

> For fear and negative emotion, thinking, read this 5 times, and then staring as high as possible at a point on ceilings or sky, keep that for 10 seconds (count from one to ten) then slowly relax and close the eyes and read several times:
>
> **I love you**
>
> **I am sorry**
>
> **Please forgive me**
>
> **Thank you!**

References:

1. 15 Best Health Benefits of Eating Papaya. (n.d.). In Wikipedia. Retrieved July 17, 2019, from https://www.gyanunlimited.com/health/papaya-benefits-and-nutritional-facts-of-papaya/5960/
2. A Level Biology. (n.d.). Factors Affecting Enzyme Activity. Retrieved July 17, 2019, from https://alevelbiology.co.uk/notes/factors-affecting-enzyme-activity/
3. AIDS. (n.d.). In Wikipedia. Retrieved July 17, 2019, from https://en.wikipedia.org/wiki/HIV/AIDS
4. Alina Wo., Bartosz W., Gerard D., Celestyna Mila-K., and Andrzej R. (2007, February 16). The effect of whole-body cryostimulation on lysosomal enzyme activity in kayakers during training. Authors. Authors and affiliations. Original Article. First Online: 16 February 2007. Retrieved July 17, 2019, from https://link.springer.com/article/10.1007/s00421-007-0404-0.
5. Andrea Kurz, MD; Daniel I. Sessler, MD; Richard Christensen, BA; Martha Dechert, BA. (n.d.). Heat Balance and Distribution during the Core-Temperature Plateau in Anesthetized Humans. Retrieved July 17, 2019, fromhttps://anesthesiology.pubs.asahq.org/article.aspx?articleid=2029234
6. Article Navigation. Influence of Dietary Lipid on Lipogenic Enzyme Activities in Coho Salmon, Oncorhynchus kisutch . (Walbaum). Huangsheng Lin Dale R. Romsos Peter I. Tack Gilbert A... Retrieved July 17, 2019, from https://academic.oup.com/jn/article-abstract/107/5/846/4769083
7. Axelrod YK, et al. Crit Care Clin. (2006). Temperature management in acute neurologic disorders. Review article. Department of Neurology. Retrieved July 17, 2019, from https://www.ncbi.nlm.nih.gov/m/pubmed/17239754/?i=6&from=/24365362/related

8. Back_pain. (n.d.). In Wikipedia. Retrieved July 17, 2019, from https://en.wikipedia.org/wiki/Back_pain
9. Baking Soda Cancer Studies and pH Medicine Published on May 2, 2012. Reference link https://drsircus.com/cancer/cancer-studies-ph-medicine/
10. Baking Soda Dos and Don'ts. Retrieved July 17, 2019, from https://www.webmd.com/a-to-z-guides/baking-soda-do-dont#1
11. Benefits and Risks of Drinking Baking Soda in Water! . (2011, June 13). Retrieved July 17, 2019, from http://doudyeissa.blogspot.com.es/2011/06/benefits-and-risks-of-drinking-baking.html
12. Berenice Hudson. (2015). EPIDEMIOLOGY. General Prevalence of Acute Pain Lifetime prevalence in general population: – Approaches 100% for acute pain leading to use of analgesics. Retrieved July 17, 2019, from https://slideplayer.com/slide/4886109/
13. Blood sugar level. (n.d.). In Wikipedia. Retrieved July 17, 2019, from https://en.m.wikipedia.org/wiki/Blood_sugar_level
14. Blood sugar regulation. (n.d.). In Wikipedia. Retrieved July 17, 2019, from https://en.m.wikipedia.org/wiki/Blood_sugar_regulation
15. Breast_cancer. (n.d.). In Wikipedia. Retrieved July 17, 2019, from https://en.wikipedia.org/wiki/Breast_cancer
16. Canceractive. (2018, September 5). Acid Bodies increase cancer risk and metastases. Retrieved July 17, 2019, from http://www.canceractive.com/cancer-active-page-link.aspx?n=1025
17. Carol DerSarkissian. (2018, February 28). Home Remedies for Nerve Pain. Retrieved July 17, 2019, from https://www.webmd.com/pain-management/nerve-pain-self-care#1
18. Carol DerSarkissian. (2018, May 3). Nonprescription Treatments for Nerve Pain. Retrieved July 17, 2019, from https://www.webmd.com/pain-management/nonprescription-treatments-nerve-pain#1
19. Carol DerSarkissian. (2018, May 3). Prescription Medications and Treatments for Nerve Pain. Retrieved July 17, 2019, from

https://www.webmd.com/pain-management/prescription-medications-treatments-nerve-pain#1
20. Catabolism. (n.d.). In Wikipedia. Retrieved July 17, 2019, from https://en.wikipedia.org/wiki/Catabolism
21. Catia G., Michele B., Marco B. T., Matteo C.,Luigi B.,and Laura G.. (2017, March 21). Venom from Cuban Blue Scorpion has tumor activating effect in hepatocellular carcinom. Retrieved July 17, 2019, from https://www.ncbi.nlm.nih.gov/pmc/articles/PMC5359575/
22. Cell_biology. (n.d.). In Wikipedia. Retrieved July 17, 2019, from https://en.wikipedia.org/wiki/Cell_biology
23. Chest_pain. (n.d.). In Wikipedia. Retrieved July 17, 2019, from https://en.wikipedia.org/wiki/Chest_pain
24. Coenzyme Q10. (n.d.). In Wikipedia. Retrieved July 17, 2019, from https://en.m.wikipedia.org/wiki/Coenzyme_Q10
25. Colleen Huber. (n.d.). Does the Baking Soda Cancer Treatment aka . (Sodium Bicarbonate) Work? Retrieved July 17, 2019, from https://natureworksbest.com/dr-tullio-simoncini-sodium-bicarbonate-cancer-treatment/
26. Corinne O'. Osborn. (2017, December 4). Can I Use Baking Soda to Treat Cancer? Retrieved July 17, 2019, from https://www.healthline.com/health/cancer/baking-soda
27. Could baking soda improve cancer treatment? Published Thursday 31 May 2018. Reference link https://www.medicalnewstoday.com/articles/321970.php
28. Cuyamaca College: Biology 230 Human Anatomy
29. David Jockers. (2016, September 23). Baking Soda: Cancer Treatment Uses for Prevention and Testing. Retrieved July 17, 2019, from https://thetruthaboutcancer.com/baking-soda-uses-cancer/
30. Diabetes. (n.d.). In Wikipedia. Retrieved July 17, 2019, from https://en.wikipedia.org/wiki/Diabetes
31. Dimitra K., Ilias V. K., Achilleas M., Sofia K., Alexandra G., and Michael I. K. (2015, January 30). Fever-Range Hyperthermia vs. Hypothermia Effect on Cancer Cell Viability, Proliferation and HSP90 Expression. Retrieved July 17, 2019, from https://www.ncbi.nlm.nih.gov/pmc/articles/PMC4312095/

32. Dr Sircus. (2012, May 2). Baking Soda Cancer Studies and pH Medicine. Retrieved July 17, 2019, from http://drsircus.com/medicine/sodium-bicarbonate-baking-soda/cancer-studies-ph-medicine
33. Effect of long-term cold exposure on antioxidant enzyme activities in a small mammal. Retrieved July 17, 2019, from https://www.sciencedirect.com/science/article/pii/S089158490 000263X
34. Effect of temperature on enzyme activity. Retrieved July 17, 2019, from http://academic.brooklyn.cuny.edu/biology/bio4fv/page/enz_act.htm
35. Ekofi Research. (2018, July 12). There is an enzyme that makes a reaction that normally takes 78 million years occur in 18 milliseconds. Retrieved July 17, 2019, from https://nitro.ekofi.science/this-enzyme-makes-a-reaction-that-normally-takes-78-million-years-occur-in-18-milliseconds/
36. Elevation Of Body Temperature In Disease. Retrieved July 17, 2019, from https://nyaspubs.onlinelibrary.wiley.com/doi/abs/10.1111/j.1749-6632.1964.tb13681.x
37. Elizabeth Mendes. (2015, September 24). Aspirin and Cancer Prevention: What the Research Really Shows. Retrieved July 17, 2019, from https://www.cancer.org/latest-news/aspirin-and-cancer-prevention-what-the-research-really-shows.html
38. Enzyme Activity. Last updatedJun 6, 2019. Retrieved July 17, 2019, from https://chem.libretexts.org/Bookshelves/Introductory_Chemistry/Book%3A_The_Basics_of_GOB_Chemistry_.(Ball_et_al.)/18%3A_Amino_Acids%2C_Proteins%2C_and_Enzymes/18.07_Enzyme_Activity
39. Enzyme Function Dependent On Temperature. Retrieved July 17, 2019, from https://www.wilsonssyndrome.com/ebook/body-function-dependent-on-body-temperature/enzyme-function-dependent-on-temperature/
40. Enzyme. (n.d.). In Wikipedia. Retrieved July 17, 2019, from https://en.wikipedia.org/wiki/Enzyme

41. Enzymes. (n.d.). In Wikipedia. Retrieved July 17, 2019, from https://www.rsc.org/Education/Teachers/Resources/cfb/enzymes.htm
42. Ethan Boldt. (2018, April 30). 33 Surprising Baking Soda Uses & Remedies. Retrieved July 17, 2019, from https://draxe.com/nutrition/article/baking-soda-uses/
43. Eva V. Osilla; Sandeep Sharma. (2019, March 16). Physiology, Temperature Regulation. Retrieved July 17, 2019, from https://www.ncbi.nlm.nih.gov/books/NBK507838/
44. Fabrizio R., Raffaele D. C., Artur F. (2015, August 18). Orthostatic Hypotension: Epidemiology, Prognosis, and Treatment. Retrieved July 17, 2019, from https://www.sciencedirect.com/science/article/pii/S073510971503939X
45. Fatma Al-Maskari. (2010, July). Lifestyle diseases: An Economic Burden on the Health Services By . Retrieved July 17, 2019, from https://unchronicle.un.org/article/lifestyle-diseases-economic-burden-health-services
46. Fatma Al-Maskari. (2010, July). Lifestyle Diseases: An Economic Burden on the Health Services. Retrieved July 17, 2019, from https://unchronicle.un.org/article/lifestyle-diseases-economic-burden-health-services
47. Fever, fever patterns and diseases called 'fever' – A review. Retrieved July 17, 2019, from https://www.sciencedirect.com/science/article/pii/S1876034111000256
48. Fever. Retrieved July 17, 2019, from https://www.mayoclinic.org/diseases-conditions/fever/symptoms-causes/syc-20352759
49. Fever: The Rules Change After a Cancer Diagnosis. Retrieved July 17, 2019, from https://www.roswellpark.org/cancertalk/201807/fever-rules-change-after-cancer-diagnosis
50. Final Recommendation Statement. Aspirin Use to Prevent Cardiovascular Disease and Colorectal Cancer: Preventive Medication. (2016, April). Retrieved July 17, 2019, from https://www.uspreventiveservicestaskforce.org/Page/Documen

t/RecommendationStatementFinal/aspirin-to-prevent-cardiovascular-disease-and-cancer
51. Five elements . (Chinese philosophy). Retrieved July 17, 2019, from https://psychology.wikia.org/wiki/Five_elements_. (Chinese_philosophy)
52. Ford, Earl S; Bergmann, Manuela M; Kroger, Janine; Schienkiewitz, Anja; Weikert, Cornelia; Boeing, Heiner. "Healthy Living Is the Best Revenge: Findings From the European Prospective Investigation Into Cancer and Nutrition-Potsdam Study", Arch Intern Med, 169 . (15) . (2009): 1355-1362.
53. Fran Kritz. (2018, Ocotober 22). Lack of Exercise Poses a Greater Health Risk Than Smoking, Diabetes, and Heart Disease - Research tracks "the relationship between extremely high fitness and mortality." Retrieved July 17, 2019, from https://www.everydayhealth.com/heart-health/lack-exercise-poses-greater-health-risk-than-smoking-diabetes-heart-disease/
54. Fran Kritz. (2018, October 22). Lack of Exercise Poses a Greater Health Risk Than Smoking, Diabetes, and Heart Disease. Research tracks "the relationship between extremely high fitness and mortality." Retrieved July 17, 2019, from https://www.everydayhealth.com/heart-health/lack-exercise-poses-greater-health-risk-than-smoking-diabetes-heart-disease/
55. Garry Egger, John Dixon. (2014), Beyond Obesity and Lifestyle: A Review of 21st Century Chronic Disease Determinants. Retrieved July 17, 2019, from https://www.hindawi.com/journals/bmri/2014/731685/
56. Glucose . (n.d.). Retrieved July 17, 2019, from https://vi.m.wikipedia.org/wiki/Glucose
57. Gomez CR. Handb Clin Neurol. (2014).Disorders of body temperature. Retrieved July 17, 2019, from https://www.ncbi.nlm.nih.gov/m/pubmed/24365362/
58. Hannah Nichols. (2019, July 4). What are the leading causes of death in the US? Retrieved July 17, 2019, from https://www.medicalnewstoday.com/articles/282929.php
59. Health Risks of an Inactive Lifestyle. Also called: Sedentary Lifestyle, Sitting Disease. Retrieved July 17, 2019, from https://medlineplus.gov/healthrisksofaninactivelifestyle.html

60. Hector Corsi. (2012,APR 25). Baking soda might have potential against cancer. Retrieved July 17, 2019, from http://digitaljournal.com/article/323645
61. Hiromi Shinya. The Enzyme Factor. Source Amazon.com
62. HIV. (n.d.). In Wikipedia. Retrieved July 17, 2019, from https://en.wikipedia.org/wiki/HIV
63. Home remedies for life. (2018, April 22). Baking Soda: 12 Benefits, Properties, Dosage And Side Effects. Retrieved July 17, 2019, from https://homeremediesforlife.com/baking-soda-benefits/
64. Hope S. R., Jeffrey V. (n.d.). Scalp Hypothermia for Preventing Alopecia. During Chemotherapy. A Systematic Review and. Meta-Analysis of Randomized Controlled Trials. Retrieved July 17, 2019, from https://www.clinical-breast-cancer.com/article/S1526-8209. (16)30543-2/pdf
65. How to Massage Your Pressure Points. By Peggy Pletcher, MS, RD, LD, CDE on March 25, 2015 — Written by Healthline Editorial Team. Retrieved July 17, 2019, from https://www.healthline.com/health/pain-relief/how-to-massage-your-pressure-points#1
66. Hyperglycemia. (n.d.). In Wikipedia. Retrieved July 17, 2019, fromhttps://en.m.wikipedia.org/wiki/Hyperglycemia
67. Hyperthermia in Cancer Treatment - . Retrieved July 17, 2019, from https://www.cancer.gov/about-cancer/treatment/types/surgery/hyperthermia-fact-sheet
68. Hyperthermia to Treat Cancer. Retrieved July 17, 2019, from https://amp.cancer.org/treatment/treatments-and-side-effects/treatment-types/hyperthermia.html
69. HYPERTHERMIA TREATMENT. Retrieved July 17, 2019, from https://www.texasoncology.com/cancer-blood-disorders/cancer-facts/hyperthermia-treatment
70. Hyperthermia: Role and Risk Factor for Cancer Treatment. Retrieved July 17, 2019, from https://www.sciencedirect.com/science/article/pii/S2078152016300724
71. Hypertriglyceridemia. (n.d.). In Wikipedia. Retrieved July 17, 2019, from https://en.wikipedia.org/wiki/Hypertriglyceridemia

72. Hypoglycemia. (n.d.). In Wikipedia. Retrieved July 17, 2019, from https://en.m.wikipedia.org/wiki/Hypoglycemia
73. Hypotension. (n.d.). In Wikipedia. Retrieved July 17, 2019, from https://en.m.wikipedia.org/wiki/Hypotension
74. Hypotension/Low Blood Pressure: Symptoms, Complications, and Treatment. (n.d.). In Wikipedia. Retrieved July 17, 2019, from https://www.practo.com/health-wiki/hypotension-low-blood-pressure-symptoms-complications-and-treatment/3/article
75. Hypothermia and cancer chemotherapy. Retrieved July 17, 2019, from https://www.ncbi.nlm.nih.gov/m/pubmed/5812564/
76. Hypothermia -Chapter 76 - Author links open overlay panelPeter J.FagenholzMDEdward A.BittnerMD, PhD. Available online 14 September 2012.
77. Hypothermia -Shelley Wells Collins. Retrieved July 17, 2019, from https://www.cancertherapyadvisor.com/home/decision-support-in-medicine/hospital-medicine/hypothermia/
78. Hypothermia. (n.d.). In Wikipedia. Retrieved July 17, 2019, from https://en.m.wikipedia.org/wiki/Hypothermia
79. Hypothermia. , in Complications in Anesthesia . (Second Edition), 2007
80. Hypothermia. Peter J. Fagenholz MD, Edward A. Bittner MD, PhD, in Critical Care Secrets . (Fifth Edition),
81. India Times. (2019, March 22). 11 Lifestyle diseases you should take seriously. Retrieved July 17, 2019, from https://timesofindia.indiatimes.com/life-style/health-fitness/health-news/11-lifestyle-diseases-you-should-take-seriously/articleshow/16419598.cms
82. Indran M, Mahmood AA, Kuppusamy UR. Protective effect of Carica papaya L leaf extract against alcohol induced acute gastric damage and blood oxidative stress in rats. West Indian Med J. Sep 2008;57. (4):323-326.
83. International Journal of Hyperthermia. Targeting therapy-resistant cancer stem cells by hyperthermia. Retrieved July 17, 2019, from https://www.tandfonline.com/doi/full/10.1080/02656736.2017.1279757

84. Introduction to Enzymes. Retrieved July 17, 2019, from http://www.worthington-biochem.com/introbiochem/tempEffects.html
85. Ivayla I Ge., Brian C., Tasaduq F., Waleed J. (3019, April). Normal Body Temperature: Systematic Review. Retrieved July 17, 2019, from https://academic.oup.com/ofid/article/6/4/ofz032/5435701
86. J. R. Beaton and , T. Orme. A NOTE ON THE EFFECTS OF HYPOTHERMIA ON ENZYME ACTIVITIES IN THE RAT. Canadian Journal of Biochemistry and Physiology, 1961, 39. (10): 1649-1652, Retrieved July 17, 2019, from https://www.nrcresearchpress.com/doi/abs/10.1139/o61-179#.XSxytOgzbIU
87. Jessie A. Key. (n.d.). Factors that Affect the Rate of Reactions. Retrieved July 17, 2019, from https://opentextbc.ca/introductorychemistry/chapter/factors-that-affect-the-rate-of-reactions-2/
88. Jose-Alberto P., Horacio K. (2017, January 30). Epidemiology, Diagnosis, and Management of Neurogenic Orthostatic Hypotension. Retrieved July 17, 2019, from https://onlinelibrary.wiley.com/doi/full/10.1002/mdc3.12478
89. Joseph West. (n.d.). Why Does Heating Interfere With the Activity of an Enzyme? Retrieved July 17, 2019, from https://sciencing.com/why-does-heating-interfere-with-the-activity-of-an-enzyme-12730636.html
90. Juárez-Rojop IE, Díaz-Zagoya JC, Ble-Castillo JL, et al. Hypoglycemic effect of Carica papaya leaves in streptozotocin-induced diabetic rats.BMC Complement Altern Med. 2012 Nov 28;12:236.
91. Julie J. Martin. (n.d.). Hypothermia. Retrieved July 17, 2019, from https://www.cancercarewny.com/content.aspx?chunkiid=99914
92. Kazem R., Connor A. E., , and Stephen M. M. (2015, March 13). The Epidemiology of Blood Pressure and Its Worldwide Management. Retrieved July 17, 2019, from

https://www.ahajournals.org/doi/full/10.1161/CIRCRESAHA.116.304723
93. Khalid S.., Rafat A. S. (2017, August 281). Papaya black seeds have beneficial anticancer effects on PC-3 prostate cancer cells. Retrieved July 17, 2019, from https://jcmtjournal.com/article/view/2224
94. Khí Công Y Đạo, Thầy Đỗ Đức Ngọc giảng về tầm quan trọng nhất của đường theo đông y . 2015. Retrieved July 17, 2019, from http://khicongydaododucngoc.blogspot.com
95. Kidney failure. (n.d.). https://en.wikipedia.org/wiki/Kidney_failure
96. Kinetics: Determination of an Enzymes Activity – Relevance. Retrieved July 17, 2019, from https://www.chem.fsu.edu/chemlab/bch4053l/enzymes/activity/index.html
97. Kris Gunnars. (2018, July 16). A Low-Carb Meal Plan and Menu to Improve Your Health. Retrieved July 17, 2019, from https://www.healthline.com/nutrition/low-carb-diet-meal-plan-and-menu
98. Laura J. Martin. (2018, July 8). Treating Nerve Pain Caused by Cancer, HIV, and Other Conditions. Retrieved July 17, 2019, from https://www.webmd.com/pain-management/treating-nerve-pain-caused-cancer-hiv
99. Leprosy. (n.d.). In Wikipedia. Retrieved July 17, 2019, from https://en.wikipedia.org/wiki/Leprosy
100. List of traditional Chinese medicines. Retrieved July 17, 2019, from https://en.m.wikipedia.org/wiki/List_of_traditional_Chinese_medicines
101. Lloyd Jenkins. (2015, June 29) . Fight Disease and Fatigue with Lemon Juice and Baking Soda. Retrieved July 17, 2019, from https://budwigcenter.com/fight-disease-and-fatigue-with-lemon-juice-and-baking-soda/
102. Matthew Lee. (2018, December 12), Metabolizing Proteins Vs. Fats. Retrieved July 17, 2019, from https://healthyeating.sfgate.com/metabolizing-proteins-vs-fats-3453.html

103. Mayer FQ, et al. Artif Organs. (2010). Effects of cryopreservation and hypothermic storage on cell viability and enzyme activity in recombinant encapsulated cells overexpressing alpha-L-iduronidase. Retrieved July 17, 2019, from https://www.ncbi.nlm.nih.gov/m/pubmed/20633158/
104. Mdhealth. (n.d.). How to Drink Baking Soda for Optimal Results. Retrieved July 17, 2019, from http://www.md-health.com/Drinking-Baking-Soda.html
105. Melinda Ratini. (2018, March 13). Unexplained Nerve Pain. Retrieved July 17, 2019, from https://www.webmd.com/pain-management/unexplained-nerve-pain-the-mystery-of-neuropathic-pain#1
106. Melinda Ratini. (2018, March 16). Nerve Pain and Nerve Damage. Retrieved July 17, 2019, from https://www.webmd.com/brain/nerve-pain-and-nerve-damage-symptoms-and-causes#1
107. Metabolic_syndrome. (n.d.). In Wikipedia. Retrieved July 17, 2019, from https://en.wikipedia.org/wiki/Metabolic_syndrome
108. Metabolism. (n.d.). In Wikipedia. Retrieved July 17, 2019, from https://en.m.wikipedia.org/wiki/Metabolism
109. Molecular mechanisms of temperature compensation in poikilotherms.. J R Hazel, and C L Prosser. Retrieved July 17, 2019, from https://www.physiology.org/doi/abs/10.1152/physrev.1974.54.3.620
110. Neuropathic pain. (n.d.). In Wikipedia. Retrieved July 17, 2019, from https://en.wikipedia.org/wiki/Neuropathic_pain
111. Ngoc D. Do. (2016, November 5). Đột phá nghiên cứu mới cho biết Làm thế nào để đảo ngược khỏi bệnh tiểu đường trong 3 tuần. Retrieved July 17, 2019, from http://khicongydaododucngoc.blogspot.com/2016/11/ot-pha-nghien-cuu-moi-cho-biet-lam-nao.html
112. Ngoc D. Do. (2016, November 5). Nhịp tim liên quan đến : Khí . (tâm thu), Huyết . (tâm trương), đường. Retrieved July 17, 2019, from http://khicongydaododucngoc.blogspot.com/2016/11/nhip-tim-lien-quan-en-khi-tam-thu-huyet_5.html

113. Ngoc D. Do. (n.d.) Chua Dau Lung : Khi Cong Tinh Do, Thay Do Duc Ngoc EIAB Germany 2014. Retrieved July 17, 2019, from http://khicongydaododucngoc.blogspot.com/
114. Nguyen TT, Parat MO, Shaw PN, et al. Traditional Aboriginal Preparation Alters the Chemical Profile of Carica papaya Leaves and Impacts on Cytotoxicity towards Human Squamous Cell Carcinoma.PLoS One. 2016;11. (2):e0147956.
115. Palma J., Kaufmann H. (2017, March 16). Epidemiology, Diagnosis, and Management of Neurogenic Orthostatic Hypotension. Retrieved July 17, 2019, from https://www.ncbi.nlm.nih.gov/pubmed/28713844
116. Parkinson disease. (n.d.). In Wikipedia. Retrieved July 17, 2019, from https://en.wikipedia.org/wiki/Parkinson%27s_disease
117. Peter J. F., Edward A. B. (2013). Hypothermia. Combination TherapyCore Temperature. Retrieved July 17, 2019, from https://www.sciencedirect.com/topics/nursing-and-health-professions/hypothermia
118. Protease inhibitor . (biology). (n.d.). In Wikipedia. Retrieved July 17, 2019, from https://en.m.wikipedia.org/wiki/Protease_inhibitor_. (biology)
119. Protein catabolism. (n.d.). In Wikipedia. Retrieved July 17, 2019, from https://en.wikipedia.org/wiki/Protein_catabolism
120. Protein metabolism. (n.d.). In Wikipedia. Retrieved July 17, 2019, from https://en.m.wikipedia.org/wiki/Protein_metabolism
121. Protein–energy malnutrition. (n.d.). In Wikipedia. Retrieved July 17, 2019, from https://en.wikipedia.org/wiki/Protein%E2%80%93energy_malnutrition
122. Proteins and Temperature. Annual Review of Physiology. Vol. 57:43-68 . (Volume publication date March 1995). Retrieved July 17, 2019, from https://doi.org/10.1146/annurev.ph.57.030195.000355.
Retrieved July 17, 2019, from https://www.annualreviews.org/doi/pdf/10.1146/annurev.ph.57.030195.000355

123. Quist Christina. (n.d). Hypothermia. Retrieved July 17, 2019, from https://www.cancertherapyadvisor.com/home/decision-support-in-medicine/hospital-medicine/hypothermia-2/
124. Sam Blanchard. (2018, May 31). Drinking baking soda could help cure cancer: Kitchen ingredient makes hard-to-reach tumour cells easier to target with drugs, study finds. Retrieved July 17, 2019, from https://www.dailymail.co.uk/health/article-5791377/Baking-soda-make-hard-reach-tumour-cells-easier-target-chemotherapy.html
125. Sandeep S., Priyanka T. B. (2019, June 20). Hypotension. Retrieved July 17, 2019, from
126. Sandi Busch. (n.d.). How Quickly Does Protein Metabolize? Retrieved July 17, 2019, from https://www.livestrong.com/article/550839-how-quickly-does-protein-metabolize/
127. Sci –News. (2018, June 6). Baking Soda Could Improve Cancer Therapy. Retrieved July 17, 2019, from http://www.sci-news.com/medicine/baking-soda-cancer-therapy-06071.html
128. Science Experiments Demonstrating How Temperature Affects Enzyme Activity. Retrieved July 17, 2019, from https://education.seattlepi.com/science-experiments-demonstrating-temperature-affects-enzyme-activity-6633.html.
129. Secondary metabolite. (n.d.). In Wikipedia. Retrieved July 17, 2019, from https://en.m.wikipedia.org/wiki/Secondary_metabolite
130. Sickle cell disease. (n.d.). In Wikipedia. Retrieved July 17, 2019, from https://en.wikipedia.org/wiki/Sickle_cell_disease
131. Sindhu R., Binod P., Sabeela B. U., Amith A., Anil K. M.,Aravind M., Sharrel R., and Ashok P. (2018, Mar). Applications of Microbial Enzymes in Food Industry. Retrieved July 17, 2019, from https://www.ncbi.nlm.nih.gov/pmc/articles/PMC5956270/

132. Suy Than : Khi Cong Tinh Do , Do Duc Ngoc EIAB Germany 2014. Retrieved July 17, 2019, from http://khicongydaododucngoc.blogspot.com/
133. Sy Kraft. (2018, August 17). Everything you need to know about hypothermia. Retrieved July 17, 2019, from https://www.medicalnewstoday.com/articles/182197.php
134. Thầy Đỗ Đức Ngọc: Nói về món ăn, thuốc uống thuộc TÌNH 2017 tại Như Tịnh Thất. Retrieved July 17, 2019, from http://khicongydaododucngoc.blogspot.com/
135. The Effects of Temperature on Enzyme Activity and Biology. Retrieved July 17, 2019, from https://sciencing.com/effects-temperature-enzyme-activity-biology-6049.html
136. Traditional Asian medicine. Retrieved July 17, 2019, from https://en.m.wikipedia.org/wiki/Traditional_Asian_medicine
137. Traditional Chinese medicine. (n.d.). In Wikipedia. Retrieved July 17, 2019, from https://en.m.wikipedia.org/wiki/Traditional_Chinese_medicine
138. Traditional medicine. (n.d.). Retrieved July 17, 2019, from https://en.m.wikipedia.org/wiki/Traditional_medicine
139. Traditional Vietnamese medicine. Retrieved July 17, 2019, from https://en.m.wikipedia.org/wiki/Traditional_Vietnamese_medicine
140. Van D. Dao. (2018, February 25). The hidden relation, clues of autism, ADHD and depression which reveals the cause and possible cure. Retrieved July 17, 2019, from http://www.awakenyouwonderfulwe.com/2018/11/the-hidden-relation-clues-of-autism_13.html.
141. Van D. Dao. (2018, March 07). Real cause of human problems: Autism, ADHD, Depression, Suicide and Stress. Retrieved July 17, 2019, from http://www.awakenyouwonderfulwe.com/2018/07/real-cause-of-human-problems-autism.html
142. Van D. Dao. (2018, May 3). Life is not paradoxical, life is art. Life is not calculated by autistic robot, life is must felt and created. Retrieved July 17, 2019, from

http://www.awakenyouwonderfulwe.com/2018/03/life-is-not-paradoxical-life-is-art.html
143. Van D. Dao. (2018, November 15). Seasonal Stress in America and World kill the most, not cold, heat or flu. Retrieved July 17, 2019, from http://www.awakenyouwonderfulwe.com/2017/09/seasonal-stress-in-america-kill-most.html.
144. Van D. Dao. (2019, Fabruary 16). Are autism, depression, ADHD, talented, mastery, poor learning, stress, seizures, drugs, violence, PTSD born or created? Retrieved July 17, 2019, from http://www.awakenyouwonderfulwe.com/2019/02/are-autism-depression-adhd-talented.html.
148. Van D. Duy. (2019, August). Ứng dụng thiền và khí công theo nguyên lý YHCT giúp tăng cường sức khỏe, phòng và chữa bệnh. Retrieved August 27, 2019, from https://edumall.vn/course/ung-dung-thien-va-khi-cong-theo-nguyen-ly-yhct-giup-tang-cuong-suc-khoe-phong-va-chua-benh.html
149. Van Duy Dao. "The Relation between Smoking, Breathing, Glycemia and the Rate of the Metabolism that Reveals the Effective Way of Controlling Body Weight and Glycemia". Acta Scientific Neurology 2.9 . (2019): 15-20.
150. Vitamin A. (n.d.). In Wikipedia. Retrieved July 17, 2019, from https://en.m.wikipedia.org/wiki/Vitamin_A
151. Vitamin C. (n.d.). In Wikipedia. Retrieved July 17, 2019, from https://en.m.wikipedia.org/wiki/Vitamin_C
152. Vitamin E. (n.d.). In Wikipedia. Retrieved July 17, 2019, from https://en.m.wikipedia.org/wiki/Vitamin_E
153. Webster Kehr. (2019, June 5). Vitamin c and baking soda cancer treatment including cancers of the digestive tract. Reference link https://www.cancertutor.com/vitc_bsoda/
154. William P. C., San P. Rd., and Jacksonville,. (2016, January 5). Thermoregulatory disorders and illness related to heat and cold stress. Retrieved July 17, 2019, from https://www.sciencedirect.com/science/article/pii/S1566070216300017

155. Worthington. (n.d.) Introduction to Enzymes. Retrieved July 17, 2019, from http://www.worthington-biochem.com/introbiochem/factors.html
156. Yin and yang. Retrieved July 17, 2019, from https://en.m.wikipedia.org/wiki/Yin_and_yang

Part II: State of Mind: Stress and Happiness.

Chapter 9: What happens in the body when we are in a happy state?

Apparently, there are four ingredients of happiness. Simon Sinek, the author of, "Leaders Eat Last" has summarized these four chemicals creating happiness. These for happiness chemicals are endorphins, dopamine, serotonin, and oxytocin. These four chemicals create a feeling of happiness.

Endorphins reduce feelings of pain. Endorphins are released when you do exercise or doing hard work. These endorphins interact with the receptors in your brain that reduce the feelings of pain. Moreover, endorphins create positive feelings in their bodies. It makes people feel healthier after exercise than before; so that some people who are familiar with exercise may addict with exercise. If we feel a little pain or tired, after joining in exercises, or fun activities, high energy activities, the endorphin will be created in the brain, it makes us feel good in the whole body. Endorphins also have sedation effects. People who work hard may feel positive and energizing and sleep well. The finding of the roles of endorphins in the brain helps people understand "the harder the work, the better people sleep." The works have paid off. Many physicians and therapist have confirmed the effect of regular exercise, regular exercise is sufficient to produce a significant reduction in depression among clinically depressed subjects.

According to Simon Sinek and scientists, another chemical for happy feelings is Dopamine. Dopamine is the chemical created when people get rewards, achieves something worthwhile. Setting goals and achieving goals motivated behavior. When we get things we want, achieve things we want, or get through project milestones, do the things on "to do list"; we have the feeling of incredible, of joy and happiness; that makes us feel good. This is the role of dopamine; create good feelings; are highly addictive. If you post a status or pictures on Facebook, you get likes, good comments, you feel good, joyful; this is the effect of dopamine. Perhaps, people who addicted to gambling addicted to the effect of dopamine; they addicted to the feelings of achieving as soon as possible. Gambling has the result quickly and instantly, within minutes, hours or a day. If they win in gambling, they will be very happy, the feelings of victory are so strong that they dare to risk all the things they have. If the results of gambling games only appear after one year, two years or ten years; all gambler may quit gambling instantly. Money or winning bring for them the feelings of happiness; they are addicted to these feelings of joy from dopamine. Especially, when people feel stressed or not joyful with other activities; they tend to find the activities created joy.

According to Dr. Ananya Mandal in News Medical Life Sciences, dopamine has some notable functions are in:

- Movement
- memory
- Pleasurable reward
- Behavior and cognition
- Attention
- Inhibition of prolactin production
- Sleep
- Mood
- Learning

Excess and deficiency of dopamine is the cause of several problems. Lacking dopamine may lead to poor learning, lack of sleep, change the mood, poor attention, poor memory, and have some strange behaviors. Parkinson's disease and drug addiction are some of the examples of problems associated with abnormal dopamine levels. The table below described some of the visible side effects of dopamine from drugs.com

Table 12: the symptoms of excessive dopamine

Excess of dopamine may cause symptoms	
- Cardiac conduction abnormalities: ventricular arrhythmia, atrial fibrillation, ectopic heartbeats - Tachycardia, angina, palpitation, bradycardia, vasoconstriction, hypotension, hypertension, - Dyspnea, - Nausea, vomiting, - Headache, anxiety, - Piloerection, and gangrene of the extremities.	
Cardiovascular	Ectopic beats, tachycardia, angina pain, palpitation, hypotension, vasoconstriction
Gastrointestinal	Nausea, vomiting
Nervous system	Headache
Respiratory	Dyspnea
Dermatologic	Piloerection
Local	Necrosis, tissue sloughing, local ischemia, and vasoconstriction
Psychiatric	Anxiety
Ocular	Mydriasis
Metabolic	Hypovolemia

Source: Dopamine side effects from https://www.drugs.com

These are the changes in the body when people feel joyful and happy because of the thinking they will win a big deal. These signs are also the visible signs of people feel happy before a good deal, an important event, before interesting trips, and before receiving a big reward. In making the deal, sale men usually pay attention to the pupils of the prospects when present the product and tell the price. If the pupils enlarge, it means that the prospects like the product despite the denial and complain about the product. Most of the time, the client are easy to accept the high price of the deal. Happy kids and students may have these signs, before the first day they enter high schools or universities, before the day they of receiving important rewards, important sports games; excessive dopamine makes them so anxious that they cannot sleep during the night before the event. With the extreme excess of dopamine, people may experience the serious side effects of dopamine: chest pain; fast, slow, or pounding heartbeats; painful or difficult urination; weakness, confusion; and weak or shallow breathing." In real life, if people feel over joyful with the sudden big rewards, the sudden surprise like winning a lottery of one million dollars they may experience chest pain, pounding heartbeats, difficult urination, shallow breathing, and weakness. When Dan Jansen, after several heartbreaking failures to capture an Olympic Gold Medal for speed skating, finally won the Gold in the 1000-meter race in the 1994 Winter Olympics in Norway, his wife was so overexcited and happy that she had to be rushed to the emergency by physicians. This is the case of excessive dopamine.

Sports are the games of dopamine in the brain of all relating people; create feelings of victory and happiness. Sports will be boring if there are no scoreboards, audiences and players only know the result when the game is finished. If there are no rewards and no scoreboards, the games will be boring and less exciting. All players perhaps will quit playing, and the number of audiences will reduce substantially under this condition. The audiences will be much more excited if they are betting the results of the games than just watching. What makes the games more worthwhile to watch? Watching the videos of the Olympic game, watchers will feel moved, touched if the players and athletes have the acts of kindness, the acts of consideration to others. In Olympic Games and Paralympic Games, audiences will feel moved with the act of kindness, act of sacrificing of players who gave up the chance of winning to come back to help others players in difficulties or in accidents. Watching these games, the audiences will feel much more motivated, more inspired because they do not only have the chemical creating from kind human behaviors, called serotonin; they also have the feeling of highest victory - the victory over the Self. Players with acts of kindness are not the selfish winners; they are the selfless winning teams - an adorable team. A boy may be fun in watching an interesting game or movie alone, or achieving a reward; this is the effect of dopamine. Interestingly, if he watches this game or movie with his beloved one, his beloved parents; or sharing the rewards to others, he will experience much more happiness, inspiration, and touching; this is the effect of serotonin.

According to Simon Sinek, scientists, and therapists, the third chemical of happiness is serotonin. Serotonin may be the best-known happiness chemical, which is the target of antidepressant medications primarily aim to increase it in the brain of depressed patients. From the web patient.info have the description of depression, "depression refers to both negative affect like blow mood and/ or absence of positive affect like loss of interest and pleasure in most activities is usually accompanied by an assortment of emotional, cognitive, physical and behavioral symptoms." Increasing the serotonin in the brain is the mechanism of common drugs treating depression: selective serotonin reuptake inhibitors (SSRIs) and serotonin and norepinephrine reuptake inhibitors (SNRIs).

Serotonin is a chemical triggered naturally by many activities. Exposure to bright light, especially sunshine, is one way to increase serotonin. This is the reason why we need sunshine, we need outdoor activities. Out-door exercise and kind behaviors stimulate the production of serotonin. Some researchers have found that doing and receiving of kindness actions can stimulate serotonin in the brain, creating a happy feeling. Good behaviors, touching actions, cooperative behaviors also help increase serotonin in brains. In a talk of Wayne Dyer, he said "when a kind action takes place, three people can get benefits from this action: the giver, the receiver, and the observer of kind action. When we watching interesting films about the effort of people, read inspiring stories about inspiring actions, we also feel moved and touched by the inspiring stories. Simon Sinek calls serotonin the leadership chemical; it provides a feeling of significance, pride, and status. It drives us to seek the recognition of others. Students feel joyful in the graduation ceremony, but students will feel of significance, pride, and status if their parents, family members are in the audiences. Most people want to do hard job "for my mom, for my dad, for my children, for my boss, for my wife" they do it to find the recognition or the praise of their beloved ones. When an employee gets a promotion, informed by a call, an email, he only has a little joy of achievement, which is the effect of dopamine; he will be motivated. On the other hand, if the employee receives an intimate handwriting letter from his admired manager, which is full of the sincere experience, emotion, and expectations, he will very happy with the feeling of significance, of belonging caused by serotonin; he will be inspired. Daren Hardy told a story about the present he gave his wife. He gave her a notebook full of notes that thank his wife, thank for her act, her consideration, her love, and her kindness; receiving the notebook, his wife said that this was the best present she ever received from him in spite the fact that last year he presented her a Mercedes car. In fact, there is a huge difference in the meaning of these happiness chemicals. Serotonin reinforces the sense of relationships within the family and group; adds high emotion of happiness to the personal emotional account; boosts the self-esteem; boosts the immune system, and boosts the allegiance; these are some of the many effects that serotonin does for every relating people.

Fourth happiness chemical is oxytocin. Women are familiar with oxytocin; the hormone produced in abundance during giving birth. Oxytocin creates intimacy and trust feeling that someone will protect you. Oxytocin is the chemical of trust. Oxytocin is primarily associated with loving touch and close relationships, touching, kissing, and caring. Mothers and children can experience the effects of oxytocin when mothers breastfeed their children. Mom, babies, lovers have serotonin when they are protected and loved. Feeling of high safety; no worry when staying naked with the spouse; put away all weapons when entering the home. Scientists have found oxytocin have good effects on autistic mice. They will take more researchers with the hope that the future can carry using oxytocin in autistic children.

In the book: "Leaders eat last" Simon Sinek described endorphins and dopamine as the chemicals of selfish, and serotonin and oxytocin are the selfless chemicals. Once we understand how our happy hormones and neurotransmitters work, we may be able to trigger them more easily than we realized. We also can easily figure out what is the feeling that our family members have when we stay with them. Physicians usually prescribe many medications to create these happy chemicals in the brain of depressive patients, autistic children, and patent with mental problems. To some extent, these medications are helpful. It would be very helpful if these patients understand the roles of happiness chemical and stress chemicals to have better approaches to their problems. Understanding these chemicals also make us understand the real causes and real drives of many human behaviors in our society: why in our modern society, many people love volunteering works, love helping others, love caring the disable; and understand the real cause for the most problem in society. On the other hand, why there are so many crimes, violence, corruption, fighting, and wars in our world. The fact is all human behaviors taken place to create happiness feelings for people. Happiness feeling comes from the perception of gaining, getting, or possessing valuable things. Saving one thousand dollars, or one million dollars, or one billion dollars in a bank account just brings the feelings of joy, significance, and safety for the owners. Possessing one house, or three houses or ten villas also just creates feelings of joy, happiness, significance, and safety for the owners. In fact, there are noble ways to create a feeling of joy, happiness, significance, connection, and safety for the human being. Mastering the art of controlling thought and feelings well will make a big change in our society, eliminate most of the chronic diseases, and reduce the burden of problems for all governments. What a wonderful world if we act in a manner that creates happy chemicals and eliminates stress chemicals in our brain and all other people's brain.

References:
Bhandari, Smitha. (2016, February 24). Exercise and depression. Retrieved July 19, 2017, from http://www.webmd .com/depression/guide/exercise-depression#1
Bouchez, Colette. (2011, October 12). Serotonin: nine questions and answers Retrieved July 19, 2017, from http://www.webmd .com/-depression/features/serotonin#1
Drugs.com. (2011, September 12). Dopamine. Retrieved July 19, 2017, from http://www.drugs.com/dopamine.html
Goldberg, Joseph. (2016, November 14).What Are SSRIs?. Retrieved July 19, 2017, from http://www.webmd.com /depression/SSRIs-myths-and-facts-about-antidepressants#1
Macgill, Markus. (2015, September 21). Oxytocin: What is it and what does it do? Retrieved July 19, 2017, from http://www .medicalnewstoday.com/-articles/275795.php
Mandal, Ananya. (2015, Oct 27). Dopamine functions. Retrieved July 19, 2017, from http://www.news-medical.net/ health/Dopamine-Functions.aspx
Scaccia, Annamaria. (2016, August 22). Serotonin: What You Need To Know. Retrieved July 19, 2017, from http://www.healthline.com/health/mental-health/serotonin# overview1
Sinek, Simon. (2014).Leaders Eat Last: Why Some Teams Pull Together and Others Don't. Portfolio/Penguin.

Chapter 10: What is happening when we are under stress?

Opposite with feelings of happiness is the feelings of stress. What chemicals circulate in our bodies when we stressed. Many studies have shown there is three main chemicals cause stress. These are adrenaline, cortisone, and norepinephrine. The three major stress hormones explained the "fight or flight" system that takes over us when we in a dangerous situation or when we are stressed. This was the survival system for our ancestors to survive well in a dangerous environment. This survival system does not help us much in safe, constant changing of our modern society. Sometimes the constant trigger of this system can cause us a lot of problems. In our daily life, sometimes the small change in life it makes a stranger, unexpected but safe thing happen to us but our survival system triggered. This makes us annoyed a lot. Constant of this activating can cause us fatigue, tired and stress a lot. For example, when you received a friend's call from the office's number late at night, your body reacts so much stressful as if there would be an attack from a tiger behind.

According to Sarah Klein (2013) from Huffingtonpost.com with the article: "Adrenaline, Cortisol, Norepinephrine: The Three Major Stress Hormones, Explained", three major stress chemicals are adrenalin, cortisol, and norepinephrine. Adrenalin is commonly known as the fight and flight chemicals produced by the adrenal glands after perceiving the threatening message from the stressful condition. These are the hormones mainly produced by adrenal glands in response to the stress situation; we may call these are stress chemicals. Imagine that you are driving your car on road, suddenly the car behind you increase speed the goes passing your car. You see that car nearly crash your car. You will have symptoms of stress hormones. Another case, you are walking on the street, suddenly there is a big black dog barking run toward you from a corner, your heart increases the beat when the dog approaching you. You will have all signs of fear, stress with stress chemicals soaring inside your body. Luckily, the dog run passes through you to chase a mouse. People may have the soaring of stress chemicals when seeing cockroaches flying if they are afraid of cockroaches when seeing snakes crawling if they are afraid of snakes when seeing policeman approaching them if they are afraid of the policeman, and when staying alone in the midnight if they are afraid of staying alone.

Cortisol, adrenalin, along with nor-epinephrine is largely responsible for the vigorous and immediate reactions when being stressed. Cortisol is a stress hormone. In survival mode, the optimal amount of cortisol can save life. Cortisol helps maintain fluid balance, increase glucose in the blood, and maintain fluid balance. On the other hand, cortisol reduces some body functions that are not crucial in the stressful condition, like reproductive drive, immunity, digestion, growth and many more functions that are no need for the survival situation. A temporary increase of cortisol is very helpful for a critical situation. People will get many serious problems when the body continuously releases cortisol. Too much cortisol can reduce substantially some body functions; which are immune system, reduce memory ability, reduce mental capacity, increase stomach problem, increase blood pressure, increase blood sugar, decrease libido, produce acne, and lead to obesity and many more problems I will describe later.

In critical condition, especially the anaphylactic shock, physicians use a large amount of adrenaline, norepinephrine, and corticosteroid to save the life of the patients. Reading the mechanism of these chemicals will help readers understand why stressed people have the signs and symptoms in this chapter. The chronic stress leads to chronically elevated levels of adrenaline, norepinephrine, and cortisol, which are the causes of many illnesses and problems in children and adults like stomach problems, intestine problems, poor memory ability, poor mental capacity, and diabetes. We can know if people are under stress or not by observing if they have signs of mental stress or physical stress. The signs of physical stress are so obvious that most people can realize. We can know by seeing the increasing heartbeats, sweating, pale skin, gray skin, and the tension of muscle in actions, which has its own motive: vigorousness, suddenness, making noise, short and quick breath, non-smoothly action, and the stiff handshake. If you pay attention closely, we can sense or see these signals from stressed people. When people are angry or stressed, they will have the signals of stress are so obvious that most of their relatives can realize. In the stressed state, you will feel a surge of energy, which you might need to run away from a dangerous situation or fight against simulations. Stressed people tend to over-react with even mild stimulations from the environment. When people are stressed or peaceful, they can radiate the pattern of stressed energy or peaceful energy to other people around. Dogs can sense the energy of opposite individuals in a blink. If you are under stress, your dog may stay away from you, lying quietly. Otherwise, when you are in happiness, your dog will go around you; a dog will play and make fun of you ceaselessly. Children can sense the energy from parents and adults more accurately than adults can. So those children can feel peaceful with a nice, calm stranger; otherwise, children will have the feel of stress with sad, negative people. After staying with stress, negative people, children may have some abnormal behaviors of stress. The mind of children - fragile creatures - can catch better and retain longer the visible and invisible stress signals than adults do. Stressed children may eat less, sleepless, and cry after seeing bad people more than previous time. Because of their weakness and dependence, children have to perfect their ability to judge other people, so that they can have the corresponding responses or send the signals to let their parents know; this is the instinct for survival of small kids - an instinct for the survival of the weak.

Let's review the effects of stress and cortisol in the article "What is cortisol?" from webmd.com to have a better understanding the symptoms on table two and the relation of stress with most of the diseases. According to researchers, too much stress can derail your body's most important functions. It can also lead to a number of health problems, including:

- Anxiety and depression
- Headaches

- Heart disease
- Memory and concentration problems
- Problems with digestion
- Trouble sleeping
- Weight gain

To some extent, these side effects are the same as the effects of excessive cortisol in the body for a long time. These potential systemic side effects of cortisone are:

- Hyperglycemia
- Insulin resistance
- Diabetes mellitus
- Osteoporosis
- Anxiety
- Depression
- Amenorrhea
- Cataracts
- Cushing's syndrome
- Glaucoma,
- And many other problems.

Source: "What is cortisol?" from webmd.com

Moreover, constant stress can lead to too much cortisol; this can cause a condition called Cushing's syndrome. It can lead to rapid weight gain, skin that bruises easily, muscle weakness, diabetes, and many other health problems.

Stress chemicals run throughout the body when we are under stress. If we are under stress for a long time, the side effects of these hormones will present apparently. How do we prove the above effects of stress chemicals on the body by the easiest way to the patients? Well, the easiest ways are looking at the side effects of these hormones or drugs in medical books. Searching the side effects of these chemicals in drug information handbook and medical website, we will easily find out these side effects. I will make detail the effects or symptoms of the stress on the body for every people to check in table 2, table 3, table 4, and table 5.

These are the information retrieved from the medical website that everybody can check it easily. So how to know if somebody is suffering stress or not?

First, by writing the emotion and thinking that they have during the day, before and after important events. Just jot it down. People will understand more about themselves by rereading it.

Second, record their changes in blood pressure and other changes of the body by smartwatch or smart devices. The fluctuation of blood pressure during the day will let therapists understand more about the patients. Before important events like dating, examining, interviewing, meeting with doctors, unwanted things, and meeting with teachers, the pattern of blood pressure. These indicators with the recording of emotion and thinking will tell more about what is happing in the mind.

Third, by closely observing and recording the physical changes in all behaviors of people like walking, dancing, smiling, paying attention, making fun, stiffness in the muscle, peaceful sleeping or fearful sleeping, peaceful eating or anxious eating, and the attitude in studying, doing, and helping. The varieties of these activities, the emotion, and attitude in these activities; all these recordings will tell more about the state of mind, the state of the body.

Table 13: Side effects of three stress chemicals

Side effects of three chemicals creating stress			
Adrenalin	Norepinephrine	Less serious side effects Cortisol	Serious side effects cortisol
Sweating	Pain, burning	Acne, dry skin, or thinning	Vision problems

		skin	
Nausea and vomiting	Numbness, weakness, or cold	Bruising or discoloration of skin	Swelling
Pale skin	Slow or uneven heart rate	Insomnia	Rapid weight gain
Feeling short of breath	Trouble breathing	Mood changes	Shortness of breath
Dizziness	Vision, speech, or balance difficulties	Increased sweating	Severe depression or unusual thoughts or behaviors
Weakness or tremors	Blue lips or fingernails	Headache	Seizures
Headache	Spotted skin	Dizziness	Bloody or tarry stools
Feeling of nervousness or anxiousness		Nausea, stomach pain	Coughing up blood
High blood pressure symptoms: severe headache, blurred vision, buzzing in your ears, anxiety, confusion, chest pain, shortness of breath, uneven heartbeat, seizure			Symptoms of pancreatitis: pain in your upper stomach that spreads to your back; nausea and vomiting; or

		fast heart rate
		Low potassium
		Dangerously high blood pressure

People who are under stress always have symptoms inside the body described in table two: side effects of three chemicals creating stress. If people usually have high levels of the stress chemicals, they will have the symptoms or diseases caused by short-term stress and long-term stress, they will have the stress symptoms in physical health and mental health. Reading the table two, ordinary people can understand the symptoms of stress explained by physicians and therapists in medical books or medical websites.

In everyday activities, people may get signs of short-term. The short-term stress can affect your body in many ways, some of them include:

Table 14: bad effects of short-term stress on body, mind, and performance

The physical symptoms of short-term stress

1. Making heartbeat faster, this may lead to increase blood pressure in short term.
2. Making breath faster
3. Making sweat more
4. Leaving with cold hands, feet, or pale skin
5. Making feel sick to your stomach
6. Making feel sick to your stomach
7. Tightening muscles or feel tense
8. Dry mouth
9. Intestine problems
10. Increasing muscle spasms, headaches, and fatigue
11. Shortness of breath

Bad effects on mind and performance of short-term stress

1. Interfering with judgment and causing to make bad decisions
2. Reducing the ability of logical thinking
3. Act irrationally and emotionally; easily fall to irrational thinking and irrational behaving.
4. Seeing normal situations as threatening
5. Reducing enjoyment in many activities, unable to laugh at funny things
6. Negative feelings: anxious, frustrated, or mad

7. Awake during sleep, nightmare or screaming during sleep with children
8. Loss of apatite
9. Making it difficult to concentrate to solve the problems and often have a distraction.
10. Feel of rejected by the group.
11. Afraid of free time, time to stay alone; like to spend time do many useless activities or kill time
12. Irritate inside
13. Unable to work, and not willing to discuss their problems with others

Children who are afraid of injection may have symptoms of short-term stress during seeing doctors or nurses in the white coat. Some pediatric center, the doctors usually wear a normal coat to diagnose for small children.

People before taking each important test, example or interview usually experience these symptoms of short-term stress. Stress makes them make the bad result, forget all knowledge they have mastered, speaks many nonsense works, have to sweat, shaking, short breathing, cramp the n stomach.

Practicing in hospital, I have seen many cases of old people taking the health check test before an important event like going abroad; they usually get the results of high blood pressure with many other normal results. They always argue that when checking at home, they have normal blood pressure. These are the signs of excessive adrenalin and norepinephrine in a stressful situation. If observe attentively, we can see many other signs of stress in old people.

The long-term stress: the detail effects of long-term stress caused by three stress chemicals are

Table 15: The effects of long-term stress

The effects of long-term stress
1. Changing appetite: eat either less or more
2. Changing sleep habits: sleep too much or sleep too little
3. Changing quality of sleep: more nightmare or screaming during sleep
4. Having anxiety behavior: twitching, fiddling, talking too much, nail biting, teeth grinding, pacing, and other repetitive habits
5. Having colds symptoms, the flu symptoms, or chills more often than healthy people do; physicians just give them medicine for symptoms with the advice of taking rest.
6. Causing illnesses: asthma, headaches, stomach problems, intestinal problems, skin problems, and pains in all body; these are problems caused by excessive stress chemicals
7. Causing many mental problems, physical problems, people experiences extreme stress may have mental diseases, and physical illness
8. Causing many anxiety behaviors, anxiety behaviors create many personal problems, familial problems, school problems, and social problems
9. Affecting sex life
10. Affecting performance, poor performance leads to poor results and poor skills. In return, they create more stress.
11. Making people feel constantly tired, and worn out

Moreover, stress is like negative energy, it may translate directly and indirectly to surrounding people. If one person in the family or community feel stressed or have symptoms of chronic stress, most of the time, surrounding people will have the symptoms of stress.

Stress state and stress chemicals make muscles much more tense than normal; after tension, the muscles become weak and spasm irregularly. The tension in neck and head muscles may cause a headache. The tension of muscles in the stomach causes stomach problems like full stomach, vomiting, and bloating. The tension of muscles in the intestine may cause irritating bowel syndrome. The tension of muscles in the back may cause back pain. People usually experience neck pain when in wrong sleep position, this pain caused by tension in neck muscles. With these kinds of pain, doctors usually give advice and prescribe some medication:

- Muscle relaxation medication with the pain of back, neck;
- Physical therapy for the pain of back, ankle, neck and many other parts of the body caused by tension of muscles;
- Acupuncture, massage, relaxation, rubbing hot pack, rubbing external medication, meditation, and hypnosis may help with these kinds of chronic pain caused by tension of muscles.
- Regular exercise strengthens the muscle to make muscle less tension so can help reduce the pain effectively.
- Anti-spasmodic medication with the pain caused by spasm of muscles in the pain of intestine routes and menstrual pain;
- Some minerals, vitamins can help so much with the people with chronic pain caused by muscle spasm. The roles of the mineral are obvious in pregnancy women, who usually get serious leg cramps because of lacking mineral in blood.
- And the painkiller medication-like: acetaminophen and other Non-steroidal Anti-Inflammatory Drugs (NSAIDs)

These treatments only help people feel at ease for a short time. They will still feel pain if the stress not diminished. Start to observe you and people around to find out the real state of mind they are usually in. If they are under stress, perhaps they need the help from you. From Mental Health America, physicians suggest ways to recognize the warning signs of stress in the body, and how to cope with stress. Readers will realize that most of the warning signs of mental illness are the effects of excessive stress chemicals. Moreover, searching list of mental disorders, and the social problems from medical journals, medical websites, you will find that all the victims of these problems have experienced symptoms of excessive stress chemicals. If taking questionnaire with all people affected these problems, we will find that they have experienced the early signs of stress for a long time. The early signs these patients are close to the severe side effects of adrenaline, norepinephrine, and cortisol. These are early signs that most professional psychiatrist, experienced people can recognize when they meet new people who have the mental problem. Experienced people may have the gut feeling, have feelings of something is not right from the ill individuals. Listening to their gut feelings, they will take further actions to get more information to have the good judgment about new people.

Table 16: The early warning signs of mental disorders are also the symptoms of stress

Mental disorders	The early signs for a long time (from side effects of stress chemicals)
Anxiety Disorders	Acne, dry skin, or thinning skin
Suicide	Blue lips or fingernails
Parkinson's disease	Bruising or discoloration of the skin
Attention Deficit Hyperactivity Disorder (ADHD)	Dizziness
	Feeling of nervousness or anxiousness
Autism	Feeling short of breath
Bipolar Disorder	Headache
Depression	Hypertension
	Insomnia
Eating Disorders	Mood changes, anxious, lack of focus
Generalized Anxiety Disorder	
Obsessive-Compulsive Disorder	Nausea, vomiting, stomach pain
	Numbness, weakness, or cold
	Pain, burning
Panic Disorder	Pale skin or spotted skin
Post-Traumatic Stress Disorder	Slow or uneven heart rate
	Sweating
	Trouble breathing
Schizophrenia,	Vision, speech, or balance difficulties
	Weakness or tremors

If paying attention to the patients with mental problems, through the diagnosing process, we can easily find out these early symptoms have appeared for a long time. The stress symptoms indicate that these patients have experienced stress for a long time. Physicians can find a lot of early signs of stress in all victims long before they get mental problems, health problems, or social problems.

From the effect of stress chemicals on the body, individuals have the different environment of living with a lot of varieties that reduce or worsen the effect of stress so that they got different outcomes from chronic stress. These outcomes can cover all diseases in the list of mental problems, and physical problems of adult and children in society. If the statisticians make statistics to figure the relationship between stress and most of the problems people have, they will find out the cause of all problems in human beings. Before they can prove it, it will clarify how and why stress can create the worst destruction of human beings.

Some statistics such as the top ten diseases in the USA are quite the same as the top ten diseases in most developed countries. The highest standard of living in developed countries, to some extent, does not make people happier than people in poor countries. Their paradox is despite the highest standard of living, they have spent a huge amount of money for treating and preventing diseases but many diseases seem out of controlled. Their health problems, mental problems, and social problems are the biggest threat to the budget of countries. Most people live in developing countries know western living via television may think that these westerners are living in heaven.

The paradox of developed countries does not lie in genes, food, air, skin color, the daily problems, or daily difficulties they meet. Most of their problems come from their lifestyle living. Their thorny question is the rich and successful men live in abundances do not have fewer health problems, mental problems, and social problems than most people live in poor countries have. The paradox of diseases and problems goes against all the expectations and assumptions of the scientists. The fact is some rich people with poor lifestyle living can feel more stressed than ordinary people do. Moreover, ordinary people with a high style of living are happier than rich ones with a bad style of living.

The fifteen most common causes of death in the United States

Source How Stuff Works:

1. Diseases of the heart
2. Malignant tumors
3. Cerebrovascular diseases
4. Chronic lower respiratory diseases
5. Accidents (unintentional injuries)
6. Diabetes mellitus
7. Influenza and pneumonia
8. Alzheimer's disease
9. Nephritis, nephrotic syndrome, and nephrosis
10. Septicemia (blood poisoning)
11. Suicide
12. Chronic liver disease and cirrhosis
13. Primary hypertension and hypertensive renal disease
14. Parkinson's disease (tied)
15. Homicide

The list of top eight health problems in people aged 15-64, in the EU, 2011 from Eurostat Statistics Explained.

The first is problems with back and neck; the second are heart, blood pressure, or circulation problems; third are problems with legs and feet; the fourth are problems with arms and hands; the fifth is chest or breathing problems, including asthma and bronchitis; the sixth is a severe headache such as a migraine; the seventh is diabetes; and the eighth is depression.

When practitioners examine these patients, they will easily find the early signs of stress, which patients have experienced many times for a long time. These early signs caused by stress chemicals included in table two, these are the most symptoms of stress that we can find in many patients. These early effects, interacting with the environment and with the ability of individuals can cause various health problems and social problems. Moreover, the interaction of these factors can create varieties in the seriousness of problems. With each cluster of specific signs from the symptoms of stress, there will have a matching definition of the cluster in the glossary of diseases. Depend on the variation of symptoms, physicians and experts may use the word "syndrome" to describe the large cluster of symptoms. The table 6 below is retrieved from table 2:

Table 17: The most symptoms of stress that we can find in many patients

The most symptoms of stress that we can find in many patients			
Sweating	Pain, burning	Acne, dry skin, or thinning skin	Vision problems
Nausea and vomiting	Numbness, weakness, or cold	Bruising or discoloration of skin	Swelling
Pale skin	Slow or uneven heart rate	Insomnia	Rapid weight gain
Feeling short of breath	Trouble breathing	Mood changes	Shortness of breath
Dizziness	Vision, speech, or balance difficulties	Increased sweating	Severe depression or unusual thoughts or behaviors
Weakness or tremors	Blue lips or	Headache	Seizures

	fingernails		
Headache	Spotted skin	Dizziness	Bloody or tarry stools
Feeling of anxiousness	High blood pressure symptoms	Nausea, stomach pain	Coughing up blood
Feeling of anxiousness		Dangerously high blood pressure	Symptoms of pancreatitis
Hypertension			Low potassium

The most popular health problem is the cold, reading effect of stress on table two and table three, people will know why some group of people usually gets the cold more often than other people get. Reading these symptoms of cold on many public websites, and medical books, you will realize that the cold is very similar to the side effect of adrenaline and norepinephrine, cortisol described in table two. In my gut feeling, these flu symptoms are the symptoms of stress. People suffering stress will experience the symptoms of the flu very often. According to the recording the book Blink, "The wife will get more cold than normal if her spouse views her with contempt." These cold patients do need taking rest, relaxing, practicing calm the mind, good nutrition, and without medication.

Let see the effects of stress on the mice in the article: "Fighting stress with adenosine antagonists" from Scientific American. According to the researchers, during development, animals are very susceptible to stress, and the hippocampus is still developing its connections. Hippocampus best known for its role in memory and spatial navigation, it is also extremely important in emotional responses. The striking fact in the article is the authors used a long-established early life stress model called Maternal Separation." The baby rats separated from their mother for an amount of time every day during early development; it is not all day of separation, just a three hours stint every day of separation and this can cause symptoms of chronic stress". The authors have recorded that the baby rats were more anxious and they show cognitive impairment.

In memory tests like the Morris water maze: "rat would swim in a big tank filled with milky water so that they cannot see the bottom. There is a hidden platform in one quadrant of the maze, where they can stand." The researchers found that those rats do poorly with this memory test. These baby rats like dark, enclosed spaces. The separation has caused stress in the baby rats. The authors have found the corticosterone levels in plasma higher than normal rats; a hormone released in response to stress. These baby rats only have stressed as babies, but they remain pretty stress as mature. The stress in early life has made these rats lack critical skills and view many normal things as threats. I think that the lack of skill and misinterpret the environment make these rats have chronic stress. In my opinion, these conditions are not only true with rats; it is the truth with other mammal animals and human being also.

Even worse, after constant of stress, constant of releasing cortisol, your body will not make enough cortisol and other chemicals for normal functions. Constant stress can make the imbalance of hormones in the body. Imbalance of some critical hormones in the body can make the imbalance of the other hormones. All hormones in the body are regulating each other to make the body in a good function. So that the imbalance caused by chronic stress may make the body severely out of balanced, and causes some systemic problems in the body.

Some factors can reduce cortisol in the body can find from Wikipedia, these are also the way that therapists usually recommend patients to apply to reduce the symptoms

· Magnesium supplementation decreases serum cortisol levels after aerobic exercise

· Omega-3 fatty acids have a dose-dependent effect in slightly reducing cortisol release influenced by mental stress

· Music therapy can reduce cortisol levels in certain situations.

· Massage therapy can reduce cortisol.

· Laughing and the experience of humor can lower cortisol levels.

· Regular dancing leads to significant decreases in salivary cortisol concentrations

· High-dosage treatment with ascorbic acid (vitamin C) has been shown to decrease circulating cortisol levels during and shortly after the treatment period.

Working in the healthcare sector, I usually the pattern of problems with some families: the father with cardiovascular diseases; mother with mental problems: anxiety, insomnia, and depression; and young kids have stomach problems or the intestine problems. I hope that the statisticians can prove the relationship between these problems.

I will conclude the side effects of stress chemicals with two tables of the six potential diseases, which are unknown the causes at present by scientists: Cushing's syndrome, adrenal insufficiency, congenital adrenal hyperplasia, epilepsy, fibromyalgia, and depression. We will easily see the familiarity in these diseases with stress. Connecting all the dot of information in this chapter, we will know what is the real cause of all the problems that all people in all rich countries and poor countries suffer?

Table 18: The symptoms of Cushing's syndrome, adrenal insufficiency, and congenital adrenal hyperplasia

The symptoms of diseases		
Cushing's syndrome	**Adrenal insufficiency**	**Congenital adrenal hyperplasia (CAH)**
Rapid weight gain	Hypoglycemia	Vomiting due to salt-wasting leading to dehydration
Moodiness, irritability, or depression	Dehydration	Functional and average sized penis in cases involving extreme virilization (but no sperm)
Muscle and bone weakness	Weight loss	Ambiguous genitalia, in some infants, such that it can be initially difficult to identify external genitalia as "male" or "female"
Memory and attention dysfunction	Disorientation	Early pubic hair and rapid growth in childhood
Osteoporosis	Weakness	Precocious puberty
Diabetes mellitus	Tiredness	Failure of puberty may occur (sexual

		infantilism: absent or delayed puberty)
Hypertension	Dizziness	Menstrual irregularity in adolescence
Immune suppression	Low blood pressure	Excessive facial hair, virilization,
Sleep disturbances	Orthostatic hypotension	Infertility due to anovulation
Menstrual disorders such as amenorrhea in women	Cardiovascular collapse	Clitoromegaly, enlarged clitoris and shallow vagina
Decreased fertility in men	Muscle aches	
Hirsutism	Nausea and vomiting	
Baldness	Diarrhea	
Hypercholesterolemia	Goiter	
	Vitiligo	

Some of the presumed causes of these three illnesses are:

The cause of Cushing's syndrome: brain changes such as cerebral atrophy may occur. This atrophy is associated with areas of high glucocorticoid receptor concentrations such as the hippocampus and correlates with psychopathological changes.

The cause of Causes of acute adrenal insufficiency: may be a sudden withdrawal of long-term corticosteroid therapy and stress in patients with underlying chronic adrenal insufficiency.

The cause of congenital adrenal hyperplasia (CAH): cortisol is an adrenal steroid hormone that is required for normal endocrine function. Production begins in the second month of fetal life. Poor cortisol production is a hallmark of most forms of

CAH. Inefficient cortisol production results in rising levels of Adrenocorticotropic hormone (ACTH), because cortisol feeds back to inhibit ACTH production, so the loss of cortisol results in increased ACTH. This increased ACTH stimulation induces overgrowth (hyperplasia) and overactivity of the steroid-producing cells of the adrenal cortex. The defects causing adrenal hyperplasia are congenital.

Table 19: The symptoms of epilepsy, fibromyalgia, and depression

The Symptoms of diseases		
Epilepsy	**Fibromyalgia**	**Depression**
Temporary confusion	Pain	Difficulty concentrating, remembering details, and making decisions
A staring spell	Anxiety	Fatigue and decreased energy
Uncontrollable jerking movements of the arms and legs	Concentration and memory problems known as "fibro fog"	Feelings of guilt, worthlessness, and/or helplessness
Loss of consciousness or awareness	Depression	Feelings of hopelessness and/or pessimism
Psychic symptoms	Fatigue	Insomnia, early-morning wakefulness, or excessive sleeping
Simple partial seizures	Headaches	Irritability, restlessness
Complex partial seizures	Irritable bowel syndrome	Loss of interest in activities or hobbies once pleasurable, including sex
Absence	Morning	Overeating or appetite loss

seizures: a brief loss of awareness	stiffness	
Tonic seizures: stiffness of muscles: back, arms, legs may cause to fall down	Painful menstrual cramps	Persistent aches or pains, headaches, cramps, or digestive problems that do not ease even with treatment
Atonic seizures: loss of muscle control, suddenly collapse, fall down	Sleep problems	Persistent sad, anxious, or "empty" feelings
Clonic seizures: repeated, rhythmic, jerking muscle movements.	Numbness, and tingling in hands, arms, feet, and legs	Thoughts of suicide, suicide attempts
Myoclonic seizures: sudden brief jerks, twitches of arms and legs	Tender points	
Tonic-clonic seizures: abrupt loss of consciousness, body stiffening, shaking, loss of bladder control or biting tongue	Urinary symptoms, such as pain or frequency	

Some of the common conditions lead to these health problems: genetic abnormality, head trauma, stroke, brain injury, brain tumors, birth defects, infectious diseases, prenatal injury, and developmental disorders. The reason researchers think about these causes are most of these patients have a problem in the brain; the patient's brain is dysfunctional. I will suggest a new theory about the brain-mind-body to clarify these problems. The root of these problems is the abnormal brain caused by constant stress.

In fact, the changes in the patient's body by stress chemicals are the symptoms that most traditional oriental doctors can perceive when diagnosis patients. Theory and practice of oriental medicine are so profound that it helps oriental physicians to have a precise diagnosis of the diseases. It is very difficult to make the modern doctors trust the diagnosis of diseases just by feeling the pulse of patients. The oriental therapist can know exactly whether the woman is pregnant or not just by feeling the pulse. With the perception of modern doctors, it is hard to trust these treatments. According to oriental medicine, patients do not have a single chronic disease at one organ; they may have systemic problems, which caused by the countless chemicals in the body. This is the reason why using oriental treatments and non-medication therapies have a good result for some chronic patients. In some cases, these treatments bring unbelievable effects in removing many chronic diseases that are hardly understandable by the paradigm of western medicine. Oriental physicians do not use the medicine have a direct effect on the organ with symptoms in the body, they may use many herbs to create good effects on the mind, and other organs to treat some chronic diseases.

Mastering the effects of stress and happiness state, the power of the brain, the characters of the mind, the laws in the universe, and the potential of human beings can help us understand all the phenomena around us. All phenomena happen to someone and created by someone are follow the law of thinking. Systemic effects are the answer to many problems in the body, family, organization, country, and the entire world. These effects compound over time and cannot be solved by one crucial treatment. All well-known therapists, masters of religion, mentors, coaches, leaders, keynote speakers, trainers, and parents using the non-medication treatment, non-violent intervention, non-hurting changes, and non-complicating methods are the people who can create changes in the people and create changes in the world. If we do not change our old mindset caused the problems, we will not understand the way of treating. The kept secrets of great men are flexible approaches based on understanding. Their powerful tools are observed and adjust their thinking according to love, compassion, gratitude, respect, consideration, positive attitude, taking responsibility, patience, humbleness, contemplation, patience, simplicity, listening, understanding and life-long learning. These are the principles, ethics, the science of achievement and happiness that taught by great men, religious leaders, philosophers, and authors: "If you seek, you shall find".

References:

American Psychological Association. (2006, February 23). *Stress weakens the immune system*. Retrieved July 19, 2017, from http://www.apa.org/research/action/immu-ne.aspx

Blahd, William. (2016, December 23). *What Is Cortisol?*. Retrieved July 19, 2017, from http://www.webmd.com/a-to-z-guides/what-is-cortisol#1

Cortisol. (n.d.). In Wikipedia. Retrieved July 17, 2017, from http://en.wikipedia.org /wiki/Cortisol

Cunha, P. John. (2016, September 16). Adrenalin Side Effects Center. Retrieved July 19, 2017, from http://www.rxlist.com/adrenalin-side-effects-drug-center.htm

Davies, H., Dorfman, M., Fons, M., Hawkins, D., Hintz, M., Lundgren. L., ... Theunissen, S. (n.d.). Fifteen most common causes of death in the United States. Retrieved July 19, 2017, from http://health.howstuffworks.com/diseases-conditions/death-dying/15-most-common-causes-of-death-in-the-United-states.htm

Epileptic seizure. (n.d.). In Wikipedia. Retrieved July 10, 2017, from http://en. wikipedia.org /wiki/Epileptic_seizure

Eurostat Statistics Explained (2015, June 16) Prevalence of longstanding health problems or diseases in people aged 15-64, by age group, in the EU, 2011. Retrieved July 19, 2017, from http://ec.europa.eu/eurostat/statistics-explained/index.php

Goldberg, Joseph. (2016, April 09). Symptoms of depression. Retrieved July 19, 2017, from http://www.webmd.com/depression/guide/detecting-depression#1

Holland, Kimberly. (2016, November 4). Everything you need to know about the common cold. Retrieved July 19, 2017, from http://www.healthline.com/ health/cold-flu/cold

Klein, Sarah. (2013, April 19). Adrenaline, cortisol, norepinephrine: the three major stress hormones, explained. Retrieved July 19, 2017, from http://www. huffingtonpost.com/2013/04/19/adrenaline-cortisol-stress-hormones_n_3112800.html

Marks, Julie. (2014, September 3).What Is Norepinephrine (Levophed)? Retrieved July 19, 2017, from http://www.everydayhealth.com/drugs/norepinephrine #sideeffects

Marks, Lynn.(2015, August 18). What is Cortisone (Cortone Acetate)? Retrieved July 19, 2017, from http://www.everydayhealth.com/drugs/cortisone

Mayo Clinic Staff. (2015, November 06). Epilepsy. Retrieved July 19, 2017, from http://www.mayoclinic.org/diseases-conditions/epilepsy/symptoms-causes/dxc-20117207

Mental Health America.(n.d.). Mental Illness and the family: Recognizing warning signs and how to cope. Retrieved July 19, 2017, from http://www.mentalhealth-america.net/recognizing-warning-signs

Mountain State Centers for Independent Living. (n.d.). Understanding and dealing with stress. Retrieved July 19, 2017, from http://www.mtstcil.org/skills/stress-deal.html

Ratini, Melinda. (2016, July 30). Fibromyalgia Symptoms. Retrieved July 19, 2017, from http://www.webmd.com/fibromyalgia/guide/fibromyalgia-symptoms#1-3

Sargis, M. Robert. (2015, April 8). An overview of the adrenal glands:

Sargis, M. Robert. An Overview of the Adrenal Glands, Beyond Fight or Flight. Retrieved July 19, 2017, from http://www.endocrineweb.com/endocrinology /overview-adrenal-glands

Scicurious. (2013, June 10). Fighting stress with adenosine antagonists. Retrieved July 19, 2017, from http://blogs.scientificamerican.com/scicurious-brain/fighting-stress-with-adenosine-antagonists/

Awaken you wonderful we

Part III: The Potential of Brain: Intuitive Mind and Gut Feelings

Chapter 11: How people and experts talk about gut feelings?

The gut feelings are the feelings that we can sense about any changes in our body in a critical situation. The most outstanding ability of experts and outliers is gut feelings. The outliers can sense strange feelings - gut feelings when dealing with difficult problems or in a critical situation. Listening to gut feelings help them a lot in dealing with the problems and avoid the risks. Katy Cowan has some advice to take advantages of gut feelings from "When to trust your gut feelings in business" in Creativeboom.com

When you first meet someone and when you are considering a new partnership. The first impression is the clearest perception of a stranger. Be alert, open, and analytical of everyone you meet. Always read between the lines of what they are saying. Take precaution with the irritating gut feelings, especially when the strangers want to ask so many private questions.

Katy Cowan also advice to pay attention to gut feelings when you are sending work over to a client to approve when someone phones your office when you are considering a new client, and when you are in a business meeting. Trust and listen to your gut feelings.

Carolyn Gregoire from Huffingtonpost.com recommended "ten things highly intuitive people do differently" to get the most of gut feeling

· They listen to that inner voice.

· They take time for solitude.

· They create: creativity appears when the mind functions intuitively.

· They practice mindfulness.

· They observe everything.

· They listen to their bodies.

· They connect deeply with others.

· They pay attention to their dreams.

· They enjoy plenty of downtimes.

· They mindfully let go of negative emotions

These ten things are also some of the activities that meditator practice every day. All of these things and techniques of meditation is to boost the quality of thinking by quiet the mind. Most well-trained people can sense the gut feelings in critical situations. According to them, there is something strange happens inside their bodies, but they do not know what it is and why it happens? Strange, transient feelings are slightly like transient chills, transient pain in the neck, slight pain in stomach, slightly sweating in hands or transient joy or warm feelings. In the book Blink of Malcolm Gladwell, the author writes many critical situations about the gut feelings of many experts. The book left in my mind one question to answer: "How and why do we have gut feelings?"

If review all the signs of gut feelings, we will find that all signs of gut feelings are the effects of happy chemicals and stress chemical: dopamine, serotonin, oxytocin, adrenaline, noradrenaline, and cortisol. Reading table 1: the symptoms of excessive dopamine; and table 6: the most symptoms of stress that we can find in many patients, we will have a clear understanding of gut feelings. Gut feelings come from listening to the tiny changes in the body. The gut feeling is transient in a tiny second. People feel it transiently but do not cognitively understand it. The reason that we cannot understand gut feelings is gut feelings is the function of emotional mind operated by amygdala in limbic system; on the other hand, understanding is the function of thinking mind operates by the cerebral cortex. If we do not practice to quiet the mind by mindfulness or meditation, we will rarely establish good connections between these parts of the brain; poor connections make the brain function badly, especially, in the critical situation. If people do not have a tranquil mind, do not have good connections among many parts of the brain owing to a thousand hours of establishing the connection, they rarely get the best function of the brain. The more people train the mind and body, the better they can understand the feelings they have in each circumstance. Gut feelings are the proof of our mind that the unconscious mind can sense something wrong and send the signals to the body but the conscious mind does not know it. In critical situations, the human mind can perceive a large amount of information from environment then create many conditioned changes inside the mind (thinking), brain (chemicals) and body (physical signals) so silently that most of the time we do not know the changes if we do not pay attention. If we train our mind well by vigorous thinking and practicing to establish good connections, our potential mind will help us a lot in difficult situations. Outliers have the best judgment with gut feelings and sharp thinking owning for the good quality of connections among many parts of brain and body. Time to create well connections inside the brain is ten thousand hours, according to Malcolm Gladwell. The number of ten thousand hours of practicing has created many disagreements. I just want to clarify the term "ten thousand hours of practicing" into "ten thousand hours of establishing connections in the brain when people are in good state." Establishing the connection inside the brain can come from practicing, or thinking, or both of them. Engineers, workers, warriors, and boxers mainly create the connections by practicing, they spent time on thinking to improve the work. However, great philosophers and gurus spend most of the time in the process of thinking to establish the dots of information in the brain and connection between parts of brains. Some of them are Buddhism, Socrates, Plato, Peter Drucker, Lao Tzu, and many others.

    The one who uses both practicing and thinking to establish the connections in mind will reach the top of the world in that areas like the leaders, generals, Olympic gold medalists, martial art masters. If anyone has the feeling of anger, hatred, tiredness, or stress - the bad state of mind – all the time, the connections established inside brain will be the low quantity and poor quality; they will hardly to become the outliers.

If individuals do not master the mind, they will be the victims of the potential mind with irrational thinking and emotional behaviors. Uncontrolled mind with bad thoughts is the sources of all stress that people meet. Chronic stress with excessive stress chemicals is the sources of all miseries that human being is bearing. Next sections, we will find out more about how and why human beings have gut feelings.

References:
Cowan, Katy. (2011, March 29). *When to trust your gut feelings in business*. Retrieved July 19, 2017, from http://www.creativeboom.com/tips/when-to-trust-your-gut-feelings-in-business/

Gladwell, Malcolm. (2008). *Outliers: the story of success*. New York: Little, Brown, and Co.

Gladwell, Malcom. (2005). *Blink: The power of thinking without thinking*. New York: Little, Brown, and Co.

Gregoire, Carolyn. (2015, April 28). *Ten things highly intuitive people do differently*. Retrieved July 19, 2017, from http://www.huffingtonpost.com/2014/03/19/the-habits-of-highly-intu_n_4958778.html

Chapter 12: Review the structure of the human brain

The power and potential of the human brain help us understand part of potential human abilities. The Brain contains approximately 100 billion cells, each one of which connects to 1000 other brain cells making a total of 100,000 billion connections. When some parts of the brain are activated, there will be more blood flow to these parts, there will be the electrical signals moving toward and backward between neurons; a lot of ions, brain chemicals, energy, and enzymes take part in the activation of the brain. The products of brain activations are all functions of mind as consciousness, imagination, memory, executive, cognitive, logical thinking, imaginative thinking, control kinesthetic, hearing, visualization; and the waste chemicals. When a pulse of electricity reaches a junction called a synapse, it causes a neurotransmitter chemical released to binds to receptors on other cells and thereby alters their electrical activity. Scientists can detect the activation of the brain by electroencephalography (EEG). The Psychologists study all the functions of the mind created by the brain. Terms, words, concepts, definitions, and labels are the products of the mind. The mind draws out the characters of phenomena into words, terms, definitions, and concepts. The forming of words, terminology, and definitions helps to upgrade the human mind to a high level of thinking. With words, terms, and definitions, the modern human mind works much more effective than the ancient human mind did. Terminology is the study of terms and their use. Doctors, therapists, and trainers are the people who work with outcomes or problems of mind and brain on the body. Philosophers, spiritual leaders are the mind influencers who direct the way of thinking and shape the patterns of thinking of the people.

The human brain has tremendous potentiality. It has evolved for millions of years, helped human beings from the weakest animals in the world to dominate the world. In ancient times the brain's function was mainly helped our ancestors to survive the fight and flight mechanism as other animals. The weak ancient people united for promoting their mutual safety. United ancient people stood, divided ancient people would fall. Our ancestors have learned the best lessons from nature to survive and take control of living. Uniting made ancient people had more safety and more free time to observe, think, plan, and perpetuate the useful information. Over time, the human brain has evolved substantially into a most complex structure in the world. The limbic system controls the emotion, short-term memory and all autonomic functions of our body. To understand the autonomic function, let think about a cupcake you eat. Do you control the salivation in the mouth? No! Do you think about squirting stomach acid on the food? No! Do you think about turn the food into glucose and fat that your body can use? No! Do you think about transferring the glucose and fat into the bloodstream? No! Do you think about of using or storing the glucose and fat from food? No! Do you think of turning the leftover food into bowls? No! All of these autonomic functions happen silently inside our bodies that we do not know about it at all.

When you see a lemon, smell lemon's juices, listening someone tells a story of eating a lemon or see someone eating slices of lemon: you will saliva and feel the sour flavor of lemon in your mouth. Countless changes inside your body appear as conditioned responses, which you do not know and cannot control.

The automatic system includes the sympathetic and parasympathetic. Most of the autonomic functions controlled by the limbic system, which includes cingulate gyrus, corpus callosum, fornix, thalamus, mammillary body, hypothalamus, hippocampus, amygdala, olfactory bulb, dentate gyrus, supracallosal gyrus, and parahippocampal gyrus.

The important part of the human brain is cerebral cortex, which accounts for 85% of the brain mass, includes occipital lobe, parietal lobe, frontal lobe, temporal lobe. The cerebral cortex controls the cognitive functions of the brain like executive, cognitive, personality, thinking with logic and imagination, control kinesthetic, hearing, and visual. Cerebral cortex forms many special abilities of conscious thinking like memory, imagination, consciousness, and mental content. Cerebral cortex starts to understand what happens inside the brain and it starts to describe all phenomena inside the brain by all human senses.

Memory is the ability to preserve, retain, and subsequently recall, knowledge, information, or experience.

Imagination is the activity of generating or evoking novel situations, images, ideas in the mind.

Consciousness is an aspect of the mind generally thought to comprise qualities such as subjectivity, sentience, and the ability to perceive the relationship between oneself and one's environment.

Mental contents include thoughts, concepts, memories, emotions, percepts, and intentions.

Human beings have two kinds of thinking: rational thinking mostly controlled by the cerebral cortex, which is perceivable or understandable by the conscious mind; and irrational thinking mostly controlled by the limbic system, which may be perceived and recognized by the conscious mind only small part. Most people usually wrongly think that they think and do rationally and consciously. The fact is in many psychologists figure out that most people act irrationally and emotionally, especially in the critical emotional situations. To some extent, most of the activities of human mind and the human body are influenced by autonomic functions, irrational thinking and emotion so silently that they do not know at all unless do they practice mindfulness.

References:
Brain. (n.d.). In Wikipedia. Retrieved July 17, 2017, from http://en.wikipedia.org/wiki/Brain
Electroencephalography. (n.d.). In Wikipedia. Retrieved July 17, 2017, from http://en.wikipedia.org/wiki/Electroencephalography

Goleman, Daniel. (1995). *Emotional intelligence.* New York: Bantam.
Mind. (n.d.). In Wikipedia. Retrieved July 17, 2017, from http://en.wikipedia.org/ wiki/Mind

Chapter 13: Multiple Intelligence

The development of many parts of the brain forms different skills. Intelligence, to some extent, is the ability to master a set of specific skills. According to Howard Gardner - a developmental psychologist, human beings have multiple intelligences. Some of the intelligence:

The first is musical-rhythmic and harmonic. People are highly sensitive to sounds, rhythms, tones, and music. People with high musical intelligence normally have a good pitch, able to sing, play musical instruments, and compose music.

The second is visual-spatial. This area deals with spatial judgment and the ability to visualize with the mind's eye.

The third is the verbal-linguistic. People with high verbal-linguistic intelligence display a facility with words and languages. They are typically good at reading, writing, telling stories, and memorizing words along with dates.

The fourth is the logical-mathematical. This area has to do with logic, abstractions, reasoning, numbers, and critical thinking. This also has to do with having the capacity to understand the underlying principles of some kind of causal system. Logical reasoning is close to general intelligence or IQ, which are most valuable in schools. Teachers in developing countries mainly teach and judge students based on this intelligence.

The fifth is bodily- kinesthetic. The core elements of the bodily-kinesthetic intelligence are control of one's bodily motions and the capacity to handle objects skillfully, and physical actions. People with this intelligence are generally good at physical activities such as sports, dance, acting, and traveling.

The sixth is interpersonal. Individuals with have high interpersonal intelligence characterized by their sensitivity to others' moods, feelings, temperaments, motivations, and their ability to cooperate in order to work as part of a group. Those with high interpersonal intelligence communicate effectively and empathize easily with others. They often enjoy discussion and debate. Gardner believes that careers that suit those with high interpersonal intelligence include salespersons, politicians, managers, teachers, lecturers, counselors, and social workers. Observing people will see small kids, especially girls, have good interpersonal intelligence. People totally lose this intelligence when they become angry or stress. Angry people are like self-centered people. They do not pay much attention to others' moods, feelings, temperaments, and motivations.

Seventh is intrapersonal. This intelligence has to do with introspective and self-reflective capacities. This refers to having a deep understanding of the self; what one's strengths or weaknesses are; what makes one unique, and being able to predict one's own reactions or emotions. Monks, religious leaders, philosophers, and meditation practitioners are the masters of this intelligence.

You can imagine a class with seven children with seven kinds of intelligence. How can we judge, compare or give a grade to these students? How can we judge correctly our students; who in the next ten or twenty years will become doctors, engineers, entrepreneurs, politicians, painters, actors, singers, and Olympic athletes. Life is too complicated with million varieties to have a correct judgment about any students.

I could not imagine how teachers can give correct grades and comments for students in class about their talent and success in life. Especially each of students has talent like one of the successful men in history such as Thomas Edison, Henry Ford, Abraham Lincoln, Albert Einstein, Benjamin Franklin, Mozart, Charles Darwin, Ralph Waldo Emerson, David Beckham, Napoleon Hill, Brian Tracy, Steve Job, Michael Schumacher, Nick Vujicic, Helen Keller, Celine Dion, Paulo Coelho, Mother Teresa, Dalai Lama, and Jim Rohn. How the teacher can give a good judgment about the talent of these people when they are was five years old, ten years old, or twenty years old. Most of their teachers did not know anything at all about the success of these people. They will seriously wrong if they give bad assumptions about their students then treat their children according to their wrong assumptions. In fact, most of the students in classes today will success as one of these men in the future. How do I know this? Firstly, I base on the percentages of successful people in society; these people also were the small kids like kids in all class. Secondly, reading the biographies of these successful people, knowing their strengths, weaknesses, family, and disadvantages, I cannot guess they will achieve worthwhile achievements or creating changes in the world. I think in the next 10, 20, 30, and 40 years, many of our kids, many of our students will achieve unbelievable worthwhile achievements, create changes in the world, leave their legacies, or at least help us when we become the old, the ill and the poor. We, the old, the young, kids, students are interdependent. No one has to bear or suffer anything from others. All individuals have the right and obligation to treat others well for their own sake, and others' sake.

Judging our children is same like give the overall grade for a class of animals with dog, cat, fish, eagle, rabbit, lion, and buffalo. All animals have to study and test with subjects: running, swimming, jumping, flying, and climbing then give overall comment about the ability of each animal. Thinking of these successful men in history and these animals, we will realize that we are extremely wrong to spend most of the time and resources to judge our children and students. Even worse, these bad judgments are more harm than good; it may become the destiny of children. Wrong understanding of parents and teachers can hurt the children. The fact is the more an individual practicing the kinds of intelligence, the more they master them. To success in modern society, individuals must master as many types of intelligence as possible. Individuals must take enough practicing, thinking, and working enough amount of time to master these types of intelligence and skills.

References:
Gardner Practice, Basic Books., Howard (1993), Multiple Intelligences.

Chapter 14: Immeasurable phenomena in one single fact

There are countless phenomena in just one single event. One single event happens to us can create countless changes as responses in our body that we do not know at all. The changes as conditioned responses in the human body depend on the characters and varieties of subject, event, and environment.

How potential the human brain is will never know. Each fact has countless varieties; the quantity and quality of varieties perceived by the brain depend on the ability of each individual. Inside the mind, these varieties interact with each other to create millions of phenomena, in returns, these phenomena interact and transform to million other phenomena that human being can never know.

Luckily, people can sense, can have the gut feeling about the phenomena. The fact is that most of the Holy spirits, all angels, great men, the God, the Buddha, and great philosophers in all in temples and pagodas were the real people in history. They had the strengths and weaknesses as many other ordinary people until one day they could gain a new level of understanding in the mind and have the transformation in the connections and communication between neurons inside their brain through training. There is no magic formula for extreme success except massive practicing.

How much information can our brain receive each day is immeasurable. How will talented people be if they spend the time to digest this information by quiet contemplating? Look back to history, we can have the answer about how talented people are, how potential people might become. In fact, every second our brain absorbs perceives and digests a million varieties from the body and from the outside environment automatically, with and without the noticing of the conscious mind. One single event or single object has countless frequencies in it that modern technology cannot describe it exactly. Seeing, watching, or re-experiencing an explosion by modern technology, observers only perceive tiny information about the real fact. They will never have the same perception as the participants because of countless varieties in the smell, emotion, the pain, the noise, the temperature, the crying, the shouting, the blood, the burn, the ashes, the weather, the electromagnetic field, the humidity, etc...

> "No man ever steps in the same river twice, for it's not the same river and he's not the same man." **Heraclitus**
>
> "No one ever has delicious taste twice with the same food, for it is not the same food and he is not the same man"
>
> "No man ever tastes the sweetness of the first kiss twice with the same girl, for the girl is not the same and he is not the same man."
>
> "No one ever smokes one taste twice with the same cigarette, for it is not the same cigarette: countless unrecognized differences; and he is not the same man because of countless changes in the body, emotion, thinking, health, state of mind and the environment; so he can never create the same conditioned responses."

With shallow looking, we may not know much about the differences between the two similar objects. With deep looking, deep understanding we may perceive the big differences from similar events, repeated events, the twin brothers, the real flowers with the plastic flowers. Strangers do not know the differences between twin brothers as their parents or their relatives; twin brothers have many differences, the strangers do not know but the differences still exist. Most of the time, the parents of twin brothers can know exactly what the child is going home just by hearing the sound of opening the door.

Our unconscious mind constantly helps us perceive the countless information, understand the differences then make some judgments, and create conditioned responses inside our body. If a spy and his friend - an ordinary man- come to a party, they will have totally different perceptions about the joy of party, the taste of food; especially, the safety and danger of the party.

It is true with a father and young son, if they go to a garden with sand, bugs, chickens, cats, and dogs, the perception, and joy of the young child are much different with the perception of the father. Most of the time, our conscious mind cannot know these judgments about the environment and countless unconscious responses to the environment unless we pay close attention. Each of perception of environment leads to emotion, actions, and results. Rarely the two people have the same perception of the same event.

Why many times is it very difficult to express our feelings in words? Why do we have feelings and emotions long before we understand what is happening? The answer is the structure of the brain and the function of the mind. The structure and activation of brain summarized well in the book Emotional intelligence of Daniel Goleman, the finding of Joseph Ledoux, and the sleep, the brain waves from Wikipedia.

According to Daniel Goleman, human being proceed up the phylogenetic scale from reptile to rhesus to human, the sheer mass of the neo-cortex increases; with that increase comes a geometric rise in the interconnections in brain circuitry. The larger the number of such connections, the greater the range of possible responses is. The neocortex allows for the subtlety and complexity of emotional life, such as the ability to have feelings about our feelings. There is more complex of the neocortex and limbic system in humans than in other species suggesting why human beings are able to display a far greater range of reactions to our emotions and more nuanced. The limbic structures do most of the brain's learning and remembering, and the amygdala is the specialist for emotional matters. Without an amygdala, people seemed to have lost all recognition of feeling, as well as any feeling about feelings. The amygdala acts as a storehouse of emotional memory. Joseph LeDoux, a neuroscientist at the Center for Neural Science at New York University, has discovered the key role of the amygdala in the emotional brain.

Incoming signals from the senses let the amygdala scan every experience for trouble based on people's obsessed desires; with one kind of question in mind, the most primitive: "Is this something I hate? Does that hurt me? Is something I fear? Does something destroy our property? Something destroys our safety?" If "Yes"—the amygdala reacts instantaneously, like a neural tripwire, telegraphing a message of crisis to all parts of the brain. When it sounds an alarm of fear, it sends urgent messages to every major part of the brain: it triggers the secretion of the body's fight-or-flight hormones, mobilizes the centers for movement, and activates the cardiovascular system, the muscles, and the gut. Other circuits from the amygdala signal the secretion of emergency dollops of the hormone norepinephrine to heighten the reactivity of key brain areas. Simultaneously, cortical memory systems are shuffled to retrieve any knowledge relevant to the emergency at hand, taking precedence over other strands of thought.

Daniel Goleman explained, the traditional assumption most scientists believe is a visual signal first goes from the retina to the thalamus, where is translated into the language of the brain. The message goes to the visual cortex, where is analyzed and assessed for the meaning and appropriate response; if that response is emotional, a signal goes to the amygdala to activate the emotional centers. But Joseph Ledoux has found a smaller portion of the original signal goes straight from the thalamus to the amygdala in a quicker transmission, allowing a faster but less precise response. Thus the amygdala can trigger an emotional response before the cortical centers have fully understood what is happening. Ledoux's research has shown that sensory signals from the eye or ear travel first in the brain to the thalamus; then the small part of the signal across a single synapse to the amygdala, second signal from the thalamus routed to the neocortex - the thinking brain. This small branching allows the amygdala to begin to respond long before the neo-cortex. The neo-cortex mulls information through several levels of brain circuits before it fully perceives and finally initiates its more finely tailored response.

Owning for the finding of Ledoux's research, we can gain a revolutionary understanding of our emotional life, and understand why most of the time emotion mind is overwhelm conscious mind in human behavior. According to Ledoux, there is a small bundle of neurons that leads directly from the thalamus to the amygdala, in addition to the larger path leads directly from the thalamus to the neocortex. This smaller and shorter pathway allows the amygdala to receive some direct inputs from the senses and start a response before information fully registered by the neocortex. The amygdala can trigger an emotional response via this emergency route even as a parallel reverberating circuit begins between the amygdala and neocortex. LeDoux found "anatomically the emotional system can act independently of the neocortex, and some emotional reactions and emotional memories can be formed without any conscious, cognitive participation at all." The amygdala can house memories and response repertoires that we enact without quite realizing why we do so because the shortcut from thalamus to amygdala completely bypasses the neocortex. This bypass seems to allow the amygdala to be a repository for emotional impressions and memories that we have never known about in full awareness.

The finding of LeDoux, the precious finding to prove for the theory of conscious mind and subconscious mind of Freud, can explain how powerful subconscious mind is, can explain many strange phenomena and mysterious events in the human world. In fact, the small bundle of neurons that leads directly from the thalamus to the amygdala and the independence of forming the impressions, responses of the amygdala over the time can create a huge repository for emotional memories.

How deep the impressions and memories are stored in the amygdala and limbic system? We can never measure or imagine exactly how deep it is. Because there are billions of living cells in the body, each changing in each cell can send out the signals of changing caught by the autonomic nervous system. Receiving the signals, the autonomic nervous system creates corresponding responses. Some cells can create signals strong enough that might be caught by the amygdala and limbic system then the automatic nervous system can create the conditioned responses, but these signals are not strong enough to be recognized by the conscious mind. Because of the short connection between thalamus to the amygdala, the amygdala can perceive the signals below the absolute threshold of seeing, below the absolute threshold of hearing, below the absolute threshold of feelings, below the absolute threshold of tasting, below the absolute threshold of irritating - these are called the subliminal messages. The finding of LeDoux and the explanation of Daniel Goleman is the greatest importance of understanding the mind and.

How deep is the subconscious mind? We will never know because human brain not only perceives information through eyes and ears, but also it receives information from billion cells in the body; all of these processes are done by the autonomic nervous system. For example, the cells in skin, mouth, and tongue can feel the frequencies of temperature, pressure, humidity, tastes, density, and many other characters of objects, the surrounding environment and inside itself. Then these cells send the signals to the autonomic nervous system in the brain. Owning for the small connection between thalamus to the amygdala, the eyes can catch many signals of images that we do not consciously know, and the ears can catch many auditory signals that we do not consciously know. In facts, each second the mind can perceive so much information that we cannot know how much it is. We may perceive the moment with phenomena has specific energy, which is out of our perception in words and conscious thinking. The signals from the living cells in the body are so small that only the amygdala and many parts of the limbic system can catch and have corresponding responses without any noticing of our conscious thinking.

Many times, our autonomic nervous system sends out conditioned responses that we do not consciously know. With the strong responses, we may sense some strange feelings inside the body, these feelings called gut feelings. There are many kinds of research done by scientists to measure the responses and changes in the body with the flashes of images; the images are flashed so fast that the participants do not know what it is but the researchers can measure the small changes in the body of participants with sophisticated machines. Moreover, researchers, psychologists, and trainers can measure the influences of subliminal signals to the decision of participants in the moment of blink and in the lifetime. Many of these researchers described well in the book Blink of Malcolm Gladwell.

Old men said: "Sometimes looking back to little things in my life, I suddenly realize that they are not the little things anymore." These little things may left marks in subconscious mind then control our behaviors that we do not consciously know.

> "Sometimes looking back to little things in my life, I suddenly realize that they are not the little things anymore."

The role of the hippocampus is recognizing the signals, and the role of the amygdala is remembering the impression of the signals. The hippocampus remembers the dry facts; the amygdala retains the emotional flavor that goes with those facts. The imprint of memory is strong with a high degree of emotional arousal. That is why we are more likely to remember where we went on a first date, remember the impression during childhood, and remember what we were doing when we heard the news of the death of a relative. The more intense the amygdala arousal, the stronger the imprint; the experiences that scare or thrill us the most are among our most indelible memories. A special system for emotional memories makes excellent sense in evolution ensuring that animals would have particularly vivid memories of what threatens or pleases them to have the corresponding responses.

It is time to change the old concept that the heart controls the emotion. The old concept said the heart controls the emotion, especially people usually advice that in love we: "Should You Follow Your Heart, Not Your Head". This concept is totally based on the fact that most of the time with the high emotion we usually have some obvious changes in the heartbeat like tachycardia, angina, palpitation, bradycardia, vasoconstriction, hypotension, and hypertension. In addition to slow or uneven heart rate, trouble breathing, speech balance difficulties, nervousness, anxiety, and mydriasis. The amygdala will form the judgments and emotions with information it receives. With each emotion, the brain stimulates to create the corresponding stress and happiness chemicals that induce the changes in the heart. The heart is the organ that we can easily observe its activity with the physical signs like the heartbeat, the rhythm, and the blood pressure. Any changes of emotion in the brain are easily observed by the change the heartbeat and blood pressure. This is the reason that we can easily match the changes of emotion with the changes of the heartbeat, this leads to the wrong assumption that the heart controls the emotion. Some situations of high emotion are:

- With a couple, they will feel joyful, happy and thrilled when dating, talking and staying near each other. They cannot conceal the happiness. The signs of happiness are most obvious in the heart.

- When a girl sees, thinks or hears about a man that she loves, she will have the signs of shyness and the obvious signals are in her heart.

- When a man struck by the ideal concepts or the breakthrough ideas for his obsessed problems. He can feel the changes in the heart with the obvious signs above.

- The woman may fear with increase heartbeat if she sees her ex-husband who used to beat her.

- Before important events, important check-ups, or important tests the un-experienced people may have feelings of anxiety and nervousness with the obvious changes in the heartbeat.

The change of emotion caused by the amygdala belongs to the autonomic nervous system and does not belong to the conscious mind. Most of the time, these individuals cannot conceal these changes inside the body by their conscious mind. Even worse, some of these changes in the heartbeat and blood pressure can make people fail in some health check-up before important events. Some people even take lowering blood pressure medication before the health check-up still have high blood pressure during the check-up. This is proof that the changing in heartbeat and blood pressure, before important events, not caused by the heart, but caused by the head. In fact, in the emergency room in the hospital, doctors usually use the sedative medication in addition to other medications to stable the mind and to reduce the complication of the stress chemicals to the organs like the heart, blood pressure, and stomach. The fact is experienced people such as policemen, spies, soldiers, and politicians are the masters in controlling the emotion, concealing and suppressing the changes caused by the emotional mind. We will discuss later the way of controlling the emotional mind.

References:
Goleman, Daniel. (1995). Emotional intelligence. New York: Bantam.
LeDoux JE. (1996).The Emotional Brain. New York: Simon and Schuster

Chapter 15: Mirror neuron, sleep, and EEG

Scientists use electroencephalography (EEG) to observe the activity of the brain during the activation of neuron cells in the brain.

EEG Frequency bands

Band	Frequency (Hz)
Delta	< 4
Theta	≥ 4 and < 8
Alpha	≥ 8 and < 14
Beta	≥ 14
Gamma	> 32

Scientists find that during REM (Rapid eye movement) sleep, the brain of human and all created beings is activating as same as the awaken state. Moreover, in NREM (Non-Rapid eye movement) sleep or deep sleep, some parts of the brain still silently activating. Many theories support that these two types of sleep work to consolidate memory, to reach the new quality of connections between neurons and different areas of the brain for specific functions.

The first time of practice and study any new skill, the brain has high brainwave like the beta wave and gamma waves. It means that the brain has to take a lot of effort to establish the connection and exchange information among many areas of the brain to control the body's activities. The more individuals practice, the more of connections established between different areas of the brain and the better of exchanging information. The more quantity of connections inside the brain makes the better quality of the brain's function and less energy for function. Enough quantity of connection leads to the giant leap in quality of the brain's function and quality of thinking.

"There comes a time when the mind takes a higher plane of knowledge but can never prove how it got there."

Albert Einstein

After taking the action, in REM sleep the brain reactivates the areas of the brain involving in the behavior. The involved areas: pre-motor and visual cortex areas are active during REM sleep. Scientists suggest that this process strengthen the connections between areas of the brain. In non-REM sleep, the brain enhances declarative memory. During deep NREM sleep, also called slow wave sleep, activity in the cortex takes the form of large synchronized waves, whereas in the waking state it is noisy and desynchronized.

The hippocampal neocortical dialog refers to the very structured interactions during SWS (slow wave sleep) between groups of neurons called ensembles in the hippocampus and neocortex. In EEG, the sharp wave patterns dominate the hippocampus during SWS and neuron populations in the hippocampus participate in organized bursts during this phase. These observations, combined with the knowledge that the hippocampus plays a role in short to medium term memory whereas the cortex plays a role in long-term memory, have led to the hypothesis that the hippocampal-neocortical dialog might be a mechanism through which the hippocampus transfers information to the cortex. Thus, the hippocampal-neocortical dialog said to play a role in memory consolidation during sleep.

Moreover, the fact is there are many patients with chronic diseases, with unknown causes and cannot be treated, usually, have problems with genotype and brain structure. Combined these understanding, I think the activity of the brain, limbic system, and the autonomic nervous system will create some changes in the gene, brain, and body as the dots to store information. Creating dots in the body are done well during the sleep state.

With the finding of mirror neurons and its functions for learning by Eldon Taylor, it is time to forget the advice that best of learning is by doing and by experience.

"By three methods we may learn wisdom: First, by reflection, which is noblest; second, by imitation, which is easiest; and third by experience, which is the bitterest."

Confucius

Owning for mirror neurons, we have the innate ability to mirror and assimilate the desirable thoughts, feelings, and inspiration of others. Mirror neurons allow us to tune into, link-up, and reflect - within our mind - the thoughts, feelings, and energies of people we love and admire, and those who we find fascinating and inspirational. Mirror neurons help individuals adopt new skill fast to their heroes and adapt well to the new environment. The children growing up in one commune will not only have the accent of that area but also have all habits, behaviors, and way of thinking of that commune unconsciously. Mirror neurons simply mirror and allow us to assimilate energetically the behavior of people we are holding in our minds. Hence, if we obsessively think about a person who we do not like, then we are linking-up with him, reflecting his mind, and energetically assimilating his feelings into ours ... making his psychic and emotional realities a part of ours.

Knowing how our mirror neurons work, we are free to decide who we want to connect with, feel, and absorb. We also know the ones we have been connecting with and assimilating; as their thoughts, feelings, and subtle energies are blended into our own. The brain's mirroring ability is the best proof that most of us are the products of the living environment.

Interestingly, mirror neurons are a certain type of brain cells that activated when a person performs an action and also when he observes, hears and even reads about the same action performed by another person. These neurons actually "mirror" the behavior of another person, as though the observer was performing the action himself. That is, the mirror neurons in an observer's brain replicate the electrical signals and brain chemistry of the person that he is observing or even reading about. New brain imaging from UCLA (University of California, Los Angeles) demonstrates that specialized brain cells, known as mirror neurons, activate both when people observe the actions of others and when they simply read sentences describing the same action. When we read a book, these specialized cells respond as if we are actually doing what the book character is doing. This is the way of we absorb the information from the environment we interact with; this learning is conscious or unconscious, with or without noticing of the conscious mind, but the information is stored deep in unconscious mind and control all of our behaviors.

References:
Alpha wave. (n.d.). In Wikipedia. Retrieved July 17, 2017, from http://en.wikipedia. -org/wiki /Alpha_wave

Beta wave. (n.d.). In Wikipedia. Retrieved July 17, 2017, from http://en.wikipedia.-org/wiki/Beta_wave

Delta wave. (n.d.). In Wikipedia. Retrieved July 17, 2017, from http://en.wikipedia.-org/wiki/Delta_wave

Electroencephalography.(n.d.). In Wikipedia. Retrieved July 17, 2017, from http://en.-wikipedia.org/wiki/ Electroencephalography

Gamma wave. (n.d.). In Wikipedia. Retrieved July 17, 2017, from http://en.wikipedia.-org/wiki/Gamma_wave

Mind. (n.d.). In Wikipedia. Retrieved July 17, 2017, from http://en.wikipedia.-org/wiki/Mind

Mu wave. (n.d.). In Wikipedia. Retrieved July 17, 2017, from http://en.wikipedia.-org/wiki/Mu_wave

Neuroscience of sleep. In Wikipedia. Retrieved July 17, 2017, from http://en.wikipedia.-org/wiki/Neuroscience _of_sleep

Rapid eye movement sleep. In Wikipedia. Retrieved July 17, 2017, from http://en.-wikipedia.org/wiki/ Rapid_eye_movement_sleep

Theta wave. (n.d.). In Wikipedia. Retrieved July 17, 2017, from http://en.wikipedia.-org/wiki/Theta_wave

Part IV: Hologram: Brain, Mind, Body, Physical Heath, and Ego

Chapter 16: New understanding of telepathy

The other mysterious of the brain is the communicating information between brain cells; scientists also have not really understood. Many researchers may be familiar with the experiment: late in the 1990s, Russian scientists made an experiment with a female rabbit and her newborn eight kits. The experiment described well in Notunique.ca by Jerry.

A group of Russian scientists in late 1990s made an experiment with a female rabbit and her newborn eight kits near seashore where a submarine was also ready to go deep and far away inside the sea. The mother rabbit was tied at a platform on the beach and then and put to sleep with an injectable sedative with the full arrangements for measuring the blood pressure, blood sugar, blood adrenaline, and some other biochemical parameters of her blood also.

The eight kits of the mother rabbit put in the submarine. Without starting the engine of the submarine, the scientists slit the throat of one of the kits, and the kit died. As soon as the kit died inside the submarine, the unconscious mother at the seashore showed an increase in the blood pressure, sugar content, and anger-raising adrenaline hormone.

Then the engine of the submarine was started, the submarine traveled to a place several miles away from the site of the experiment. Then another of the kits was slaughtered. As soon the second child of the mother rabbit died, the unconscious mother turned more agitated, and her biochemical parameters showed further enhanced readings. In the same manner, while the submarine was covering a distance of hundreds of kilometers, the remaining kits of the mother were also slaughtered one-by-one, but each time when the child was killed the unconscious mother turned more and more agitated and restless with increased readings of the biochemical parameters. And as soon as the last of the eight kits of the mother rabbit was killed, several hundred kilometers away from the unconscious mother, she suddenly regained consciousness and started crying with grief as if she had got a full realization that her kits were no more in this world. The grief-stricken hapless mother started showing enormously increased blood pressure, blood sugar, and blood adrenaline, and then she suddenly collapsed and died.

This is not popular publishing, but it gives a lot of meaning for the scientists who research telepathy and communicating information between neurons and parenthood connected individuals. The experiment may help us understand that in some circumstances some people may have gut feelings, transient pain, slightly throbbing around the eyes when our relatives are in danger, died or killed. If we do not understand these events, we may think that there is the Holy Spirit and Great Power helps us to have incredible abilities in the crucial circumstances. People in every country have their own religion and their own ritual with their own Holy Spirits. They easily believe all strange good or bad things happen to them is the intention of their Holy Spirit or gosh

There is a way of communicating information in the world that people have not yet fully known. The signal the mother rabbit perceived about the kits is by the subconscious mind and the changes in the body are by the autonomic nervous system. The strength of signals is highest when:

- There is a strong bond among subjects; here is the bond of mother and kits.
- The mother rabbit obsessed with the safety of the rabbit kits; if rabbit kits were mature, scientists would not saw any changes in biochemical parameters.
- The mother rabbit put at sedative state, the conscious mind put to rest so the unconscious mind and autonomic nervous system are in the highest state of alertness to focus on obsessed desires. I think If the mother rabbit were chasing objects or doing other activities, scientists would not notice the big changes in

biochemical parameters; they might be observed a little lack of concentration.

- The changes in biochemical parameters of the mother rabbit can be sensitive to atropine (atropine sensitive). Putting mother rabbit to sleep with an injectable sedative is the same as the first stage anesthetization in human for operation. In anesthesia, physicians use many medications, affecting the cortex and autonomic nervous system, to control the conscious responses and unconscious responses of the patients during the operation.

- In fact, physicians and scientists have observed that the wishes or the pray of relatives have some good effects on recovering of patients, even the patients do not know at all about the wishes or actions of their relatives. It means that there is another way of communicating information among individuals that scientists do not fully know.

According to Michio Kaku, quantum teleportation already exists, he thinks within a decade we will teleport the first molecule. Humans we have already achieved this at an atomic level, but unfortunately, it takes a lot of energy with the giant sophisticated machines to entangled particles. Quantum entanglement permits links to be made between atoms, with their information being directed to others further away. In particular, the entangled particles are linked in such a way that the action of one openly affects the others, even if they are parted over huge distances. Quantum teleportation triggers big question for scientists that the speed of sending back and forth information between particles is faster than the speed of light. According to Michio Kaku, physicists at the University of Geneva achieved teleportation by teleporting the quantum state of a photon to a crystal over 25 km of optical fiber. Dr. Kaku said teleportation is actually possible; it does come with a set of decent problems that would need to be solved.

In the future, scientists will have a deep understanding of the telepathy of human being and perhaps creature beings also. The neuron cells in the human brain of an individual and the brains of individuals with strong bonds have gained the ability to use telepathy communication. Telepathy communication is the function of the autonomic nervous system so that only well-trained people with quite a mind can understand the perceived information. The more people train themselves, the stronger bonds between individuals, the better telepathy communication is.

We do not see the connection but there always have invisible connections between the beings. Especially, the deepest connection created by love and parenting hood, and science has not found how deep and how strong love can make. Doctors will never dare to make an operation for a mother who is anxious about the safety of her children. With an anxious mother, physician have to calm down her anxiety by love, support and breathing exercise, then they have to use sedative medications to make her totally calm before the operation.

Around everybody, there is the invisible field but it contains the invisible energy that the science has not fully known or detected. This energy can be sensed by the intuition. The more trained powerful men, there stronger the energy around them are. Just sitting next to a good man, bad man, religious leader, warm leaders, greedy leaders, people can have the gut feeling about these people in a blink. People change, environment changes but these invisible energies may still linger on that we do not know, but we can sense. Cover the eyes and ears of a group of people and take them to the churches, pagodas, universities, battlefields, war zone, hysterical community, stressed families, and happy families they will have gut feelings in the bodies; interestingly, the varieties of their bodies may according to the environments that they do not consciously know. Western therapists do not see the flow of invisible energy run through the body, but Eastern therapists can sense and feel it. So that in Eastern countries, therapists use a lot of alternative medicine to treat chronic diseases, some of them are acupressure, acupuncture, affirmative prayer, aromatherapy, autosuggestion. In Eastern philosophy, mind and brain is the kind of the body.

Readers can test about the invisible around their hand

The first way is by hanging a ring by a thin thread above your palm then slightly swing the thread, the rings will move in a specific pattern according to the energy on your palm. The most obvious signs are there the big different moving pattern of the ring over the boy's palm and girl's palm.

The second way is to place the opened palms parallel in front of the body then you slightly move the palms backward and forward, far away then move back several times, do not touch the two palms together. The more you move your hand back and forth, the stronger you feel there is an invisible force pushes your palms away. If you do in the strong wind, you will not sense the force clearly.

References:
Anthony, Sebastian. (2014, September 3). The first human brain-to-brain interface has been created. In the future, will we all be linked telepathically?. Retrieved July 19, 2017, from http://www.extremetech.com/extreme/188883-the-first-human-brain-to-brain-interface-has-been-created-in-the-future-will-we-all-be-linked-telepathically

Astn, Peter. (n.d.). A powerful rabbit experiment [Blog post]. Retrieved July 19, 2017, from http://www.notunique.ca/content/blog/a-powerful-rabbit-experiment

Carter,Craig.(n.d.). Religion is a myth: some random thoughts [Blog post]. Retrieved July 19, 2017, from http://www.notunique.ca/content/blog/religion-is-a-myth-some-random-thoughts.shtml

Iozzio, Corinne. (2014, October 2). Scientists prove that telepathic communication is within reach. Retrieved July 19, 2017, from http://www.smithsonianmag.com/innovation/scientists-prove-that-telepathic-communication-is-within-reach-180952868/

Mei, Amanda. (2015, November 4). Science or science fiction? Telepathy and mind control. Retrieved July 19, 2017, from http://www.yalescientific-.org/2015/11/science-or-science-fiction-telepathy-and-mind-control/

Physics Astronomy. (2015, September 9). Michio Kaku: "Star Trek-style teleportation IS possible and we could be beaming to other planets within decades". Retrieved July 19, 2017, from http://www.physics-astronomy.com/2015/09/michio-kaku-star-trek-style.html#.WW3eGJA2vZ4

Sage, Crystal. (2009, January 02). Mirror neurons and telepathy[Online forum comment]. archived at http://www.unexplained-mysteries.com/forum/topic/143723-mirror-neurons-and-telepathy/

Sartori, Mauro. (2015, March 9). Brain-to-brain interfaces: the science of telepathy. Retrieved July 19, 2017, from http://theconversation.com/brain-to-brain-interfaces-the-science-of-telepathy-37926

Chapter 17: The universe is a gigantic and splendidly detailed hologram of interconnected phenomena

I will summarize some experiments and finding of scientists for a theory that the world is a hologram, so is the human brain. Thank for the writing of Michael Talbot "Does Objective Reality Exist, or is the Universe a Phantasm?" He has summarized well the complicated theory of hologram. Michael Talbot was the author of "The Holographic Universe".

In 1982, a remarkable event took place. At the University of Paris, a research team led by physicist Alain Aspect performed the most important experiments of the 20th century. Aspect and his team discovered that under certain circumstances subatomic particles such as electrons are able to communicate instantaneously with each other regardless of the distance separating them. It does not matter whether they are 10 feet or 10 billion miles apart. Somehow, each particle always seems to know what the other is doing.

The problem with this finding is that it violates Einstein's long-held tenet that no communication can travel faster than the speed of light. Since traveling faster than the speed of light is tantamount to breaking the time barrier, so it is not accepted by most scientists, but this finding has inspired others to offer many radical explanations for some mysterious event around the world. I hope that one day the scientists can prove this theory of instantaneous communication.

University of London physicist David Bohm believes Aspect's findings imply that objective reality does not exist, that despite its apparent solidity the universe is at heart a phantasm, a gigantic and splendidly detailed hologram.

To understand why Bohm makes this startling assertion, we must first understand a little about holograms. A hologram is a three-dimensional photograph made with the aid of a laser. To make a hologram, the object to be photographed is first bathed in the light of a laser beam. Then a second laser beam is bounced off the reflected light of the first and the resulting interference pattern is captured on film. When the film is developed, it looks like a meaningless swirl of light and dark lines. But as soon as the developed film is illuminated by another laser beam, a three-dimensional image of the original object appears. The three-dimensionality of such images is not the only remarkable characteristic of holograms. If a hologram of a rose is cut in half and then illuminated by a laser, each half will still be found to contain the entire image of the rose. Indeed, even if the halves are divided again, each snippet of film will always be found to contain a smaller but intact version of the original image. Unlike normal photographs, every part of a hologram contains all the information possessed by the whole.

> "The whole in every part
>
> Every part contains the whole
>
> One in all and all in one"

Eastern philosophers said: "whole in every part" and "every part contains the whole"; the nature of a hologram provides us with an entirely new way of understanding organization and order.

According to Bohm, the reason subatomic particles are able to remain in contact with one another regardless of the distance separating them not caused by sending some sort of mysterious signal back and forth; but because of their separateness is an illusion. He argues that at some deeper level of reality such particles are not individual entities, but are actually extensions of the same fundamental something. Bohm says this is precisely what is going on between the subatomic particles in Aspect's experiment. According to Bohm, the apparent faster-than-light connection between subatomic particles is really telling us that there is a deeper level of reality we are not privy to, a more complex dimension beyond our own that is analogous to the aquarium. He adds we view objects such as subatomic particles as separate from one another because we are seeing only a portion of their reality. Such particles are not separate "parts", but facets of a deeper and more underlying unity that is ultimate wholeness as holographic, and indivisible as the previously mentioned rose. Since everything in physical reality is comprised of these "eidolons", the universe is itself a projection, a hologram.

In addition to its phantomlike nature, such a universe would possess other rather startling features. If the apparent separateness of subatomic particles is illusory, it means that at a deeper level of reality all things in the universe are infinitely interconnected. Perhaps most religious leaders in the world perceived the infinite interconnection of all things in the universe so that they all behaved differently compare to most of the ordinary people. Moreover, all the principles they taught people contained love, fairness, kindness, and respect. The theory of Big Bag gives us understand that the electrons in a carbon atom in the human brain are connected to the subatomic particles that comprise every salmon that swims, every heart that beats, and every star that shimmers in the sky. Everything interpenetrates everything. There is no separate self, there is no I, no you; all things are in the infinite interconnection of all things in the universe. All apportionments are of necessity artificial and all of nature is ultimately a seamless web.

Why human beings seek a way to categorize, pigeonhole, and subdivide the various phenomena of the universe? Categorizing all phenomena and combination of phenomena in the universe into specific concepts, which are perceivable by five senses is human nature. This is the big evolution of the human brain, which the huge information about the universe is concrete, and effectively and effortlessly communicated to other individuals. By categorizing and subdividing the huge information, huge phenomena into words forming concepts, definitions, nouns, verbs, adjectives; human brain can easily absorb information and mix this information to create many more new phenomena, many more new invention from the previous information. To illustration, most of the ordinary people live in the twenty-first century easy understand the concepts of an airplane, Mercedes car, Toyota car, Ford car, the Sun, the Earth, computer, television, and smartphone; just hearing the word television, modern people can have detail perception in mind. However, it would take months or years and thousands of books to explain one of these concepts to the scientists of fifteenth-century or scientists of eighteen century; even we would fail to explain normal functions or characters of these things for them. Because there were no perceivable concepts in eighteenth-century which have the same meaning with the concepts of the twenty-first century, and there were so many wrong religious concepts controlled the perceiving of natural phenomena. The lack of right understanding the phenomena created a lot of difficulties for scientists in the eighteenth century, some scientists even died to prove the new concepts for the governors; which turnout are obvious to the student of the twenty-first century. Categorizing and subdividing phenomena into words and concepts helps reduce the burden on the mind and brain from overloading information for cognitive thinking and cognitive behaviors. Concepts, words, and definitions are the products of conscious thinking to try to categorize phenomena into perceivable things. Gradually, owning for better understanding, the perception of people about these concepts may change substantially. Scientists in the twenty-first century are freely explaining and talking about some religious taboos of the eighteenth century.

From some simple phenomena, these phenomena freely interact with each other create many more phenomena. Compound over time, the interaction of some simple phenomena can immense phenomena. These phenomena interconnect into a seamless web.

The interaction of phenomena is the best explanation for the forming of the universe and the best explanation for the creating of living on earth. The earth only had only some inorganic elements described in Mendeleev's periodic table around four billion years ago. The names of these inorganic elements are the perceptions of the human mind to concrete the characters or the combination of specific phenomena inside inorganic elements. These inorganic elements freely interacted have created organic elements. Immense phenomena created over billions of years.

Over a billion years, some simple form of life included human being created from the chemical reactions that produced many of the simpler organic compounds, including nucleobase and amino acids.

Bohm is not the only researcher who has found evidence that the universe is a hologram. Working independently in the field of brain research, Standford neurophysiologist Karl Pribram has also become persuaded of the holographic nature of reality. Pribram was drawn to the holographic model by the puzzle of how and where memories are stored in the brain. For decades, numerous studies have shown that rather than being confined to a specific location, memories are dispersed throughout the brain. In a series of landmark experiments in the 1920s, brain scientist Karl Lashley found that no matter what portion of a rat's brain he removed he was unable to eradicate its memory of how to perform complex tasks it had learned prior to surgery. The only problem was that no one was able to come up with a mechanism that might explain this curious "whole in every part" nature of memory storage excepting adopting the theory of Hologram. Pribram believes memories are encoded not in neurons, or small groupings of neurons, but in patterns of nerve impulses that crisscross the entire brain in the same way that patterns of laser light interference crisscross the entire area of a piece of film containing a holographic image. He believes the brain is itself a hologram.

Pribram's theory also explains how the human brain can store so many memories in so little space. Similarly, it has been discovered that in addition to their other capabilities, holograms possess an astounding capacity for information storage simply by changing the angle at which the two lasers strike a piece of photographic film, it is possible to record many different images on the same surface. It has been demonstrated that one cubic centimeter of film can hold as many as 10 billion bits of information.

You can test the concept of the hologram by observing the mind and thinking, what comes to your mind when your friend says the word "dog" "wolf" and "smartphone." You do not have to clumsily sort back through some gigantic and cerebral alphabetic file to arrive at an answer. Instead, associations of all senses about these words pop into your head instantly. Indeed, one of the most amazing things about the human thinking process is that every piece of information seems instantly cross-correlated with every other piece of information. This is another feature intrinsic to the hologram. Because every portion of a hologram interconnects with every other portion, it is perhaps nature's supreme example of a cross-correlated system. Another is how the brain is able to translate the avalanche of frequencies it receives via the senses like light frequencies, sound frequencies, temperature frequencies, humidity frequencies and so on, into the concrete world of our perceptions. Encoding and decoding frequencies are precisely what a hologram does best. Hologram functions as a sort of lens, a translating device able to convert an apparently meaningless blur of frequencies into a coherent image, and coherent words.

Researchers have discovered, for instance, that our visual systems are sensitive to sound frequencies. In fact, the cells in our bodies are sensitive to a broad range of known frequencies and unknown frequencies. Such findings suggest that it is only in the holographic domain of consciousness that such frequencies sorted out and divided into conventional perceptions.

In a universe in which individual brains are actually indivisible portions of the greater hologram and everything is infinitely interconnected, telepathy may merely be the accessing of the holographic level. It is obviously much easier to understand how information can travel from the mind of individual 'A' to that of individual 'B' at a far distance point and helps to understand a number of unsolved puzzles in psychology.

In particular, Stanislav Grof feels the holographic paradigm offers a model for understanding many of the baffling phenomena experienced by individuals during altered states of consciousness. In the 1950s, while conducting research into the beliefs of LSD (Lysergic acid diethylamide) as a psychotherapeutic tool, Grof had one female patient who suddenly became convinced she had assumed the identity of a female of a species of prehistoric reptile. During the course of her hallucination, she not only gave a richly detailed description of what it felt like but noted that the portion of the male of the species' anatomy was a patch of colored scales on the side of its head. After confirming with a zoologist, Grof was startled that although the woman had no prior knowledge about such things she knew it exactly. During the course of his research, Grof encountered examples of patients regressing and identifying with virtually every species on the evolutionary tree. He also had patients who appeared to tap into some sort of collective or racial unconscious. In other categories of experience, individuals gave persuasive accounts of out-of-body journeys, of precognitive glimpses of the future, of regressions into apparent past-life incarnations. In later research, Grof found the same range of phenomena manifested in therapy sessions, which did not involve the use of drugs. As Grof noted, if the mind is actually part of a continuum, a labyrinth that is connected not only to every other mind that exists or has existed, but also to every atom, organism, and region in the vastness of space and time itself.

Such a turnabout in the way we view biological structures has caused researchers to point out that medicine and our understanding of the healing process also be transformed by the holographic paradigm. If the apparent physical structure of the body is but a holographic projection of consciousness, it becomes clear that each of us is much more responsible for our health than current medical wisdom allows. What we now view as miraculous remissions of disease may actually be due to changes in consciousness, which in turn effect changes in the hologram of the body. Similarly, controversial new healing techniques such as education, visualization, affirmation, meditation, imagination, hypnotherapy, subliminal messages may work so well as treatment with medicine because, in the holographic domain of thought, outside is ultimate as real as inside. All authors of personal development confirm the power of thinking. To understand the role of thought in people life, you can find these books.

- *"As a man thinketh"* of James Allen

- *"The strangest secret*" of Earl Nightingale

- *"Thi*nk and grow rich" or *"Hill's golden rules"* of Napoleon Hill

- *"The power of positive thinking"* of Norman Vincent Peale

"As above so below

As within so without"

The fact is non-medicine healing techniques are very effective in treating chronic diseases, which are untreated by modern medicine. Moreover, these healing techniques have created many myths and miracles of recovering with many seriously ill patients. Understanding the hologram of thoughts, all myths, all religious belief, and all religious concepts will no longer seem so mysterious as before.

Adopting the theory of hologram, we can understand the teaching of Buddha. In the book, "Old path, white path" of Zen Master Thich Nhat Hanh, Buddhism is no longer a mysterious religion, Buddhism becomes applicable in daily life for every people to have a good life. The book is the story of Buddha as an ordinary man gained enlightenment, and contains many teachings of Buddha. People find Buddha statue in pagodas usually is in a gesture of Zen sitting. Buddha was a prince gained enlightenment by vigorous practicing of meditation.

Buddha's teaching instructs people to focus powers of concentration to look deeply at their body. They will see that each cell of their body was like a drop of water in an endlessly flowing river of birth, existence, death, and they will not find anything in the body that remained unchanged or certain that can be said to contain a separate self.

Intermingled with the river of their body was the river of feelings in which every feeling is a drop of water. These drops also jostle with one another in a process of birth, existence, and death. Some feelings were pleasant, some unpleasant, and some neutral, but all of their feelings were impermanent: they appear and disappear just like the cells of his body. Look deeper, we will find the river of perceptions, which flowed alongside the rivers of body and feelings. The drops in the river of perceptions intermingle and influence each other in their process of birth, existence, and death. If one's perceptions are accurate, reality reveals itself with ease; but if one's perceptions were erroneous, the reality is veiled. People will be caught in endless suffering because of their erroneous perceptions: they believed that which is impermanent is permanent, that which is without self-contains self, that which has no birth and death has birth and death, and they divided that which is inseparable into parts.

Following the teaching of focusing concentration to observe the body of Buddha, we will find that our awareness on the mental states, which are the sources of suffering: fear, anger, hatred, arrogance, jealousy, greed, and ignorance. Mindful awareness of people is like a bright sun to illuminate the nature of all these negative mental states. People will be enlightened that they all arise due to ignorance. They are the opposite of mindfulness.

Buddha taught that the key to liberation is to break through ignorance and to enter deeply into the heart of reality and attain direct experience of it. Such knowledge would not be the knowledge of the intellect, but of direct experience, of understanding.

Buddha's teaching helps us gain understanding by looking at a pippala leaf. With a pippala leaf in hand, looking deeply at the pippala leaf, we can clearly see the presence of the sun, stars, earth, water, cloud, rain, and space. Lacking any of these like lacking the sun, without light and warmth, the leaf could not exist.

In fact, at that very moment, the entire universe existed in that leaf. The reality of the leaf is a wondrous miracle. If paying attention, you will see in your child, there are countless presences of you, your spouse, your teachers, your relatives, your place of birth, your education, your thoughts, your anger, your cheating, your mistakes, your wounds, your childhood, your books, your emotion, your friends, your countries, your managers, and your presidents. All of these presences are the dots that influence your life and your child's life. We all live under the hologram of countless phenomena. Each small changing in each of countless phenomena, the hologram will change. It means we are not the same; we are the holograms of countless compounded phenomena. Our body embeds all information of these phenomena that we do not consciously know.

> You are the result of the thoughts you have. The more good thoughts you have the more your good life is.
>
> "Good thoughts good fruits
>
> Bad thoughts bad fruits"
>
> Quality of life is measured by the quality of thoughts. The environment will shape the thoughts. Jim Rhon taught: "you are the average of the five people you spend with." People you spend time with, the environment you live in, the things you read will shape your thoughts.
>
> Show feed your mind with good thought by:
>
> + Choosing good people to spend time with,
>
> + Choosing the good kinds of stuff to read,
>
> + And taking care of your thoughts with needed correction.

Though we ordinarily think that a leaf is born in the springtime, Buddha taught us to see that it had been there for a long, long time in the sunlight, the clouds, the tree, and in ourselves. Seeing that the leaf had never been born, we could see that we ourselves too had never been born. Both the leaf and we have simply manifested—we have never been born and are incapable of ever dying. With this insight, ideas of birth and death, appearance and disappearance dissolved, and the true face of the leaf and our own true face revealed themselves. This insight is the same as the insight of Lao Tzu.

Practicing more, we can see that the presence of any one phenomenon made possible the existence of all other phenomena. One includes all, and all are contained in one. The leaf and our body are one. Neither possessed a separate, permanent self.

Neither could exist independently from the rest of the universe. Seeing the interdependent nature of all phenomena, Buddha taught that we could see the empty nature of all phenomena—that all things are empty of a separate, isolated self.

Buddha and Lao Tzu taught the key to liberation lay in these two principles of interdependence and non-self. With the practice of meditation, we can see these two principles. Clouds drift across the sky, forming a white background to the translucent pippala leaf. Clouds are one manifestation; rain is another. Clouds also are not born, so that it would not die. If the clouds understood that, Buddha taught, surely they will sing joyfully as they fall down as rain onto the mountains, forests, and rice fields.

We are interdependence for our happiness

"Long and short contrast each other,

Above and below rest upon each other,

High and low rest upon each other,

Difficult and easy complement each other,

Voice and sound harmonize each other,

Front and back follow one another,

Husband and wife complete each other,

Father and son rest upon each other,

Leaders and followers follow one another,

No students no teachers,

They rest upon each other.

Things named and known based on its contrasts

Synergize to create phenomena

Creating the life and creating happiness

Things are neither birth nor death,

Neither production nor destruction,

> Neither one nor many,
> Neither inner nor outer,
> Neither large nor small,
> And neither impure nor pure.
> All concepts are distinctions created by the intellect
> To support for thinking and interacting
> Things are interdependent.
> Problems come from stubbornly attach to concepts."

Buddha taught with the illuminating the rivers of our body, feelings, perceptions, mental formations, and consciousness, we can understand that impermanence and emptiness of self-are the very conditions necessary for life. Our feelings, perceptions, mental formations, and consciousness are just the illuminating of surrounding phenomena with our senses in our brain; in return, we create many more phenomena by our thinking, speaking and behaving. Without impermanence and emptiness of self, nothing could grow or develop. If a grain of rice does not have the nature of impermanence and emptiness of self, it cannot grow into a rice plant. If clouds are not empty of self and impermanent, they cannot transform into rain. Without impermanent and non-ego, a child can never grow into an adult.

> "To accept life means to accept impermanence and emptiness of self. The source of suffering is a false belief in permanence and the existence of separate selves"

Thus, Buddha taught, "to accept life means to accept impermanence and emptiness of self. The source of suffering is a false belief in permanence and the existence of separate selves. Seeing this, one understands that there is neither birth nor death, neither one nor many, neither inner nor outer, neither large nor small, and neither impure nor pure. All such concepts are false distinctions created by the intellect. If one penetrates into the empty nature of all things, one will transcend all mental barriers, and be liberated from the cycle of suffering." This teaching of

Buddha is very similar to the teaching of Lao Tzu, I think that there were many other teaching had the same insight into human history. Fortunately, Buddha pointed the way for people to meditate and train to gain such insight. Reaping knowledge and enlightenment from direct experience; these are the fruits that Lao Tzu showed us with just one single poem: "Te-Tao Ching".

The real world around us

1. Phenomena are constant:
They are described in the teaching of Lao Tzu
Look, it cannot be seen - it is beyond form.
Listen, it cannot be heard - it is beyond sound.
Grasp, it cannot be held - it is intangible.
These three are indefinable;
Therefore, they are joined in one.
It returns to nothingness.
The form of the formless,
The image of the imageless,
It is called indefinable and beyond imagination.

2. How do we know the phenomena?
By its outstanding characters
Outstanding characters are
Yield and overcome,
Bend and be straight,
Empty and be full,
Wear out and be new,
Have little and gain,
Have much and be confused.
That which shrinks
Must first expand.
That which fails
Must first be strong
That which is cast down
Must first be raised.
Before receiving
There must be giving.
Begin by sciences

But masters love arts.

3. As above so blow
As within so without
As the causes, so the effects
As the effect, therefore, the cause
This is called the perception of the nature of things.
Soft and weak overcome hard and strong.
Inside and outside has a strong bond.

4. It is two faces of appearance and essence
One gets by seeing, hearing and sensing
With cognitive thinking
And logical thinking.
Other is get by feeling like gut feeling
With emotional thinking
And rational thinking
They have a close relation.
Like Yin and Yang.

5. In fact, things are one
Separated by thinking of human beings
Crystallizing phenomena into simple specific things
Words and definitions are born.
Good for thinking and developing
Understanding and communicating

6. Unfortunately:
Same words have different perceptions
Same events have different understandings
And different feelings
By all people
Employers and employees
Generals and soldiers
Brothers and sisters
The blind and the deaf
The rich and the poor
The young and the old

You and me.

7. Therefore:
Extreme danger goes with the attachment
Self-destruction goes with possessing or egotizing.
Problems are born
Wars and fighting are inevitable
Constantly and endlessly
Diseases and illnesses are flourishing
Constantly and endlessly
In spite of hopeless actions
And vigorous quick-fixes.

8. Life is funny
Life is great
Live closely
And in mindfulness for understanding.

Yin and Yang theory

Taijitu.

These phenomena have characters the same as energy. To understand it, it is better to be felt than grasped, use the unconscious mind rather than conscious mind. In Eastern philosophy, the characters of these phenomena and energy are well described in Yin and Yang theory. In Chinese philosophy, the rhythm of life, which pulsates through the universe, is the action of complementary principles Yin and Yang. The symbol for Yin Yang is called the Taijitu. Yin and Yang can be seen as the two opposite characters in one phenomenon; Yin and Yan rest upon each other, Yin and Yan interchange with each other. In Yin there is the seed of Yan, in Yan, there is the seed. The taijitu symbol has been found in more than one culture and over the years has come to represent Taoism. The symmetrical disposition of the dark Yin and the light Yang suggests cyclical changes.

Yin is the below, within, inside, invisible, quiet, female, intuitive, receiving the force that is associated with earth. The earth is the source of life; it provides us with what we need to survive.

Yang is the above, without, outside, appearance, strong, male, creative, giving force that is associated with heaven. The heaven above us is always in motion and brings about change.

When Yin reaches its climax, it recedes in favor of Yang, then after Yang reaches its climax it recedes in favor of Yin. This is the eternal cycle. The dots inside the white and black halves indicate that within each is the seed of the other. Yin cannot exist without Yang and vice versa.

Basic Concepts Defining the Nature of Yin Yang

Neither Yin nor Yang is absolute. Nothing is completely Yin or completely Yang. Each aspect contains the beginning point for the other aspect. For example, day becomes night and the night becomes day...Yin and Yang are interdependent upon each other so that the definition of one requires the definition for the other to be complete.

Yin Yang is not static. The nature of Yin and Yang flows and changes with time. A simple example is thinking about how the day gradually flows into the night. However, the length of day and night are changing. As the earth ages, its spin is slowing causing the length of day and night to get longer. Day and night are not static entities. Sometimes changes in the relationship between Yin and Yang can be dramatic where one aspect can literally just transform into the other. As an example: some species of fish have females that transform quickly into males when the population of males isn't enough.

The summation of Yin and Yang form a whole. One effect of this is: as one aspect increases the other decreases to maintain the overall balance of the whole.

The balance of Yin-Yang can be skewed due to outside influences. Four possible imbalances exist:

Deficiency Yang

Deficiency Yin
Excess Yang
Excess Yin

These imbalances can be paired: so an excess of Yin can also simulate a Yang deficiency and vice versa. An example of this concept is especially important for Chinese healing practices

Yin Yang can be subdivided into additional Yin and Yang aspects. For example, a Yang aspect of Heat: can be further subdivided into a Yin warm or Yang burning.

This is only the start. You can dig into Yin Yang in an infinite manner due to its relative nature.

The ideal state of things in the physical universe, as well as in the world of humans, is a state of harmony represented by the balance of Yin and Yang in body and mind.

Table 20: Yin and Yang in all phenomena

Yin	Yang
Body Mind Spirit Health Art of living: as... so...	
Causes	Effects
Below	Above
Within	Without
Inside	Outside
Invisible	Visible
Mind, character	Appearance
Quiet	Strong
Female	Male
Intuitive	Creative
Receiving force	Giving force
Subconscious mind	Conscious mind
Thinking	Behaving
Irrational thinking	Rational thinking

Peace inside	Peace outside
Mind	Body
Spiritual life	Physical life
Intuition	Intellect
Passive, Static	Active, Dynamic
Conservative	Innovative
Soft	Hard
Contraction	Expansion
Psychological	Physical
Astral World	Visible World

PHENOMENA IN UNIVERSE ENVIRONMENT

Night, Dark	Day, Light
Rain, Water, Cold	Fire, Heat
Winter, Autumn	Summer, Spring
Odd Numbers	Even Numbers
The Moon	The Sun
North, West	South, East
Right, Down	Left, Up
Decreasing	Increasing
Traditional	Reformative
Valley	Mountain
River	Desert
Curve	Straight Line
Solidifying	Dissolving
Tiger	Dragon
Kidneys, Heart	Bladder
Liver, Lungs	Intestines, Skin

All things else are changing. All things else are the illuminating of specific phenomena. Nothing is constant, in static, there is the seed of motion. The source of suffering is a false belief in the permanence and the existence of separate selves. Wrong pursuing, the permanence of separate self, has created vicious phenomena in the world. The bodies with the selves have disappeared but the created phenomena are still constant. To understand these, let use your imagination to play the game with the question of if then.

The first is Socrates:

1. Who is Socrates?

"He was a philosopher two centuries ago" - it means he died. So who is the owner of the philosophy, the knowledge that philosophers in most universities are studying?

"Socrates's ideas, concepts" - but he died?

2. What is the image of Socrates' face?

The fact is his face dissolved in the dust, but all philosophers can perceive his face in mind, which influenced by his picture on the philosophy books.

3. What would we have called Socrates if his mother named him Sacrato? Or when he was matured he changed his name to Sacrato? All the works he did were the same, perhaps human beings would have recorded in all the books with the name of Sacrato without any concern.

4. How could friends of Socrates perceive exactly about Socrates?

- When Socrates was one year old, how did he look like, how his neighbors thought about him?

- When Socrates was five years old, how did he look like, how his neighbors thought about him?

- When Socrates was twenty years old, how did he look like, how his neighbors thought about him?

- When he was fifty years old, how did he look like how his neighbors thought about him?

They may saw him in the appearance, his voices, his thinking, his feelings, his characters, his attitude, his work, the feeling he made for them. These were changing day after day.

If we could ask the people who lived the same time with Socrates, we would get thousands of different answers about him, these lead to thousands of perceptions about him. From his wife, his disciples, his governors, and the rich in Athens, we would find out some people loved, some people protected, some people hated, some people did not care, and some people killed him when he was old.

We will never get the concreted perception about Socrates even if we ask the two philosophers in one university.

The second is Jim Rhon:

1. Who is Jim Rhon?

"He was a philosopher of business and personal development, he was born 1930 and died 2009" - it means he died, it means ended. So who is the owner of the theories, knowledge that people all over the world are studying from him?

"Socrates's ideas, concepts" - but he died?

2. What is the image of Jim Rhon's face?

The fact is his face dissolved in the dust, but many people could perceive his face in mind based on the recording video about him when he was 40 years old, 60 years old, 70 years old. Most of the time, the perception of his face changed.

3. What would we have called Jim Rhon if his mother named him Jimmy Ron? Or when he was matured he liked that name so much that he changed his name to Jimmy Ron before was

successful? All the works he did were the same, perhaps human beings would be recorded in all books with the name of Jimmy Ron without any concern.

4. How could friends of Jim Rhon perceive exactly about him?

- When Jim Rhon was one year old, how did he look like, how his neighbors thought about him?

- When Jim Rhon was five years old, how did he look like, how his neighbors thought about him?

- When Jim Rhon was twenty years old, how did he look like, how his neighbors thought about him?

- When Jim Rhon was fifty years old, how did he look like how his neighbors thought about him?

They may know him in the appearances, his voices, his thinking, his feelings, his characters, his attitude, his works, the feeling he made for them. These things are changing day by day.

If we ask the people who lived with Jim Rhon, we would get thousands of different answers about him, these lead to thousands of perceptions about him. From his wife, his ex-wife, his disciples, his governors, the businessmen, we would find out some people loved, some people protected, some people hated, some did not care about him.

We will never get the concreted perception about Jim Rohn even if we ask his two children, his two students, and his ex-wife. Even with sophisticated technology, we will never have the concrete perception of him.

The third is Adolf Hitler.

1. Who is Adolf Hitler? (1889 - 1945)

He was a German politician from 1933 to 1945. He was a dictator". Most people did not agree with the concept that he died in 1945. Even the name Adolf Hitler had its old history, if some factors changed in his family, humankind would have different dictators' name. Why so many people still have the full perception of the name Adolf Hitler? They still have the perception of his appearance, actions, and emotions with the name.

2. What is the image of Adolf Hitler's face?

What was the exact image of him when he was an infant (1889-19890), adolescence, a soldier during World War I, or the politician. There will be no exact images. It is continuous perceptions about him.

3. How could friends of Adolf Hitler perceive exactly about him?

- When Adolf Hitler was one year old, how did he look like, how his neighbors thought about him?

- When Adolf Hitler was five years old, how did he look like, how his neighbors thought about him?

- When Adolf Hitler was twenty years old, how did he look like, how his neighbors thought about him?

- When Adolf Hitler was fifty years old, how did he look like how his neighbors, his soldiers thought about him?

Nobody had the same perception about him, even the historians living during the war. The boys played with him, the soldiers fought with him in World War I. The German soldiers fought for him in World War II, the soldiers died for him, and the soldiers fought against him. We will get a flow of perceptions, which changes constantly and depends on so many varieties.

The fact is that when he was four years old, he nearly drowned in an icy river; he saved by the son of his house owner. Would four-year-old Hitler become a dictator? Nobody could know. I think that even the innocent four-year-old Hitler did not know he would become a dictator also.

We will never get the concreted perception of Adolf Hitler. Even with sophisticated technology, we will never have the concrete perception of him. Most people have had a bad feeling of disgusting and fear during and after World War II. Even hearing the word Adolf Hitler has created a lot of fear in listeners. What would happen to the world if Adolf Hitler had given a different name to his parents?

The fourth is Michael Jackson.

1. Was he a black man or a white man?

2. Was he happy or not happy?

3. What about his property when he was alive: trousers, pants, hats, houses, cars, pictures, images…are these still on his own?

We will never get the concreted perception about the name Michael Jackson. All we know about him is just the hologram of all our perception of the phenomena he created.

The fifth is the kings, heroes, and warriors

Who are Pharaoh, Emperor Qin Shi Huang, Adolf Hitler, Napoleon Bonaparte, Alexander III, and Genghis Khan?

1. Were they great kings, to you, to their peoples, to their slaves, to their spouses, to their children?

2. Which did they leave? Was it legacy or tragedies for life, admiration or fear, peace or war, happiness or stress?

3. Were they really representative of God? Where did God, Holy Spirits stand for when the war has taken place?

To the victims, slavers, the poor, the sufferers… the God, Holy Spirit were stood for the good belief that they stand for or hope for, to keep them safe, to make them feel sure or certain about life, to make them have hope, the power to suffer the tragedy put on them.

To the warriors, the kings, and the rulers… they believed the representative of God, they had the right to kill or save anybody. The fights, killed or murdered someone else for the God's side or their Holy Spirit's side.

4. What did the things they think "eternity"? From which they had sacrificed thousand or million people to create and protect for their eternity.

The fact all of us have a relatively specific perception about these characters in history, this perception changing gradually. They were visible of million phenomena; they were the effects of million causes. In return, they created millions of other phenomena or causes in life. Each phenomenon happened to them was the effect of previous phenomena, also the cause of changing inside them; and then create thoughts, words, and actions. Each of these can cause many phenomena in life.

The sixth is you.

1. Who are you? Which of the following are constant in you: the appearance, the voices, the thinking, the feelings, the characters, the attitude, the work?

2. Which of you is constant: body, feelings, perceptions, mental formations, and consciousness? Are they the same between you, your spouse, and your children?

3. What is your possession? Your children, your houses, your cars, your name, your address, your position in work, your job, your money, your fame, your idols, your God, your Holy Spirit, your spiritual costume, etc… which of these are constant over time?

- What is your response if someone makes harm to each of these things?

- Why do you have this response?

The seventh is an imagined story.

Imagine a story happen to characters. Please answer the questions: who are they? What do they have? Why do they have that, and why not?

In a Miss USA contest, three candidates for the crown standing to wait for the results are Elizabeth Brown, Elizabeth Maxwell, and Victoria Tracy. The master of ceremonies slowly announces loud "The Miss USA is …. Elizabeth… Brown…." (Who is the most anxious and disappointed during hearing the announcement?) Elizabeth Brown is walking to the center of the stadium to taking crown, suddenly the there is a loud voice from Sarah Williams - who has just released from prison - in the front row of audiences: "She is not Elizabeth Brown, she is my daughter. Her name is Elizabeth Williams." The conference hall is quiet to let her explain. She explains: "it was the mistake of the doctors and nurses in the hospital where I delivered my child twenty years ago that make me lost her, a beloved child. I have found her for twenty years." Audiences start to bandy about Miss Elizabeth Brown and the bad reputation she may make because of her bad unknown origin. A rich and powerful man takes advantage of this chaos to give the title of Miss USA for Victoria Tracy; because of his influence, the board of examiners agrees with him. The perceptions about everything in the contest of all people have changed since Sarah Williams raised her voice.

All the perception of a title, an individual may change because of million phenomena. The illuminating of these phenomena created our perception. Because of all the things we think we know about the situation is the hologram of relating phenomena, there are no definite things in that situation. Thousands of people in stadiums or billions of people watching The 2014 FIFA World Cup Final match between Germany - Argentina had different point of views about the game, players, and decision of referees. Because of million different accumulated phenomena during lifetime, so that no one had the same view, emotion or the same frequency of emotion when watching the game.

The fact is there have been a lot of withdrawing the rewards, the Olympic medals, or the degrees of many people because of the later investigation found out they have cheated in the contest. In corrupt countries, some men can have an influence on the result of the investigation. I do not care about the act of investigation or contest. I only care about the perception of relating people, the titles, the fame, and the names of these people; what is its characters, is it constant or changing with the perception of other people? What made the rewards, who made the rewards and what affected the rewards? With a lot of imagining question: If... then...I find that these titles, fame, possession, and names are the meeting of phenomena caused by the mind of human being. It is the result of illuminating of countless phenomena, it is not constant; in return, rewards, fame, and medals are the cause of countless other phenomena that effect to other people.

Nothing is certain, nothing is static; things are the solidifying and dissolving of countless phenomena; the decreasing and increasing of phenomena. Thing is not born, also not died, they are constantly changing from perceivable to unperceivable of the human mind. We are in the hologram with the seamless web phenomena.

References:

Hanh, Thich Nhat. (1987).Old path white clouds: Walking in the footsteps of the Buddha. Parallax press.

Hitler, Adolf. In Wikipedia. Retrieved July 17, 2017, from http://en.wikipedia-.org/wiki/Adolf_Hitler

Is our universe a Hologram? In 1982 a little known but epic event occurred at the University of Paris [Web log post]. (2011, September 29). Retrieved July 19, 2017, from http://www.dailygalaxy.com/my_weblog/2011/09/is-our-universe-a-holo -gram-in-1982-a-little-known-but-epic-event-occurred-at-the-University-of-paris.html

Lao Tsu. The Tao Te Ching. Translated by Gia-Fu Feng and Jane English. Vintage Books, 1972.

Talbot, Michael (n.d.). The Holographic universe. Retrieved July 19, 2017, from http://www.rense.com/general69/holoff.htm

Talbot, Michael (n.d.). The Universe as a Hologram. Retrieved July 19, 2017, from http://www.mindbodyneurofeedback.com/content/resources-articles/universe-hologram

What is Yin Yang?. (n.d.). Retrieved July 19, 2017, from http://personaltao.com /teachings /questions/what-is-yin-yang/

Chapter 18: New philosophy of relation between brain, mind, body, physical health, ego

By deep reflection, you will see there is no Ego, nothing constant inside you. You are the illuminating of the rivers of your body, body, feelings, perceptions, mental formations, and consciousness. They are constantly changing, nothing stays the same. You can sense the direction of changing, your destiny by the phenomena you created and the phenomena you received. The phenomena are beyond form, beyond sound, and intangible, which cannot listen, cannot see, and cannot be grasped. The right degree of illuminating of these phenomena created the physical object that you may see, hear, and grasp. In the same environment, the things you see, hear, and grasp may be different to your relatives, your friends, and your brothers. The phenomena are subjective, but the belief, the state of mind and the emotion of us decide which side we view these phenomena. Small changes of view side may make us have a totally different perception. All of the human beings are under the hologram of phenomena around us. Each of us has a slightly different point of view so that our perception may be different or contrast to others.

The emotion and belief system affected our perception of the environment the most. There are many kinds of research show that human beings easily fall into the trap of irrational thinking. The book Blink of Malcolm Gladwell and other Irrational Thinking books show many kinds of research that help us understand how easily we fall into the trap of irrational thinking and emotional thinking.

From the belief system, the emotion, and point of view, we process the perceived information like:

"Sow a thought reap a feeling

Sow a feeling reap an action

> Sow an action reap a habit
>
> Sow a habit reap a character
>
> Sow a character reap a destiny."

Thought, emotion, action, habit, character, and destiny are the names of one phenomenon, which is a human being. Destiny is the summation of all the results and perceptions of life. The root of destiny is the thought so people need to care for thoughts to have health, wealth, peace, and happiness. The relations between these factors are as subtle as Yin and Yang. There is nothing exists separately; they are interdependent on each other.

Each thought, action, habit, and character we sow not only are the effects of million input phenomena but also are the causes of countless other output phenomena. Human beings are powerful creatures because of thought. The two powerful laws that control human being are the "law of thought" and "law of cause and effect." We do not understand all the phenomena go in and out ourselves, but we may have good gut feelings about the quality of these phenomena. Under the influence of mind and law of causes and effect, countless laws and rules have been created to take advantage of mind and cause and effect. From the causes at present, we may sense the effects in future; and from the effects at present, we may sense the previous causes.

If the brain is in a bad state, we may reap ill thought, we may reap an ill action, and gradually, we may reap ill fate.

Some people may have the brain in a good state, but they have a bad point of views for viewing the situation. They will get bad thoughts; they may nourish the bad thoughts long enough that create strong emotion. From negative emotion, they may reap bad actions, bad behaviors, bad characters, and ill fate.

Some people have the brain in a good state and perceive good thoughts form environment. But they are not really strong enough to maintain the good state of the brain and good mental state before the changing of the environment with million phenomena interacting back and forth between them and the environment. So that they may reap bad emotions, over time, the bad emotions lead to bad action, bad habits, and character and ill fate.

Some people have the brain in a good state, sharp mind, and good actions. Unfortunately, the good state of brain, mind, and good actions are not strong enough to endure with changing of an environment to create a good habit. They may infect bad habit because of the negative consequences of interdependence between mind, body, and environment. Gradually they get ill fate.

Only small people train themselves well enough that they gain good state of the brain, nourishing sharp mind, and patiently taking good action to reap good habits, and good characters. Gradually, they reap good destiny.

On the way to success, people need to have endurance, patience, and discipline enough to sow the seeds of goodness in every thought, and action. Then continue to protect the good seeds before million phenomena from an environment to reap a good habit, good character, and good destiny. The best tools for them are the principles that guide them to confront with million phenomena around them. Most ordinary people do not have principles of action so that they easily exhausted with the confronting of countless phenomena as pressure and difficulties so that they are easily tempted with temporary joy. Lao Tzu taught to have a good life, people need to have patience, compassion, and simplicity; he did not talk about intelligence at all as most of the modern people think.

There is no separate self, no constant ego or constant spirit. We are the illuminating of the interaction between phenomena we meet and we create. We live in the seamless web on cause and effect we created. Each response we take is the effect of countless previous phenomena, and from that response, we create many other phenomena. We are changing every day as the hologram of compound phenomena. Phenomena are stable, but we are changing because we are the illuminating of compounded phenomena.

The longtime after the death of great spiritual leaders, good kings or bad kings, the dictators, good philosophers or bad philosophers, human being are still getting benefits or enduring the burdens they left. The inspiration, from the action of great spiritual leaders thousand years ago, still has an effect in modern life. And the fear they created a thousand years ago still embeds in modern life. The phenomena they created may available in the spiritual life, the religious customs, the philosophy, the genome, and deep in the subconscious mind of modern people. If we do not train ourselves well, if we do not pay attention, we will be the victims of bad phenomena. We can see our brain in the structures of the brain, the activation of the brain, the EEG waves, and other devices to see the brain are in good state or not. We can know our mental ability and our mind by the mind is a set of cognitive faculties including consciousness, perception, thinking, judgment, and memory. By defining this set, we can know our mind is in the good state or bad state.

When the conscious mind is obsessed with these ideas with the highest emotion and by repetition, the subconscious mind will adopt these ideas without any rejection. The ideas relating to survival, joy, safety, health, and happiness will embed in the mind of people with the highest feeling of fear and joy. Confronting with the strange and unknown natural phenomena: storm, thunderstorm, birth, and death, hurricane, flood, drought, diseases, pandemic, mysterious event, fragile people look to for their leaders. Any strange behaviors taught by the most influential people of the commune to bring food, safety, and health may become the mysterious customs if repeated many times. These strange behaviors may become the ritual customs, religious customs. In the human history, the belief of people of the community with the religious customs was so strong that they sacrificed virgin girls, people, women, or their children in the ritual customs without any hesitation. With the strong belief of bringing safety, health, abundance, and protection they did not have any concern with sacrificing people, fighting and creating human miseries in their ritual customs. Reading the strange religious customs, the strange burial customs, and ritual customs, we will see how stupid, how crucial some of these ritual customs were.

Moreover, the state of the brain, the quality of conscious and unconscious mind, will create the quality of spiritual life and the quality of physical health. The brain, the mind, and physical health are the interdependent factors. In the brain, there is the reflection of mind and body; in the body, there is the reflective quality of the brain and mind. There is no mind can stay separate the brain and body." This is because of that is. That is because of this is." The interdependency described in many laws of life: the law of cause and effect, law of attraction, law of thinking, law of believing, and Yin and Yang philosophy. In a human being, the development of brain gives birth to the human mind; in return, the human mind is the most powerful factor that decides and corrects slowly the structure of the brain, mental health, and physical health. Buddha, Jesus, and many spiritual leaders, philosophers, trainers and educators all give advice that we should pay attention in protecting the mind, pay attention in feeding the mind, pay attention to the quality of thinking to have a good life.

What happens if you have good thoughts about bad events? What are your emotion, and your actions?

What happens if you have bad thoughts about good events? What are your emotion and your actions?

Can you see the differences? We are the only creatures that we can master our destiny.

Mind, body, health, life, and environment.

> Environment feeds the mind
> People choose to feed the mind.
> Good feeding to the mind creates good thought
> The good thought creates the good belief,
> The good belief creates the good mind,
> The good mind creates good gene
> The good mind creates many other conditions
> Visible or invisible
> These good conditions are perfect for good brain
> These conditions are perfect for good health.
> And in reverse,
> These are the interdependent factors

They are interdependent with the phenomena from the environment
And interdependent with the phenomena they created.
They operate with the law of cause and effect
Belong to other laws and principles in the universe
Follow the Yin and Yang theory.
Nothing is independent
Things are interdependent, empty, and selfless.
Emptiness means things rely on each other to illuminate
Phenomena rely on each other to coexist or non-exist
Appear and disappear.

Questions to ponder to help people gain wisdom and enlightenment

> - Who are you?
>
> - Where is the person that you had when you were one year old?
>
> - What language do you speak? Why do you speak your language?
>
> - What religious are you? What makes your religion, your friend's religion and your cousin's religion different? Why do you believe and trust totally in you are religious?
>
> - Where is the person that you had when you were five years old?
>
> - Where are your old concepts, the old belief you had during childhood?
>
> - You are a successful man. What happens if the misjudging of the court will make you become a prisoner in the next five months? Perhaps you will lose all: properties, houses, cars, family, your spouse, your children, your good

> attitude, your good work, your reputation, your pride, your happiness. A coming accident will take all of you. So what is the remaining?
>
> - You have a Ph.D. degree in business administration; you are a good lecturer in a university." You think therefore you are" as Descartes said.
>
> - What you will become, what will remain if tonight's sleep you get a stroke, the stroke make injury in your brain, affect your cognitive thinking, and you forget all basic information, even worse you may lose the ability to control of the normal behaviors like walking, talking, and urinating.
>
> - Will stroke accidentally happen or the result of the accumulation of bad phenomena before?

The story of selflessness and emptiness:

An imagine story: a rich and healthy man was spending time and money to build a beautiful villa, and giant mausoleum for him when he dies. One year after finishing the villa and mausoleum, he got a stroke. The stroke made him forgetting all things, losing all cognitive behaviors, losing all of his cognitive thinking, and becoming paralyzed. He had to lie in bed all day, fed by tubes. He has lived in a persistent vegetative state, also known as "unresponsive wakefulness syndrome", for ten years in his villa. All of his properties have been sold to have money for healthcare. When he dies, his body only has skin and skeleton, all of his relatives cannot find any similarity between the dead body and his picture when he was a healthy man; even the characters have changed drastically. According to the follow the testament, People put the dead body in the mausoleum.

- Who lived in the villa for ten years? Was that person the same as a rich, healthy man building villa and mausoleum? Why you make the answer?
- Where was the rich and healthy man?
- Did the stroke accidentally happen to him?

- Could people forecast the stroke?
- What do people really put into the mausoleum?

Answer these questions, ponder with the imaginative stories, we will find out the truth about life, about self, about constant things. Best of all we will find out the relation between body, mind, physical health, behaviors, environment, and countless phenomena received and created by the individual.

Chapter 19: Outliers: a new level of brain, mind, physical body, and health

The combination of training, practicing, studying, and thinking creates the connections between neurons in the brain. When having enough connections, the brain can function well with the least effort; scientists may get EEG with the alpha wave instead of the beta wave with the sophisticated activities that individuals have mastered. The brain will work very effectively with less energy and less effort for when they master sophisticated activities compare with the first time of acting.

Malcolm Gladwell suggested that people should spend ten thousand hours of using the mind to become outliers. To this point, the mind can see, hear, and feel the signals from the environment than the normal mind cannot see, hear or feel. The brain of outliers works much more effective and much more silently. Some Zen monks can control the activation of the brain to have the most effective brain's function. In the function of the brain, it is not the vigorousness or the band of oscillations or the constant of activation of brain cells that makes the best brain function; it is the rhythm, the harmony of every part of the brain, the smooth cooperation of every relating parts of the brain to make the best function of brain.

The brain cells are too weak, too fragile before any tension or any injury to the body; the brain cells need the condition of biological homeostasis to develop well. Protected by a skull, the brain well protected from the physical injury. Unfortunately, the stressed state with stress chemicals is the hazard to homeostasis that may harm the brain cells and structure of the brain. Especially stress during early childhood can create irreversible damages to the structure of the brain. These damages make parts of brain act out of normal biological rhythm; in response to these damages, the brain may overdevelop the cells, the mass in some the parts of the brain to restore some vital functions of the brain. The damages and the abnormalities in the structure of the brain may cause abnormalities in EEG, in hormonal imbalances, in cognitive mind, in behaviors, physical health, etc... these called the systemic problems or the syndrome of illnesses. The facts to prove these ideas is there are too many patients, with chronic diseases that are untreatable, have abnormal structures in the brain, have abnormal EEG, have an abnormal gene, have problems with cognitive thinking, have problems in interacting in family members, society, have big changes in appearance... They all have one same problem is they constantly become stressed.

Theta brainwave has seen in meditation. Theta wave has been associated with reports of relaxed, meditative, and creative states. Zen-trained meditation masters produce noticeably more alpha waves during meditation. Some people who practice a type of deep meditation called Yoga Nidra (*Sleep yoga*) can remain conscious while in deep sleep with the delta wave.

People can be trained to create gamma waves or a new level of brain and mind. According to the Gama wave in Wikipedia, a study has been taken place by scientists in an American university. Scientists have observed eight Tibetan Buddhist monks, who took long-term meditation. Simultaneously they compared the brain activity of the monks to a group of novice meditation practitioners. In a normal meditative state, both groups were shown to have similar brain activity. However, when the monks were told to generate an objective feeling of compassion during meditation, their brain activity began to fire in a rhythmic, coherent manner, suggesting neuronal structures were firing in harmony. This was observed at a frequency of 25-40 Hz, the rhythm of gamma waves. These gamma-band oscillations in the monk's brain signals were the largest seen in humans, apart from those in states such as seizures.

Interestingly, the gamma-band oscillations were scant in novice meditation practitioners. A number of rhythmic signals did appear to strengthen in beginner meditation practitioners with further experience in the exercise. The strengthening of gamma rhythmic signals did imply that the aptitude for one to produce gamma-band rhythm is trainable. This may indicate that the brain of the monks and patients with seizures has the strongest electrical activity but in a different manner due to mind practicing and brain injury.

Some mysterious abilities of well-trained people are proof that the human mind can have so much more potential to reach and we have not known how much potential of our mind. Examples of people who claim to have developed some extraordinary abilities. Perhaps we are evolving into a world of zero limits. Here are the examples from three websites, where you can view to see the extraordinary abilities that ordinary people may have.

X-Ray Vision: Natasha Demkina is a Russian woman who claims to be able to see into peoples' bodies. Just like an X-ray machine, she is able to detect problems inside of people and diagnose them.

Super language abilities: Harold Williams was able to speak 58 different languages.

Eagle Vision (20 times more acute than the rest of us): Veronica Seider holds the world record for being able to see the smallest object without assistance from technology.

Sonar Vision (like Bats or Dolphins): Ben Underwood is blind, both of his eyes were removed (cancer) when he was three. Yet, he plays basketball, rides on a bicycle, and lives a quite normal life. He taught himself to use echolocation to navigate around the world. He uses sound. Ben makes a short click sound that bounces back from objects.

Sensory abilities and the recognition of music: Arthur Lintgen is an American physicist who can look at phonograph records and recognize the song. He says he is able to look at the grooves and recognize the song recorded. He can also tell if the song is being played loud or quiet based on his ability to focus in on the little details of the records.

Photographic memory: Stephen Wiltshire is a British architectural artist who can look at a landscape once and then draw it with perfect accuracy.

Iceman: Wim Hof claims it has enhanced his immune system; and that he does not suffer any bad effects from this ice dips.

Super Human Reflexes: Isao Machii is a Japanese Iaido master who has the quickest reflexes in the world. He holds many world records for his quick sword skills

The Lion Whisperer: Animal behaviorist Kevin Richardson says he relies on instinct to win the hearts and form an intimate bond with the lions.

Monks generating magical heat energy from their bodies

Experts have been studying Buddhist monks for more than 20 years, trying to figure out just how in the hell they're doing what they do. By using a meditation technique called Tum-mo, these monks can lower their metabolism by 64 percent. Normal people's metabolism only drops 10 to 15 percent when you sleep. But far more awesome than that, the monks can also increase the temperatures of their fingers and toes by 17 degrees. No one knows how.

The woman who can laugh at a peak volume of 110 decibels: Jittarat laugh with the volume of 110 decibels. The noise is the same as the noise of a rock band event.

The man who claps as loud as a Helicopter: Zhang Quan, 70, is a Chinese man can clap his hands nearly as loud as a helicopter. His claps apparently measured 107 decibels - three decibels lower than whirling helicopter blades.

There are many extraordinary abilities of human beings, known or unknown to the writers and readers, which are hard to understand by temporary science. People often use myths, God, Holy Spirit to explain these extraordinary abilities. Mastering your mind, you will never know how potential your abilities are. Thousand heroes, Superman or Holy Spirits of the human kind once time they were ordinary people.

References:
Cowart, R. Kirsten. (2014, August 30). Sixteen people with real superpowers. Retrieved July 19, 2017, from http://thespiritscience.net/2014/08/30/16-people-with-real-super-powers/

Gamma wave. (n.d.). In Wikipedia. Retrieved July 17, 2017, from http://en.wikipedia.org/wiki/Gamma_wave

Gladwell, Malcolm (2005). Blink: The Power of Thinking Without Thinking. New York: Little, Brown

Gladwell, Malcolm (2005). Blink: The Power of Thinking Without Thinking. New York: Little, Brown

Gladwell, Malcolm (2008). Outliers. New York: Little, Brown & Co

Gladwell, Malcolm (2008). Outliers. New York: Little, Brown & Co

Real-life superheroes: ten people with incredible abilities. (2007, November 27). Retrieved July 19, 2017, from http://www.oddee.com/item_91848.aspx

Ten extraordinary people with weird superpowers. (n.d.). Retrieved July 19, 2017, from http://www.mindpowernews.com/RealSuperpowers.htm

Part V: Conditioned Responses

Chapter 20: All the things we have are the results of conditioned responses

> "Results do not come from the environment, but from the responses.
>
> Responses come from thoughts and emotion.
>
> Feed the mind with good food, the mind will create good thought
>
> Feed the mind with rubbish, the mind creates rubbishy thought
>
> The best way is to care to feed the mind if to have a good life"

*** *** ***

When information and signals come to mind, our conscious mind focuses on analyzing the patterns of signals and information. The process of analyzing mobilize a lot of energy, the concentration, all senses, experiences, the known knowledge, the deepest desires and the feelings to draw out the patterns of information. After perceiving clearly the characters of information, the conscious mind sends the pattern of information to the unconscious mind to remember. It will be the material for subconscious mind use when they need to make a decision.

People can create the behaviors or habits of other people by reward and punishment. In Pavlov's dogs, the dogs have conditioned with the conditioned response by the ringing the bell and feeding food. Pavlov has rung the bell before feeding the dogs. After several times, the dogs have conditioned with the responses. Next time, he only rung the bell but not fed the dogs, the dogs still salivated. The mind of the dogs has remembered the pattern of condition so well that just hearing the small part of the condition the dogs had the conditioned responses.

In fact, we can create conditioned response to our children, workers, employees and other people by reward and punishment. Moreover, the condition is much more complicated than our understanding, because the condition put on other people has so much more varieties and frequencies than we can imagine. There are millions of phenomena in one condition, which we use to condition responses to other people. Our neo-cortex only catches the perceivable information from the condition, but our limbic system can catch much more information form the condition that we do not know. All the information caught by neocortex and the limbic system can stimulate the conditioned responses inside the body. The conditioned responses help people and animals to adapt well to the environment, help people and animals to survive in the environment. Moreover, with the development of brain and mind, the conditioned responses directed to satisfying the needs of the human being to bring the feeling joy and happiness for them. The brain and mind function well and effectively owing to the condition responses. Unfortunately, the conscious mind only knows very little about the conditioned responses stored in the brain structure, the conscious mind and the subconscious mind. People can consciously know these conditioned responses by mindfulness or observe the changes in the body before the changing of environment. To this point, we can know that many other conscious responses or unconscious responses are the conditioned responses people gain throughout the life. The pattern of responses and information about the environment may be available in brain, cell, body, genome, habit, and environment; and the information accumulated by one generation is heritable. The facts, which prove that the previous information that individuals met lie in the brain, cell, body, genome, and environment, is the chronic diseases, chronic health problems and social problems available around us. Scientists have made many investigations into chronic diseases and mental diseases; they have found that the patients with these diseases have problems or abnormalities in the structures of brain, cells, body, genome, habit. These abnormalities are not only the results of the previous problem but also the causes of later serious problems.

Gut feelings are conditioned responses. The mind makes the judgment about phenomena in the environment; then it silently sends the corresponding conditioned responses about the environment for us via autonomic nervous systems without any noticing of the conscious mind. In danger situation, the autonomic nervous system has made some changes in our body long before we consciously know what is happening.

Allergy is also the conditioned responses of the patient to the specific allergens despite patients known or unknown about the allergens. Allergy controlled by the autonomic nervous system.

Homesick is also conditioned responses. People who live far away from home can have the feeling of homesick if they meet part of the condition like the new year festival, the union day, the changing to cold temperature like Christmas in Western countries; and Tet festival (lunar new year) in the north of Vietnam; the changing of decoration on the road, listening the festival songs. Any of the perceivable signals or imperceptible signals created a happy feeling at home can create a feeling of homesick.

Only adults grew up in the countryside can have the strong feelings, the surge of high emotion when seeing, watching videos or pictures, or hearing the familiar sounds from their countryside that make them miss countryside. During childhood, they have met millions of phenomena in the countryside with strong feelings. The pattern of phenomena and feelings are stored in the subconscious mind. During their lifetime, they may relive the childhood memory and have the feeling of missing homeland whenever the limbic system catches any phenomena similar to the phenomena during their childhood. Vietnamese often have the feeling of missing home when seeing the images of children playing in rural Vietnam like playing marbles, tug of war, mandarin square capturing, Bermuda grass fighting, skipping rope, playing with water at the village well, swimming in the river with buffalos, riding buffalos, playing on paddy field.

People in every country in the world also have the feeling of homesick where they grew up if they meet part of the condition, which has created the feeling of joy and happiness for them.

It is the same as the adults or old people live abroad, seeing, hearing, meeting any familiar things can make them have the feeling of missing their countries.

The interesting novels, poems, songs, films, and fictions can create high emotion in some specific readers. The fictions and songs written for wartime created the strongest feeling or vibration for the old people who had lived during the war and fought in the war. In peacetime, these fictions, poems, and songs do not create much emotion in the pupils, students and the youth as the experienced people. On the other hand, romantic novels, romantic films attract a lot of young audiences but rarely attract old audiences. Because the emotion, feelings as the conditioned responses caused by these products in young readers and in old readers are not at the same level as the different group of people.

Anger, fear, stress, happiness, and all other emotions are the conditioned responses of the body controlled by the nervous system, most of the time the autonomic nervous system will dominate the body and behaviors with strong emotion if we lack awareness or mindfulness. Understanding conditioned responses can help scientists understand the behavioral psychology. The first kiss in love has total different feeling and taste with the last kiss in anger.

With the addictions like opium addicts, chess addicts, gambling addicts, smoking addicts, game addicts, monetary addicts, sexual addicts, reward addicts, fame addicts, drinking addicts or food addicts, these people will have the condition responses in the body by autonomic nervous system when they see, hear, smell, or sense some of the signals related to satisfying addiction. This is the reason if we want to make the addicts quitting the addicted habit, we should put them in the new supporting environment and help them stay away from the environment where had the condition relating to addiction. The conditioned responses caused by addicted patterns are the strong negative feeling of irritating, tingling, sad, anger, bored, pain, changing of behaviors, changing of emotions, extreme pain or loss of consciousness like crazy if the attack of addiction is not satisfied. They have the symptoms relating to excessive activation of the autonomic nervous system, the conscious mind is absent under the strong attack of addiction.

Religious customs, taboos, and spiritual rituals have the strongest influences on its disciples. Following or violating religious custom will create the strongest feeling in people's mind as the conditioned responses. Some people even become hysterical if they violate their taboos or religious traditional customs. Even though, they and their friends, cousins in the same building have totally different opinions and behaviors in their own religion.

Punishment and reward can create conditioned responses. With the baby being beaten by his father when the father goes out for work if someone threatens the baby that if he does not sit and play in the boring safety, his father will beat him. The words of threatening, beating can trigger all the previous painful feeling in the kid because of conditioned responses so real that the kid is scared to sit and play in safety unnaturally. The fear has made the kid to suppress the instinct of playing, learning, trying and curiosity.

Being beating or punishing for the rebelling behaviors that teachers, parents, and managers do not like can create the painful conditioned responses in the sufferers. So that each time the good chances come, the chances demand little of challenge, courage, and uncertainty. The children who were punished severely may hesitate or feel chill when taking chances. Gut feelings, small talk, and conditioned responses will prevent him from taking a risk. Because of pain and fear, they like to stay in the comfort zone.

The taste of eating same food is never the same because of the taste is the sum up of countless conditions. Seeing, smelling, imagining, or hearing can trigger the conditioned responses as real as that people are eating. Enough of repetition with emotion, we can create conditioned responses for ourselves and others.

The sweet kiss and disgust kiss: depend on the opinion of the receivers about the partners. They fall in love is the sweet kiss. But if they get married, experiencing enough of crying, blaming, kicking, beating and shouting, the kiss may become painful or disgust because of countless conditioned changes inside the body.

Having sex ends with conditioned responses ejaculation. Ejaculation is the conditioned response. Masturbation also ends with ejaculation without sex partners. Famers usually make a male animal to masturbate to take its spermatozoon. Doctors in Andrology usually make an order for male patients to masturbate to take the spermatozoon for needed tests. Scratching, warmness, touching, kissing, visualizing, sound, pressing, moving, and emotional feelings, all participate in the forming conditioned ejaculation.

Visualization in the mind the exciting experiences or painful experiences vividly in sound, images, colors, words, environment, the atmosphere can make the people relive the previous moment. Participants may have some changes in the body as if they re-experience the situation. These changes in the body are the conditioned responses in the body created by focusing on the direction of the mind.

Chapter 21: Beliefs, religions, taboos and conditioned responses

> The more we read and visit other countries and other people the more we know that we have different perceptions about taboos, customs, and religious rituals. If there is an object that you and a group of people see as taboos, by searching on the internet, we may find that this object is the ritual object of other people. Why do human beings have so much different in the concepts of taboos, religious customs, and festivals? The only right answer for this is thinking. No matter what you do in your festivals or taboos, if you strongly believe it will bring luck, health, and happiness, you will feel good with the joining in festivals.
>
> Trainers and therapists use all the techniques to bring back good thoughts and right beliefs for their participants.

Religious customs has the strongest influences on their disciples. Following or violating religious custom will create the strongest feeling in people's mind as the conditioned responses.

Let answer the following questions to have a better understanding of religions.

- Where were you born?

- Which religion are you? Why do you have that religion? Why do you love your religion? Why do you follow your religious rituals?

- Why do you think your belief in your religions is different than your friend's belief?

- Are you a Christian, Muslim, Buddhist, Hindu, Protestant, Catholic, Jewish or Atheist?

- Where do you usually go to church, mosque, synagogue, pagoda or temple?

- Do you believe in God? Do you believe in life after death? Do you believe in reincarnation? And why do you believe that?

- Do you think that your religious belief is the belief you chose? Or have you been conditioned with your religious belief?

- What happened with your religious belief if you were born in China, Vietnam, United State, Israel, Australia, Korea, or Singapore?

- Would you still have the same religious belief as the major people in the community of these countries or still have the same religion as the present?

I usually wonder about these kinds of questions. The fact is I were born in the north of Vietnam, I am an Atheist. I have adopted the ancestor worship custom from my parents and my relatives since my childhood. In my traditional custom, there is the mixing of Ancestor worship, Buddhism, Chinese religion, Taoism, and Confucianism. We do all of these traditional customs on New Year Eve, Mid-Autumn festival, region festival, town festival, worship in pagoda and worship in temple; and the spirit of traditional custom available in many other important events, and important places like: giving birth, welcoming new baby, worship ancestors, commencement ceremony of building or projects, wedding ceremony, working, departures, and in funeral. All of us do all these traditional custom without any concerning or hesitating. We have our set of own taboos and set of acting to fit with traditional custom - which is quite strange to the foreigners.

Here are some of our taboos in Vietnam that foreigners with the nickname Travellingkid and other foreigners discussed in the https://www.lonelyplanet.com. As a Vietnamese, I confirm that these sayings are the taboos in Vietnam.

- When visiting a graveyard, people place incense sticks on the tomb of their loved ones and on every tomb around in the area, regardless who's in those tombs.

- The bed headboard in the house can point to any direction but out to the street because only the coffin head points out to the street. The Vietnamese often do the funeral in their homes

- On Fifth, fourteenth, and twenty-third of the months on Lunar Calendar are bad days to travel or to do anything major. The Vietnamese never never never travel far on those days. Never never never never open a business in those days. No one in Vietnam can answer me WHY. (Perhaps he was too shocked with the think he encountered in Vietnam)

- When two people in a family died within 100 days from each other, that is a very bad sign for the family because there will be more death in a very short time after that. - I have witnessed a family spent all their saving - and even borrowed money - on several elaborate rituals to expel the bad spell.

- You should never touch anybody's head, nor point the soles of the feet at other people. Both are bad manners.

- Every three years of the lunar calendar, a leap month is added to bring it back into line with the solar calendar. Weddings and new contracts are banned due to bad luck superstition during leap months, but dead people must be buried.

- An Australian friend recently had a design problem when designing his bathroom: his Vietnamese wife insisted that the mirrors in the bathroom must not face the bedroom.

> - A girl often (99%) does not get married within a year after the death of her father or her mother. Any prearrangement has to be postponed.
>
> - Other person responded: I think it applies to guys, too. The death of a grandparent would mean no marriage for grandchildren within a year.
>
> - Travellingkid responded: Just a bit off the subject, in the article posted by one person, the author said: Confucius preaches, "Tam nhân đồng hành tất tổn nhất nhân" (Three men traveling will unavoidably lose one) - This is a wrong quote. The right quote is: "Tam nhân đồng hành tất hữu ngã sư." Meaning: Three men traveling together, one is the mentor. That means every person that you encounter, there is at least one thing in him for you to learn.

Source: https://www.lonelyplanet.com.

Confucius teaching is the philosophy that all Vietnamese practice in everyday life. Vietnamese are influenced by ideas of some philosophers in history.

Food and luck, we can eat many foods, but some foods we should not eat at the beginning of the lunar month. We only should eat some foods at the end of the lunar month if we want to avoid bad luck. The taboos change from region to region and religion to religion. It is much funnier that recently, most students have the belief not eating a banana before exams because they may fail like slipping on banana cover; even we make worship with the banana. It is better for them to eat some beans because beans in Vietnamese spelled "đỗ", which has the same homophone with "Passing"; and students can eat chicken but they do eat duck, eggs, or squid before an important exam.

Other like Taking photos of three, perhaps it is relating to the story of three Kitchen Gods. No one can give the correct answer for when, where and why these taboos and traditional customs appeared, but these taboos and concepts are silently controlling all of our behavior.

Understanding the conditioned responses, we can explain all the behaviors of people around us. When children are young, they study by observing and practicing. Then they will remember the things that should do with the feeling of safety, joy, excitement, and happiness. On the other hand, they will remember the things that should not do with the feeling of danger, pain, loss, and stress. They have formed the things that should do and should not do. Every day, they feed their mind with the stories, the myths, misinterpretation of the old teaching, which are the examples of good rewards, gaining with the obeying of should list and of bad punishment, or severe loss with the activity of disobeying should list. They feed their mind consciously or unconsciously with the information from the surrounding environment. The things that should or should not do now become the things that have to do and have not to do to bring for them survival and safety. The concepts like should list and should not list adopted during childhood now may become the belief or strong belief in religious belief. Their unconscious mind and conscious mind embed the set of religious belief. The unconscious mind and religious belief control all other activities. People also introduce their adopted religious belief as a private possession, become part of their life. The traditional custom and religious belief now become the part of their life, if the subconscious mind or limbic system can detect any things go against their religious belief, they may become upset, irritating, or even get mad to protect these beliefs; sometime they may fight with other, kill others or sacrifice themselves to protect the adopted belief. Each of thing that should do or has to do in the teaching of traditional custom and religious now become part of their life, they may unconsciously spend all things they have to protect that should do a thing. Each of thing in should list seems like an invisible net put on them. The more of things in should list, the thicker and the stronger the invisible net of the web. The invisible web control all thinking and behaviors of people, and control all the process of thinking and working of the conscious mind and unconscious mind. The invisible web may distort all the view and perception of these people about the environment and event happened to them in the direction of supporting the belief. The mind blindly becomes a good servant for the strong belief. If these people do any things against their traditional or religious customs, they may become anxious, worried, irritated and stressed by the arousal of the autonomic nervous system with the symptoms described in table two "Side effects of three chemicals creating stress".

Let see some of the examples to illustrate:
If two people in a family die within 100 days from each other, and the people in this family do not spend a large amount of money on several elaborate rituals to expel the bad spell. Most of the time, they will reinterpret any difficulties, problems as the indication of not making rituals to expel the bad spell. More often, they will feel uncomfortable, ill, tired, irritated; they will have more nightmare, and sometime they may get hallucination. Adopted the custom or taboo, they have the strong belief that the result of violating the traditional custom and taboos will appear soon. In fact, if people obsessed with taboos, the law of belief and law attraction will attract proofs to confirm the taboos. Obsessing with the taboos, the mind is conditioning to direct all of its power to prove what said in taboos. This is the reason why all of the people who violated their religious belief and traditional custom will meet the problems in health, work and life.

If before an important exam, students eat meals with egg, banana and duck meat, some of them will be more nervous than the student eat other food.

I want to use the story: "tying up a cat in a monastery" as an explanation for many of human rituals, taboos or beliefs." When the spiritual teacher and his disciples began their evening meditation, the cat lived in the monastery made such a noise that it distracted them. So the teacher ordered his disciples to tie up the cat during the evening practice. Years later, when the teacher died, the cat continued to be tied up during the meditation session. When the cat eventually died, another cat was brought to the monastery and be tied up during the meditation session. Even centuries later, learned descendants of the spiritual teacher wrote scholarly treatises about the religious significance of tying up a cat for meditation practice." To some extent, this story can help us to understand the origins of our adopted belief, taboos, and rituals. Most of us as human beings only follow these rituals without any wandering or concerning, even some of the rituals may cause pain, harm, and loss of ourselves and other people.

Let see another example, when you come to a party in Asia, you eat a slice of delicious roasted meat; it is the most deliciously sticky, glazed exterior meat that you have ever eat. So that you want to ask the receipt and the name of meat you have to eat. You ask the cook to explain to you. What will your responses when you hear the answer? Do you think that your taboos, your religious belief or your belief have an influence on your response after hearing?

The cook answers, the meat is:

- Pork

- Beef

- Lamb

- Dog meat

Do you recognize any responses in your organs? As personal research into the belief, I guess that:

If your religion is Hinduism, you will vomit or have strange taste in the mouth when hearing that meat is beef. You will have the feeling of nausea, irritation, and discomfort with belief that you have committed a guilty.

If your religion is Islam, you will vomit or have strange taste in the mouth when hearing that meat is pork. You will have the feeling of nausea, irritation, and discomfort with belief that you have committed a guilty.

If your religion is Christianity, you were born and raised in Europe or America; you may vomit or have strange taste in the mouth when hearing that meat is dog meat. You will have the feeling of nausea, irritation, and discomfort with belief that you have committed a guilty.

If your religion is Christianity, you were born in Korea, China or Vietnam; you will feel good and tend to ask about the receipt when hearing that meat is dog meat. You do not have the feeling of nausea, irritation, and discomfort at all.

If you are a monk living in Korea, China, Vietnam, and other countries; you will vomit or have strange taste in the mouth when hearing that the food you eat made from any animal meat. You will have the feeling of nausea, irritation, and discomfort with belief that you have committed a guilty.

The fact is if you are from China, Korean, and Vietnam, you will like to eat all delicious roasted meat made from any meat from pork, beef, lamb, and dog meat. Is that the meat make people have responses when eating the meat served as food around the world? The answer is no. With the human being, the belief and feeling in eating are much more important than the food. To some extent, the belief and feeling can create the quality of eating more than the food can create. If people eat a portion of food, which is their belief or religious belief forbid or they think that this food is poisonous, they may have the symptoms of the symptoms of food poisoning. These symptoms may be nausea, vomiting, diarrhea, upset stomach, chill, and strange tastes in the mouth. With some people, the perception about the food may create many more conditioned responses than the food can create. I have heard a lot of story like that: many westerners visit Vietnam, after eating food, they like it and give a good comment about the food. However, right after people said the food made from dog meat; some of the foreigners immediately vomit and have the feeling of nausea.

Most of the people are the products of the environment, of the regional customs and regional religions that they do not know. They have conditioned to become part of their community. They may think that the adopted religions, customs, and philosophy are part of their identity. Even worse, they force others to have the same belief and religious with us. Some people even use the violence, threatening or killing to force others. A lot of wars, fighting between individual to individual, village to village, commune to commune, people to people, and countries to countries because they have the conflicting perception of reality. Worst of all is the wars between different religious, human beings are willing to sacrifice themselves and other lives to do the things that they perceive that they should do to protect their religion. Some human beings so blindly become the products of the environment that they have been conditioned by the environment with some evil actions like beating, destroying and killing other human beings to protect their belief, their tangible or intangible properties. The root cause of miseries in the world is ignorance; all miseries caused by violent actions, ignorant actions under the mask of noble purposes. The cover of noble purposes makes people so blind that the violent actions they make at home, offices, communities are the right needed action for noble purposes.

In fact, human beings can create many good conditioned responses inside the body just by imagination or focus the mind on specific subjects. This is the mechanism of many techniques and therapies like art therapy, breathing exercises, chiropractic, dance therapy, guided imagery, guided meditation, hypnosis, hypnotherapy, massage therapy, meditation, music therapy, osteopathic manipulation, prayer, progressive muscle relaxation, Tai chi, and yoga, which help people to create wanting changes in health, performances and quality of living. These therapies only bring the best result when it forces people in the way of the pursuit of knowledge to remove their ignorance. If a therapist applies one of these therapies to people, it is better if the close relative of these people to participate in the process of treatment.

Let do this exercise by cross-matching column of meat with the column of regions, belief, and religions with you and your relatives With each matching, can you figure out the corresponding responses? Doing these exercise as often as possible will help you understand the responses of other people around you. With the right understanding of the belief and conditioned responses, you can create as many changes as you want to you and others.

Table 21: food, animals, religions and conditioned responses

Meat	Religious, belief, regions	Responses
Pork	Buddhism	
Beef	Hinduism	
Lamb	Islam	
Dog meat	Taoism	
Spider	Christianity	
Kangaroos	Hinduism	
Crocodile	Westerner: American, French, Italian, Australian	
Shark Fin	Easterner: Chinese, Korean, Vietnamese, India	

Let see the traditional custom and funeral rituals to understand how strange other people believe. If people traveling a lot, they will find out that the funeral rituals varies a lot from region to region, country to country, and religion to religion. I have attended a lot of funerals for my relatives and my friend's relatives since my childhood. I have seen many strange rituals taken place. People do these different rituals without any hesitation or concern. You can follow the links below to understand how strange other people think and do with their traditions and funeral rituals.

The weird traditions and strange customs

You can review the weird traditions and strange customs and taboos around the world from "Twenty weird traditions from around the world" from lolwot.com some strange customs that you do not know:

- Whipping women on the butt (Czech Republic)

- Greeting Magpies (UK)
- Cinnamon on all the single ladies (Denmark)
- Boot tossing (Finland)
- Wife carrying contests (Finland)
- Cleaning doorknobs on 30th birthday (Germany) if the women are unmarried.
- Congratulating the entire family on one person's birthday (Netherlands)
- Teeth tossing in Greece: people throw a baby's recently liberated tooth on their roofs.
- Avoiding using red ink to write someone's name in South Korea, because the red ink was used to write down names of dead people. Therefore, it is considered a taboo to write someone's name in red.
- The Monkey Buffet Festival in Thailand
- Tomato craze in Spain: La Tomatina takes place on the last Wednesday in August. People throw tomatoes at one another in the lighthearted good fun.
- The Blackening and Henna weddings in Muslim countries: the bride's family surrounds her and paint designs on her feet, arms and hands to symbolize womanhood, provide fertility and luck to the woman. This happens two days before the wedding
- Camel wrestling in Turkey: Many spectators are delighted to watch two male camels fight
- Footbinding in China: Young girls were compelled to go through the painful process of foot binding.
- Eating The Ashes Of Loved Ones. The Yonamamo tribe of Brazil. When a person dies, his or her body is burnt. The bone and ash powder is mixed into a plantain soup that the people attending will drink. They believe that this pleases the dead soul as it finds a resting place in their bodies.

- Piercings in India: It is strange how Hindus show their devotion to the Lord through piercing their body parts including the tongue.

- Kanamara Matsuri in Japan is a fertility festival or the Penis Festival. In recent years, this festival has become really popular among foreign tourists; every year it gets bigger and bigger. Outstanding figures are the penis forms are the central theme of the event, and the penis-shaped lollipops are devoured by the young and the old.

Some Japanese customs that are shocking to foreign travelers from business insider

- In Japan, the number four is avoided at all cost. The number four is avoided because it sounds very similar to the word for death pronounced by Chinese. And the number 49 is especially unlucky, as it sounds similar to the phrase which means "pain until death ". In my understanding, this is the influence of Chinese culture with these numbers and the pronunciation of these words in the Chinese-Japanese words that have the same spelling as bad luck. Vietnamese also have some same taboos relating to these numbers as Japanese.

- Tipping can be seen as insulting. Tipping is considered rude and can even be seen as a degrading.

- People will sleep on the trains with their head on your shoulder. If someone falls asleep with their head on your shoulder in Japan, it is common practice to just tolerate it.

- Pouring your own glass is considered rude. If you have poured for others, another guest will hopefully see that your drink is empty, and pour for you.

Unusual death rituals

Some unusual death rituals retrieved from "25 Unusual Death Rituals from Around the World" from http://cloudmind.info make me afraid of what other people believe about death and afterlife. I dare not to see some pictures in the article. I just rewrite some rituals that do not cause fear for the readers. Reading these funeral rituals and reviewing Vietnamese funeral rituals, I know that people around the world have different belief and perception about the death. So that they practice the funeral ritual based on the belief of right thing to do. I wonder if a Vietnamese man, a Chinese man or you die, how about if the relatives use one of these funeral rituals. What will the relatives think? What is their emotion during and after experiencing one of these rituals applied to his relatives?

Sky Burials

Tibetan Buddhist Celestial Burials "Sky Burials" — the tradition of chopping up the dead into small pieces and giving the remains to animals, particularly birds. Sometimes the body is left intact. In Buddhism, a dead body is seen as an empty vessel and is not commemorated.

Sati

Sati was a funerary practice among some Hindu communities in which recently widowed women immolated themselves on their husband's funeral pyre. The custom was seen as a voluntary act, but there were many instances in which women were forced to commit Sati. Although the practice is outlawed and illegal in today's India, yet it occurs up to the present day and is still regarded by some Hindus as the ultimate form of womanly devotion and sacrifice. Interestingly, India was not the first and only culture to adopt the tradition. Other ancient societies that practiced something similar to Sati included the Egyptians, Greeks, Goths, and Scythians.

Self-Mummification

Self-Mummification practiced seemingly exclusively by Japanese Sokushinbutsu Buddhist monks, the rite of self-mummification was intended as a means of demonstrating dedication and spirituality

Endocannibalism

The Yanomamo community in South America still eats the ash and ground bones of the deceased after cremation. The

Yanomamo tribes of Venezuela and Brazil practiced endocannibalism by mixing the ashes of the deceased with a plantain soup and then drinking it.

The chief tribesman of the West-African Junkun tribe eats the hearts of his predecessors, as a way of placing himself away from the normal society where he administers. Thus, many uncivilized tribes were known to practice this act within their communities. Today it has ceased in most places, but may continue in certain remote parts.

LifeGem - a dazzling death!

People can now wear their loved ones on their fingers. To create the shiny crystal, this American company called LifeGem takes a person's cremated remains, turns them into graphite then places it into a diamond press.

The Viking Funeral

You should not know this inhuman funeral ritual. According to the historical account of Ahmad ibn Fadlan, a 10th-century Arab Muslim writer, the ritual following the death of a chieftain was exceptionally brutal.

Ritual Finger Amputation

In West Papua, New Guinea, when a loved one passed on, the Dani people used to cut off their own fingers. This ritual is now banned but was allegedly practiced to drive away spirits as well as to use physical pain as a form of expression.

Funeral Strippers

Taiwan showgirls are known to strip for the dead during religious events in order to "appease the wandering spirits."

In China's Donghai region, funerals are actually status symbols. A dead man's reputation and honor are considered to be directly proportional to the number of people who attend his funeral. So, the relatives hire strippers to pull the crowds. The Chinese authorities have started cracking down on the practice of incessant media glare.

Famadihana - Turning of the Bones

The celebration is often held once every five or seven years and is a time of joyous family reunions. The Malagasy people of Madagascar have a celebration for the dead by exhuming the bodies and dressing them in new clothes or cloth. The spirit of the deceased joins the ancestors after the body has decomposed. Then, the Malagasy dance with the corpses around the tomb to live music.

Tana Toraja in Eastern Indonesia

Funerals in Tana Toraja, in eastern Indonesia, are epic affairs that involve an entire village and can last anywhere from a couple days to weeks. The burial ceremony has music, dance, and a feast for a number of guests. Understandably, death here is an extravagant occasion with a huge price tag. The relatives of the deceased are given a reprieve. Sacrificial water buffalo are slaughtered to carry the soul of the deceased into the afterlife. But that moment could take years. In the meantime, they are considered one "who is asleep" or a "sick man" and are placed in special rooms within the home and symbolically fed, included in the daily routines and conversations, cared for and taken out- remaining a part of their relative's lives. An actual burial takes place when the family is prepared for it and the coffin is placed in a grave, a cave, or hanging on a cliff. The Torajans do not consider physical death at the end of the line. Instead, death is considered only part of the gradual process toward "Puya," or the Land of Souls.

Torajan death ritual -"tomb sweeping,"- is taken to a morbid extreme. Depending on the village, every one to five years, families reunite to exhume the bodies of their deceased relatives, clean up the inside of their coffins, and, if the mummified bodies are in solid enough condition, give their ancestors a fresh change of clothes. Some parts of this ritual are same as the ritual in Vietnam.

Santhara or Fasting to Death

India, Santhara begins after a person decides their life has served its purpose and they are ready for spiritual purification. This practice is often seen as a form of suicide or euthanasia.

Fantasy Coffins

In Ghana, the death of a loved one is a time to mourn for them as well as a time to celebrate their life. Instead of being buried in a traditional coffin, carpenters fashion out caskets symbolizing the deceased person's life, including their character traits or status in society. Some are quite creative and made into fish, coke bottles, animals, or beer cans.

What happens if each group of people interchanges their funeral rituals with another group? Will they feel fine, at ease by switching to the funeral ritual for their relative?

References:

Do you know of any taboos in Vietnam?. (n.d.). Message posted to http://www.lonelyplanet.com/thorntree/forums/asia-south-east-asiamainland /vietnam/do-you-know- of-any-taboos-in-Vietnam

Garfors, Gunnar. (2016, December 6). Twenty-five strange customs and traditions around the World. Retrieved July 19, 2017, from http://garfors.com/2016/12/25-strange-customs-and-traditions-html/

Hostel World. (2014, August 21). The fifty weirdest foods from around the world. Retrieved July 19, 2017, from http://www.hostelworld.com/blog/the-50-weirdest-foods-from-around-the-world

Khan, Ejaz. (n.d.). Ten bizarre traditions from around the World. Retrieved July 19, 2017, from http://www.wonderslist.com/10-bizarre-traditions/

Khedkar, Anupama. (2015, June 23). Five Japanese Festivals That Are Weird, Awesome And Batshit Crazy. Retrieved July 19, 2017, from https://www.festivalsherpa.com /5-Japanese-festivals-weird-awesome-batshit-crazy/

May, T. Kate. (2013, October 1). Death is not the end: Fascinating funeral traditions from around the globe. Retrieved July 19, 2017, from http://ideas.ted.com/11-fascinating-funeral-traditions-from-around-the-globe/

Thorpe. Jr. (2015, July 15). Five interesting death and funeral rituals around the world, from Mongolia to Sweden. Retrieved July 19, 2017, from http://www.bustle.com/articles /97030-5-interesting-death-and-funeral-rituals-around-the-world-from-Mongolia-to-Sweden

Tsunagu Japan. (n.d.). Ten Strange Japanese Festivals. Retrieved July 19, 2017, from https://www.tsunagujapan.com/10-strange-japanese-festivals/

Twenty-five unusual death rituals from around the World. (n.d.). Retrieved July 19, 2017, from http://cloudmind.info/25-unusual-death-rituals-from-around-the-world/

Tying up the cat. (n.d.). Retrieved July 19, 2017, from http://www. emotionalintelligenceatwork-.com/resources/tying-up-the-cat/

Vietnamnet. (2013, February 13). Top ten taboos during Vietnamese Tet. Retrieved July 19, 2017, from http://english.vietnamnet.vn/fms/art-entertainment/66347/top-10-taboos-during-Vietnamese-tet.html

Chapter 22: Brief history of humankind

"I am not apt to follow blindly the lead of other men"

"We must, however, acknowledge, as it seems to me, that man with all his noble qualities... still bears in his bodily frame the indelible stamp of his lowly origin."

"We can allow satellites, planets, suns, universe, nay whole systems of the universe, to be governed by laws, but the smallest insect, we wish to be created at once by special act."

Charles Darwin

****

Sometimes I wonder when seeing some discussions or forums discuss God is real or not. Many modern people are still arguing about the existence of God, the ideas of God and the creation of God. Many people still believe the story of "Seven Days of Creation" to explain creation on earth. Their religious belief is so strong that they ignore all the scientific experiments proved the evolution of the world. The "Theory of evolution by Darwin" gives the human a thorough understanding of the origin of creatures and the origin of human beings. All of the applications of human beings on agriculture, medicine, biology and many other sciences based on the theory of evolution. Recently, I have met a man with bachelor degree try to convince me to believe the teaching of God in the Bible. He totally agrees with the concept of the world has been created in seven days. Moreover, he still insisted on the theory of evolution by Darwin is wrong. He is so stubborn to try to convince me what he believes. It is quite difficult for people who have two set of beliefs one for daily life and scientific life and one for religious life. The conflicting between these two beliefs sometimes make them getting stuck in problems, denying new ideas, or even creating pain for themselves and other people; bearing the conflicting is like bearing a heavy burden preventing from development. It would be great if people can combine these two beliefs into one. Science and religion are the two important parts that complement each other to create a good life. As an Atheist, perhaps I accept the theory proved by science easier than the people who obsess with the religious belief.

We live in the seamless web of phenomena so that we never find a concrete or constant thing. We use the words, symbols, or definitions to make us the process of consciousness easier. The process of consciousness like thinking, imagination, and many functions of the brain that process countless phenomena become easier with words, definition, symbols, and emotion. Words, symbols, definitions are the products of cognitive thinking, they make the mind easier to understand the situation by relating to the known things and the process of thinking is easier and much more effective. Even the words, symbols, and definitions change gradually by the raising awareness of human beings. To understand the process of thinking, let see some definitions from Wikipedia.

The thought is a mental act that allows humans to make sense of things in the world, and to represent and interpret them in ways that are significant, or which accord with their needs, attachments, goals, commitments, plans, ends, desires, etc.

Thinking involves the symbolic or semiotic mediation of ideas or data, as when we form concepts, engage in problem-solving, reasoning, and making decisions. Thinking is also deeply connected with our capacity to make and use tools; to understand cause and effect; to recognize patterns of significance; to comprehend and disclose unique contexts of experience or activity, and to respond to the world in a meaningful way.

Words that refer to similar concepts and processes include deliberation, cognition, ideation, discourse, and imagination.

Memory is the ability to preserve, retain, and subsequently recall, knowledge, information, or experience.

Imagination is the activity of generating or evoking novel situations, images, ideas or other qualia in the mind. It is a characteristically subjective activity, rather than the direct experience or the passive experience. The term is used in psychology for the process of reviving in the mind percepts of objects formerly given in sense perception.

Consciousness comprises qualities such as subjectivity, sentience, and the ability to perceive the relationship between oneself and one's environment. Some philosophers divide consciousness into phenomenal consciousness, which is the subjective experience itself, and access consciousness, which refers to the global availability of information to processing systems in the brain.

From some simple phenomena, these phenomena freely interact with each other create many more phenomena in the way of interacting. Compound over time, the interaction of some simple phenomena can immense phenomena. These phenomena interconnect into the seamless web. The interaction of phenomena is the best explanation for the forming of the universe and the best explanation for the creating of living on earth from some simple materials. The earth only had some inorganic elements described in Mendeleev's periodic table around four billion years ago. The names of these inorganic elements are the perceptions of the human mind to concrete the characters or a combination of specific phenomena inside the inorganic elements. The free interactions of these inorganic elements created organic elements. Over a billion years, some simple form of life created from the chemical reactions that produced many of the simpler organic compounds, including nucleobases and amino acids. Immense phenomena created over billions of years.

How did human beings appear? The first animals classified in the genus Homo had appeared from the evolution of small African ape ten million years ago. The process of evolution was still slowly for millions of years. Throughout more than 90% of human timeline, Homo sapiens lived in small bands as nomadic hunter-gatherers. As language became more complex, the ability to remember and communicate information resulted. Ideas could be exchanged quickly and passed down through the generations.

Cultural evolution quickly outpaced biological evolution, and history proper began.

Cosmic calendar

Looking at the cosmic calendar zoomed in one year of human beings for easier understanding of the formation of life and human beings; we will know how special human beings are. All the concepts and the name of spices, cells in the cosmic calendar are taught in high school; the subject of history and biology.

- 1st January to 6th September or the Big Bag to the 4.4 billion years ago is the forming of the Universe. The oldest rocks known on Earth are 4.4 billion years old.

Evolution of life on Earth

- Then from 14th September or 4.1 billion years ago, the evolution of life on earth began from "biotic life" found in 4.1 billion-year-old rocks in Western Australia, to first life of Prokaryotes.

· 30th September: photosynthesis began

· 29th October or 2.4 billion years ago is the oxygenation of the atmosphere, creatures can live on the surface of the earth.

· 5th December or 0.8 billion years ago started the first multicellular life.

· 7th December started the simple animals.

· 14th December: started Arthropods (ancestors of insects, arachnids)

· 17th December started the fish and Proto-amphibians

· 20th December started land plants

· 21st December started insects and seeds

· 22nd December started amphibians

· 23rd December started reptiles

· 24 December: big events: Permian-Triassic extinction event, 90% of species die out.

· 25 December or 230 million years ago started dinosaurs

- 26 December started mammals
- 27 December started birds
- 28 December started flowers
- 30 Dec, 06:24 am or 65 million years ago Cretaceous-Paleogene extinction event, Non-avian Dinosaurs Died Out

The start of human evolution is on the last day of the year of the Cosmic calendar:

- 30th December or 65 million years ago started primates
- 31 December, 6:05 am started apes
- 31 December, 2:24 pm or 12.3 million years ago, started hominids
- 31 December 10:24 pm or 2.5 million years ago started primitive humans and stone stools
- 31 December 11:44 pm or 0.4 million years ago started domestication of fire
- 31 December, 23:52 pm or 0.2 million years ago started anatomically modern humans
- 31 December, 23:55 pm 0.11 million years ago: the beginning of the most recent glacial period
- 31 Dec, 23:58 pm or 35000 years ago: started first sculpture and painting
- 31 Dec, 23:59:32 pm 12000 years ago started agriculture

Begin with human history is the last second in the New Year's Eve of the Cosmic calendar.

- 31 Dec, 23:59:33 pm or 12000 years ago: End of the Ice Age
- 31 Dec, 23:59:41 pm or 8300 years ago: the flooding of Doggerland - an area now beneath the southern North Sea that connected Great Britain to continental Europe during and after the last glacial period.
- 31 Dec, 23:59:46 pm or 6000 years ago: Chalcolithic
- 31 Dec, 23:59:47 pm or 5500 years ago: Early Bronze Age; Proto-writing; Building of Stonehenge Cursus

· 31 Dec, 23:59:48 pm or 5000 years ago: First Dynasty of Egypt, the early dynastic period in Sumer, Beginning of Indus Valley civilization.

· 31 Dec, 23:59:49 pm or 4500 years ago Alphabet, Akkadian Empire, Wheel

· 31 Dec, 23:59:51 pm or 4000 years ago: Code of Hammurabi, Middle Kingdom of Egypt

· 31 Dec, 23:59:52 pm or 3500 years ago Late Bronze Age to Early Iron Age; Minoan eruption

· 31 Dec, 23:59:53 pm or 3000 years ago Iron Age; Beginning of Classical Antiquity

· 31 Dec, 23:59:54 pm or 2500 years ago: Buddha, Mahavira, Zoroaster, Confucius, Qin Dynasty, Classical Greece, Ashokan Empire, Vedas Completed, Euclidean geometry, Archimedean Physics, Roman Republic

· 31 Dec, 23:59:55 pm or 2000 years ago Ptolemaic astronomy, Roman Empire, Christ, Invention of Numeral 0, Gupta Empire

· From 2500 years ago to 2000 years ago is the time of flourishing of philosophers, religious leaders of human beings.

· 31 Dec, 23:59:56 pm 1500 years ago Muhammad, Maya civilization, Song Dynasty, Rise of Byzantine Empire

· 31 Dec, 23:59:58 pm 1000 years ago Mongol Empire, Maratha Empire, Crusades, Christopher Columbus Voyages to the Americas, Renaissance in Europe, Classical Music to the Time of Johann Sebastian Bach

The current second of the cosmic calendar

· 31 Dec, 23:59:59 pm Modern history; the last 437.5 years before present, is the time of major inventions and creation and development of human beings.

Facts of human history reveal mysterious of humankind:

Between 8500 and 7000 BC, humans in the Fertile Crescent in the Middle East began the systematic husbandry of plants and animals: agriculture. Adopting agriculture increased productivity provided by farming allowed the population to expand. Agriculture had a major impact; humans began to affect the environment as never before. Surplus food allowed a priestly or governing class to arise, followed by an increasing division of labor. This led to Earth's first civilization at Sumer in the Middle East, between 4000 and 3000 BC. Additional civilizations quickly arose in ancient Egypt, at the Indus River valley, and in China. The invention of writing enabled complex societies to arise. Record, keeping, and libraries served as a storehouse of knowledge and increased the cultural transmission of information. Humans no longer had to spend all their time working for survival, enabling the first specialized occupations like craftsmen, merchants, priests, etc... Curiosity and education drove the pursuit of knowledge and wisdom, and various disciplines, including primitive science, arose. This, in turn, led to the emergence of increasingly larger and more complex civilizations, such as the first empires, which at times traded with one another, or fought for territory and resources.

By around 500 BC, there were advanced civilizations in the Middle East, Iran, India, China, and Greece, at times expanding, at times entering into decline. In 221 BC, China became a single polity that would grow to spread its culture throughout East Asia. The religious, philosophical, and customs of China and India have been mixing to create the religious, philosophy and customs in Eastern Asia. These mixing of religious customs and philosophy have remained in some countries in Eastern Asia. In the feudal system in Vietnam and China, if the feudal mandarins had made the big contribution to the development of the feudal system, after dying they might become the Holy Spirits just by a decree of the King. The King of feudal system decreed that the people of the community built a temple as a worship place for the loyal mandarin. After that, the people in the community have held a ceremony or regional festival every year on the date that the loyal mandarin died. Some of the regional festivals are still held by the people of the community to the present time. There are many regional festivals held every year in Vietnam, Korea, China, and Japan. These festivals are the occasions for the people to worship their Holy Spirit and their ancestors. One tradition in Asia is any death individuals, after dying their pictures will be put on the altar of the family for the family members make worship. The pictures of dead people may be put next to the pictures of Buddha and many other Holy Spirits.

The Kings in the feudal system use the religious as a tool to rule their peoples. Many myths created to make people think that the kings were the representative of God. The words of kings, the decisions, or the decrees were the imperial edicts. These imperial edicts were like the orders of God. People had to kneel to listen to the imperial edicts of kings. In Vietnamese history, a king who had made one serious wrong imperial edict to exterminate Nguyen Trai, an illustrious Vietnamese Confucian scholar, a noted poet, a skilled politician and a master strategist, along with their entire extended families, approximately one hundred people. Kings in the feudal system were powerful as God; they could make the punishment of nine familial exterminations or nine kinship exterminations; the punishment could make one hundred innocent people with little resistance. Twenty years later after the extermination of Nguyen Trai, the king Lê Thanh Tong officially pardoned Nguyen Trai, saying that he was wholly innocent in the death of King Le Thai Tong. Then Nguyen Trai was divinized; people started to build tempers to make worship Nguyen Trai as a Holy Spirit. Relating to the death of one hundred people of Nguyen's family because of the feudal governors' injustice, there was a rumor about the revenge of poisonous snake spread among the common people. Many people believed this rumor. They were so afraid of this rumor, afraid that poisonous may revenge them so that they dared not to talk about this event. Even many people in Vietnam recently still believe if the disaster happened to someone, it is maybe the revenge of the poisonous snake.

The punishment by nine exterminations was popular in ancient China, Korea, and Vietnam. The punishment by nine exterminations is usually associated with the tyrannical rulers throughout Chinese history who were prone to use inhumane methods of asserting control compare with slow slicing, or "death by ten thousand cuts". The first written account of the concept is in the Classic of History, officers would threaten their subordinates that they would exterminate their families if they refused to obey orders. Kings and yellow emperors considered God, with severe punishments or sentence punishments, the myths, belief, and philosophy, the governors had created the conditioned obey without any resistance. If people disobeyed any decisions of the yellow emperors, they would be frightening or became panicking. No one, even the richest man, the strongest man could have enough the courage to resist the orders of the kings if they wanted to have a good life.

The fundamentals of Western civilization were largely shaped in Ancient Greece with the world's first democratic government and major advances in philosophy, science, and mathematics. In Ancient Rome shaped major advances in law, government, and engineering.

The Roman Empire was Christianized by Emperor Constantine in the early fourth century and declined by the end of the fifth century.

Beginning with the seventh century, Christianization of Europe began. The teaching of different religions makes differences in the organization of pagodas and churches. In pagoda in eastern Asia, there are many statues of the holy spirits that people do not know, and the statue of Buddha, sometimes I even see the picture of a monk who has just gone, sometimes the pagodas are much more chaos than churches. There is no image of any dead people on the altars or churches. Looking for the answer, I find the commandments of God "You shall have no other gods before Me. And you shall not make idols". The fact is there is no teaching of Buddha-like this. This finding leads to the conclusion that we are the product of the things we believe.

In 610, Islam founded and quickly became the dominant religion in Western Asia. The House of Wisdom established in Abbasid-era Baghdad, Iraq. It considered having been a major intellectual center during the Islamic Golden Age, where Muslim scholars in Baghdad and Cairo flourished from the ninth to the thirteenth centuries until the Mongol sack of Baghdad in 1258 AD.

In 1054, the Great Schism between the Roman Catholic Church and the Eastern Orthodox Church led to the prominent cultural differences between Western and Eastern Europe. In the 14th century, the Renaissance began in Italy with advances in religion, art, and science. At that time, the Christian Church as a political entity lost much of its power.

In 1492, Christopher Columbus reached the Americas, initiating great changes to the new world. European civilization began to change beginning in 1500, leading to the scientific and industrial revolutions. That continent began to exert political and cultural dominance over human societies around the world.

From 1914 to 1918 the nations around the world were embroiled in World War I, and from 1939 to 1945 the nations around the world were embroiled in World War II. Established following World War I, the League of Nations was a first step in establishing international institutions to settle disputes peacefully. After failing to prevent World War II, the bloodiest conflict of humankind, the League of Nations was replaced by the United Nations. After the war, many new states were formed, declaring or being granted independence in a period of decolonization. The United States and the Soviet Union became the world's dominant superpowers for a time.

The big question, was Adolf Hitler the man created World War II? Would World War II have happened if Adolf Hitler had drowned when he was a child? Or was the War the product of disputes and conflicts of the beliefs, philosophies, and opinions among human kind of that time?

Reading the brief of human history, we may see that human beings are the creators and receivers of phenomena relating to human life. We are the servants of our own belief, customs, religion, rituals, and taboos, which are the products or opinions of previous philosophers. Each stage of human history has its own characters with the events, people and the dominating philosophy. Millions of people died in these events are just the small dots in the chapter on dominating philosophy in human history. Human beings have been conditioned so silently and sophisticatedly that we may think that our beliefs, opinions, actions, behaviors, customs, religions, rituals, and taboos are parts of their constant identities or Egos. We sometimes obsess about our beliefs, opinions, religions, rituals, and taboos so much that we may beat, threaten, or kill others if they violate one of the thoughts.

Talking about the definition of religions, I love the teaching of Muhammad Ali:

"Rivers, ponds, lakes, and streams - they all have different names, but they all contain water. Just as religions do - they all contain truths."

In my understanding, religions are the powerful belief, the belief comes from the thinking of protecting, caring, loving and giving from their Holy Spirits. All people will become equal under the caring of their Holy Spirit. With the protecting, caring, giving and loving from their God, people will feel safe to dare to work more, dream more, risk more, sacrifice more and take more action. All customs, rituals, and behavior like praying, asking, worshipping will reinforce the belief of people. Believing will make people feel safe in danger; they will more open to others, and more generous than in stressed state. Believing will activate the happy state of mind to make people take more good behaviors.

Religions in the human world, there are always the most powerful invisible forces control the behaviors of human beings. From the table some religions in the world, Can you imagine how well for you if you adopt one of these religions, or do the ideas contrasted to your religious rituals?

Can you have a clear answer to what is your religion, what is your cousin's religion, what is your friend religion, what is your spouse religion? And Why do you, your friend and your spouse have that religion?

Table 22: Some religions in the world

Religious	Description	God(s)?	Afterlife?	Holy Texts?
Ancestor worship	Belief that good relations need to be kept with tribal ancestor spirits.	Not defined	Yes	None
Buddhism	The belief that meditation and good living can break the cycle of reincarnation and result in enlightenment	Atheist	Reincarnation until escape	Multifaceted
Atheism	Either the active and extrinsic disbelief that God exists or not	Atheist	Not defined	None
Hinduism	Cultural religion of India which was historically decentralized and disparate, and not a	Polytheist	Reincarnation until escape	Multifaceted

Religious	Description	God(s)?	Afterlife?	Holy Texts?
	single belief system.			
Islam	Strict monotheism taught by Muhammad	Monotheist	Heaven or hell	Qur'an and Hadiths
Taoism	A relaxed and peaceful religion based on following and accepting the flow of life	Atheist	None	Tao Te Ching
Christianity	Belief that a single creator god had a son, Jesus Christ, born to a human mother, and that Jesus' crucifixion by the Romans brings salvation	Monotheist	Heaven or hell	The Bible
Confucianism	A collection of ethical and moral teachings	Atheist		None
Chinese religion	A varied cultural	Atheist	Reincarnation until	None

Religious	Description	God(s)?	Afterlife?	Holy Texts?
	religion practiced traditionally on a town-by-town and region-by-region basis		escape	
Heaven's Gate	Apocalyptic suicide cult who combined Biblical eschatology with New Age and ideas about UFOs. All 39 members committed suicide in San Diego, the USA in 1997	Theist	Yes	
Christian Apostolic Church in Zion	Fundamentalist Anti-science flat-earth Christian cult, who also predicted the End of the World would occur 4 different	Theist	Heaven or hell	The Bible

Religious	Description	God(s)?	Afterlife?	Holy Texts?
	times			
Raja Yoga	An astika school of Hindu philosophy based on mastering and quieting the mind, involving meditation	Polytheist		The Yoga Sutras of Patanjali
Order of the Solar Temple	Apocalyptic suicide cult, with mass suicides in Switzerland, France, and Quebec, in preparation for Jesus' second coming	Theist	Yes	The Bible and other
People's Temple	Apocalyptic suicide cult that imploded, resulting in the deaths of over 600 adults and 276 children	Theist	Heaven or hell	The Bible

Source: http://www.humanreligions.info/religions.html

Question to ponder:

Two girls are traveling through a war zone to their office for important work. They see a lot of beating, screaming, killing, bombing, blood, and dead bodies on road. One has a religious object in her hand with the thinking of being cared for and protected from Holy Spirits. Another girl is an atheist and does not have anything on hand make her has a feeling of safety.

Who will feel safer?

Who will feel stressed?

Who will work better in the office?

The relation between religion and committed suicide

Group of researchers: Lawrence RE, Oquendo MA, Stanley B. have found the relationship between religion and suicide risk: "After adjusting for social support measures, religious service attendance is not especially protective against suicidal ideation, but does protect against suicide attempts, and possibly protects against suicide."

The other group of researchers: Dervic K, Oquendo MA, Grunebaum MF, Ellis S, Burke AK, Mann JJ. Have found "Religious affiliation is associated with less suicidal behavior in depressed inpatients," after other factors were controlled, it was found that greater moral objections to suicide and lower aggression level in religiously affiliated subjects may function as protective factors against suicide attempts." To some extent, religious belief, religious values, and the belief of connection to the Holy Spirits and God, and being protected by their God reduce their stress and burden of the sufferers.

References:

Brain. (n.d.). In Wikipedia. Retrieved July 17, 2017, from http://en.wikipedia.org/wiki/Brain

Cosmic Calendar (n.d). In Wikipedia. Retrieved July 17, 2017, from https://en.wikipedia.org/wiki/Cosmic_Calendar

Crabtree, Vexen. (2013). A list of all religions and belief systems. Retrieved July 19, 2017, from http://www.humanreligions.info/religions.html

Dervic, K, et al. (2004, December)." Religious Affiliation and Suicide Attempt." The American Journal of Psychiatry., U.S. National Library of Medicine. Retrieved July 17, 2017, from www.ncbi.nlm.nih.gov/pubmed/15569904.

History of Earth. (n.d.). In Wikipedia. Retrieved July 17, 2017, from http://en.wikipedia.org/wiki/History_of_Earth

Lawrence, RE, et al. (n.d.)." Religion and Suicide Risk: A Systematic Review." Archives of Suicide Research: Official Journal of the International Academy for Suicide Research., U.S. National Library of Medicine. Retrieved July 17, 2017, from www.ncbi.nlm.nih.gov/pubmed/26192968.

List of religious populations. (n.d.). In Wikipedia. Retrieved July 17, 2017, from http://en.wikipedia.org/wiki/List_of_religious_populations

Major religious groups. (n.d.). In Wikipedia. Retrieved July 17, 2017, from http://en.wikipedia.org/wiki/Major_religious_groups

Mind. (n.d.). In Wikipedia. Retrieved July 17, 2017, from http://en.wikipedia.org/wiki/Mind

Nguyễn Trãi. (n.d.). In Wikipedia. Retrieved July 17, 2017, from http://en.wikipedia.org/wiki/wiki/Nguyễn_Trãi

Winston, George. (2014, February 9). World War 1 was not inevitable. Retrieved July 19, 2017, from http://www.warhistoryonline.com/war-articles/world-war-1-inevitable.html

Chapter 23: Obsessing with characters and concepts of living environment, we forget who we are

We are the products and the creature of living environment. As an instinct, we will feel safe, comfortable with the people same as us. Living in the familiar environment makes us have the feeling of security. Looking at how much security and safety small children want? Especially in a new environment, the children want to go with their parents or close relative to have the feeling of safety. I have observed many children had the feeling of fear, anxiety when they were in a crowd and could not find their parents. The instinct of safety is the most priority in children. If the children adopted by new parents to a new living environment, these parents should create as much as possible the protection and care for these children on some first day, the children will learn all day to adapt with the new environment. The learning is most effective when they have the feeling of safety and caring. The adopted behaviors and belief from living environment make them have the feeling of safety and joy. Gradually, they become the members of their community; they have all the same religious belief, rituals, interests, purposes, languages, accent, and many same things. These common things may be seen as the glue to create bonds in the community. People live oversea make friend easier with other people from the same country. In America, Vietnamese are easier make friend with other Vietnamese; Chinese people are easier make friend with other Chinese; Korean is easier make friend with other Korean. The common things in beliefs make them easier find out each other and make friend with each other. Many groups, clubs, organizations are formed by the people who have the same interests, belief or opinions. A family formed when a man and a woman come together. The couples have same interests, belief, and opinions about some aspect of life. They may have many joys, excitement, the feeling of care, and safety when they are in love. When they come to live together, problems may appear because of the different hidden belief between them. Living together, a lot of conflicts happen to like the idea of should do or should not do in many areas like studying, doing, saving money, spending money, buying things, giving birth. Husband has his own belief, wife has her own belief of should or should not do. If they do not have compassion or understanding, their old belief may make hurt for them and for other in spite of the love you have for other. Husband and wife do not fight or hate each other; their conflicts come from the different old belief in their mind. Especially when they have children, the difference in the lists of should do or should not do to their beloved children may make the severe conflicts in the family. When their children grow up, there will be many more conflicts because of the deepest separation of their belief system from by different condition of living. For example, the father was born in 1970 and grew up in wartime or hunger villages in the north of the country, the mother was born in 1980, grew up in a wealthy family in the south of the country, and their children were born in 2000 and 2010 and raised in the city. They will have the deepest separation in their beliefs formed by their conditioned of living. The lack of compassion, lack of understanding make them cannot solve the problems in their family; even they have asked the best advice from the best experts. Is that our consciousness, thinking, and perception about life are our properties? Are these things constant or changing? Do we choose them? Have we been conditioned these thinking by the living environment? Can we change them? Let see the influence on the consciousness, thinking, perception, behavior, and behaviors of human beings by some examples. What happened to the young babies left in the jungle and adopted by animals? These babies lack connection with human beings, lack of support for physical development, lack of love from parents so they lack social human skills. To some extent, they get the close connection, love, and care for wild animals. Under the influence of living condition, these children have learned some survival skills by imitation; the skills help them deal well with the problems in wildlife. Living with the wild animals, these children have conditioned with the responses of these wild animals. The article: "Six cases of children being raised by animals" from theweek.com will help us understand how babies have conditioned the responses from the living environment. The repeated responses in these babies by the influence of living environment have created the habits. From the adopted habits, repeated gradually, the individual will have specific adopted characters.

Raised by monkeys in Colombia

When Marina Chapman was about five years old, she was kidnapped, and was abandoned in the Colombian jungle. For some five years, she lived out in the wild, where she was taken in by a group of capuchin monkeys. The animals taught young Marina how to catch birds and rabbits with her bare hands, so she was able to survive. She rejoined the human world when she was taken by hunters and be sold to a brothel, from which she eventually escaped.

Raised by goats in Russia

In June 2012, social workers in Russia discovered a toddler who had been locked in a room with goats by his mother. The boy reportedly played and slept with the goats, but nourishment was apparently hard to come by as he weighed a third less than a typical child of his age. Doctors had tried to acclimatize the toddler to human life. They troubled with some difficulty. He refused to sleep in the cot. He tried to get underneath and sleep there. He was very scared of adults," one doctor said.

Raised by feral cats and dogs in Siberia

In 2009, welfare workers found a 5-year-old girl they called "Natasha" in a Siberian town. While technically living with her father and other relatives, Natasha was treated like one of the many dogs and feral cats that shared the space. Like her furry companions, Natasha lapped up food from bowls left on the floor. She didn't know any human words and only communicated with hisses and barks. The father was nowhere to be found when authorities rescued the girl, and Natasha has since been placed in an orphanage.

Raised by wild cats in Argentina

Argentinean police discovered an abandoned 1-year-old boy surrounded by eight wild cats in 2008. The cats reportedly kept the boy alive during the freezing winter nights by laying on top of him and even tried to lick the crusted mud from his skin. The boy was also seen eating scraps of food likely foraged by his protective brood.

Raised by wild dogs in Chile

A 10-year-old Chilean boy was found in 2001 to have been living in a cave with a pack of dogs for at least two years. The boy had already survived a rough and unstable childhood, having been abandoned by his parents and then fleeing alternative care. Alone, the child sought refuge with a pack of dogs who helped him scavenge for food and even protected him. Officials said the boy might have even drunk milk from one of the female dogs. They were like his family, a spokesman said.

Raised by wolves in India

Kamala and Amala were well known as the "wolf children." Discovered in 1920 in the jungles of Godamuri, India, the girls, aged 3 and about 8, had been living with a she-wolf and her pack. The man who found the girls, Reverend J.A.L. Singh, took them back to his orphanage, where he tried to get them accustomed to their human surroundings. While the girls made some progress over the years, both eventually came down with fatal illnesses, leaving the reverend to wonder: "if the right thing to do would have been to leave these children in the wild where I found them." Dogs, cats, cows, milk cows, and all other animals that tamed by human beings are the products of conditioned responses. The ancestors of these animals were wild animals. Human ancestors caught wild animals, fed them, and nourished from generation to generation. Since the early of life, the baby animals were feeding b the human being. These animals gradually misinterpreted human beings as their safety. Gradually, some wild animals are tamed become pets of human beings. Pets like dogs do not have a judgment that the owners are the good or bad people. The dogs only care for the people who feed them and fight for the people for people who feed them. Dogs do not care for the perception of people that other people are good or bad people, dogs have the sharp instinct; tamers use their understanding to create some condition responses with dogs like orders, communicate. Even repeating call one specific name with a dog, the dog will have some conditioned responses by matching the words, emotion, frequencies of words with the results like rewards or punishment dog gets. The tamers use the same techniques to the wild mammals in circuses or zoos. Tamers have a good understanding of the behaviors of animals. They direct the behaviors of animals to specific directions by creating conditioned responses with rewards and punishments. Gradually, the animals can perform the conditioned behaviors right after catching the signals of the condition. Some questions that make us get the right understanding, how tiny we are. Getting the right answer to all questions in this book will help you gain the right understanding of you. Asking and answering the questions about you will give you the great materials for your wisdom and enlightenment.

A. You

1. Who are you? What is your nationality? Which country, province or district do you hate the most because of the behaviors of the people in that area? Why do you hate them?

2. What happened if you were born and raised in the area you hate, would you still have the same hatred?

3. What happened if your beloved spouse, the heroes you meet are from the area that you hate, would you still have the same hatred for that area?

4. Where are the sources of the atoms like carbon, oxygen, nitrogen, and many others in your body?

We know that we grow from the combination of egg and sperm, we formed by organs, under organs are cells, under cells are chemical compounds, under compounds are the atoms, under atoms are protons, neutrons, and electrons, under protons and neutrons, are quarks. The scientists have used the most sophisticated machine to shoot the quarks and material smaller than quarks, they found nothing. Yes, it is nothing except pure energy. The world of the atom, the quanta of particles, appears so strange that we can no longer visualize what we think and talk about. The particles have a quality of complete random existence and non-existence about them; and yet the methods of quantum electrodynamics, quantum chromodynamics, and the whole of quantum mechanics provide such precise, useful, and powerful tools, that it encompasses all of the classical physical laws. If you delve into the strange world of atoms, you might start going crazy and start speaking to dogs, chickens: "Hey friends, perhaps we come from the same sources. There is no I, there is no you, there is nothing called ego. We are the rare meeting of countless phenomena. We are coming from nowhere and going nowhere. Chance of meeting are so rare that we should unite to create many more good phenomena, do not fight for the perceptions, do not fight to protect nonsense opinions. Please, stop the nonsense actions. I can understand the teachings of Buddha and Lao Tzu. They pointed us the way to enlightenment. I have the feeling we are not in Hanoi anymore. I am not sure about Asia, Earth and Solar system. Who are you, where are you, what are you doing if there is an observer observes you from the center of Milky Way? Perhaps some philosophers were right with the saying that they are the citizens of the world. Who are you? Do you stay still? Can you have clear definitions of the earth, solar system? The more we ask, the more we know little about reality. Scientists say the earth is moving about our sun in a very nearly circular orbit. It covers this route at a speed of nearly 30 kilometers per second or 67000 miles per hour. In addition, our solar system- Earth and all - whirls around the center of our galaxy at some 220 kilometers per second, or 490000 miles per hour, the speeds involved become unimaginable huge. We can never know the Earth exactly. The Earth is not static, it changes every second. Disaster will happen or the Earth will explode if the Earth stops spinning. The Earth is just like a small particle spinning with high speed in the Milky Way. The Earth contains living creatures, including human beings and countless living creatures. There are billions of star systems like the solar system in the Milky Way. Galaxy is a large system of stars held together by mutual gravitation and isolated from similar systems by vast regions of space. The Milky Way measures about 100000 light-years across and is thought to contain 200 billion stars. Scientists measure the size of Milky Way by the light-year across. How big the size of our houses, tombs, and Egyptian pyramid compare to the distance of light-second and light-year across. Human atomic bombs are too tiny if compare to the atomic reactions in the Sun? What is the effect of human atomic bombs to the solar system, and to the Milky Way? The answer is nothing! The table below will let us see how tiny we are. Let see the relative of our human being with an electron, neutron, cell, earth, solar system, and Milky Way with the criteria of size, weight, time and duration. To have a good perception about the universe, scientist use astronomical units and light year for distance, the speed of light for traveling, million years for time and solar mass for weight instead of the meter, second, kilogram to measure everything in the system. Astronomical units: 1 au = 3.0857 $*10^{16}$m Lightyear: 1 ly = 9.4607 * 10^{15}m Solar mass: $M_{\oplus}$ = 5.9722*10^{24} kg The solar system has orbital speed is 220 km/s. Solar system moves around Galactic Center, its orbital period is 225 million years Galaxy Milky Way has a spiral pattern rotation period approximately 300 million years.

Table 23: relativities between human being, cell, atom, electron, earth, solar system and the Milky Way

	Size (m)	Weight (kg)	Age (year)	Speed km/s	Spiral rotation period (year)
Milky Way	100000 ly	$10^{12}\ M_{\oplus}$	13.7 * 10^9		3 *10^8
	9.4607 *10^{20}	5.972 *10^{36}			
Solar system	30.10 AU	1.0014 $M_{\oplus}$	4.568 * 10^9	220	225 * 10^6
	4.503 *10^{12}	1.99278*10^{30}			
Earth	12.742 * 10^6	5.9722 *10^{24}		29.78	1
Man	1.7	80	70		
Cell	15 * 10^{-6}	3.5 * 10^{-12}	10/365		
Atom carbon	2.2*10^{-10}	1.998 * 10^{-26}			
Electron	2.82 * 10^{-15}	9.1094*10^{-31}		2200	
Relative compare between man					

		Times
Relativities of length	**Electron/man** is bigger than **man/solar system**	0.0044
	Cell/man is bigger than **man/solar system**	$233.7*10^5$
	Atom carbon/man is bigger than **man/solar system**	342.8
	Cell/man is bigger than **man/earth**	66
	Atom carbon/man is bigger than **earth/milky way**	9632.8
	Electron/man is bigger than **man/Milky way**	$92.3 * 10^4$
	Quark/man is bigger than **man/milky way**	$28.8 * 10^7$
The relativity of Weight	**Quark/man** is bigger than **man/milky way**	$28.8 *10^7$

To compare the relativity of the size, the size of a man with the size of the solar system is twenty million times smaller than the size of a cell to the size a man and three hundred and forty-two times smaller than the size of the carbon atom to the size of a man. The size of a man with the size of Milky Way is approximately nine hundred thousand times smaller the size of an electron with the size of a man. This is so astonishing! Just imagine with mysterious science fiction assumes there are divine spirits formed the Milky Way. These divine spirits use their own tools: astronomical units, light year, the speed of light, million years, solar mass to travel and measure. They will never know the existence of human being; even they use the highest universal power microscope. The more divine spirits use the high technology to find out what human beings really are; the more they will find out nothing. To know more about human beings, divine spirits of Milky Way have to use universal quantum mechanics, the Schrödinger equation to know about human beings. Schrödinger equation is a mathematical equation that describes the changes over time of a physical system in which quantum effects, such as wave-particle duality, are significant. I think these divine spirits will fail and never find out exactly what is the concrete in the human being, because óf their wrong assumptions about concrete particles. We as human beings always busy with the finding out our roles, missions, origin and permanence of self, and ego. These things are nonsense with the gigantic Milky Way and Universe. We are so busy that we may forget our essence. We are just tiny-tiny dust in a tiny-tiny world.

B. Other people:

1. Who are American, Indian, Chinese, Korean, Germany, and Vietnamese? What are their characters? Can you distinguish them by the ways they act, their habits, the pattern of thinking, their religions, or their accent?

2. What is the best effective way to make a newborn baby become American, Indian, Chinese, Korean, Germany, and Vietnamese?

3. Do you see it is a miracle for you if you can speak English as American, Vietnamese and Vietnamese people, Chinese as and

Chinese people? The American has the instinct about the language of English, they can distinguish small changes in sound, consonant, and stress of the world. Wow, how miracle! As a Vietnamese student, I wondered why they could have that ability, the ability that Vietnamese students cannot master if we take five years to study English. American teachers can distinguish the English sentence read by Vietnamese, Indian, or Chinese. They have instinct talent in English.

4. Which is the most effective in the way of making a man has the identities, characters, belief system or nationality of American:

· Let him live in American since the infant.

· Let him live in Vietnam until the age of five then move him to America to study and live.

· Let him live in Iraq until the age of twenty then move him to America to live and study.

· Let him live in South Korea until the age of fifty then move him to America to work and live.

· Let him live in Vietnam until he is seventy years old then move him to America to live for the rest of his life with the hope that brings him happiness.

· Can you guess who will have the feeling of missing home, what is the name of their home?

The answers or the ideas about the assumption situations will help us understand how well we are shaped by the living environment.

C. The world is a giant hologram of interdependent phenomena

International System of Units for seven base quantities, these quantities are the mutually interdependent assumptions which described the characters of phenomena of the world. These quantities are not real; they are just the assumptions of human beings about some sets of certain phenomena to help the process of communication, visualization, and contemplation more effectively.

International System of Units

Base quantity	Name	Symbol
Length	meter	M
Mass	kilogram	Kg
Time	second	S
Electric current	ampere	A
Thermodynamic temperature	Kelvin	K
Amount of substance	mole	Mol
Luminous intensity	candela	Cd

For detail with the meter, kilogram, and second One meter is the distance traveled by light in a vacuum in 1/299792458 second. One kilogram is the grave defined as being the weight of one cubic decimeter of pure water at its freezing point. One second is the duration of 9192631770 periods of the radiation corresponding to the transition between the two hyperfine levels of the ground state of the atom Caesium-133; from the second we have the assumptions of a minute, hour, day, week, month, year, decade, and century. The world is the hologram of countless phenomena. The illuminating of countless phenomena in human beings create their perceptions about world and present. The development of potential brain help perfect the cognitive thinking like remembering, recording the previous events, phenomena; and perceiving all phenomena happen inside and outside the body; and predicting the phenomena in the future from the current information. Cognitive thinking has created the perception of time along with other base quantities in the International System. All the seven base quantities are the approved premises; from these base quantities, science started to develop. In Vietnam, we are using the SI-system in every measurement. So reading any measurement in meter, liter, and kilogram are much more understandable for us than reading the measurement in other systems with qualities like an inch, gallon, and pound. It is hard to teach children and our ancestors to understand these quantities, but after understanding and using these quantities, people started to attach with the theory of time dimension. The theory of time has created a lot of debates among scientists, philosophers, and people. Countless phenomena happen in the world and universe. To know what is the gap between two phenomena in one place, people formed the concept of time. Two seconds is the amount of time for the seed drop from the tree onto the earth. Two days is the amount of time for the seed to become a small tree if the seed meets the right condition and not eaten by bugs. This is the continuous process of the meeting countless phenomena. With the observation of ordinary people, the seed, and the tree on the earth is still. But with the observation of the quantum physicists, each Plank time (5.4×10^{-44} seconds) pass by, countless changes happen inside the seed and the tree. To know the relativity of phenomena, concepts of appearing and disappearing of the events, people have created the time scale and calendar. Time is just the conceptualization of the mind to help the mind understand the countless surrounding phenomena. All human assumptions, human conceptualizations are to help the mind function more effectively in the world of countless phenomena. Time is not a reality, but a concept or a measure." Time is an interdependent factor. In time, there is the existence of length, mass, motion, electric, temperature, amount of substance, and luminous intensity. Time, currency, money, fame, possession, properties, countless other definitions, base quantities are just the conceptualizations of the mind to help the mind work effectively. These are the assumptions change constantly based on the understanding of human beings. Forget about time dimension and time travel. Can you imagine that if you jump on a time machine then go back to yesterday to see you of yesterday? It means that there will be billions of cells, atoms, and electrons to duplicate by just one simple action. It violates the law of cause and effect or the law of compounding phenomena. Scientists have encountered how hard to create entangled atoms but they have never created the two similar atoms. How can a time machine create billions of atoms in just a blink of an eye? In fact, the carbon atoms, nitrogen atoms, calcium atoms, oxygen atoms, and all atoms of our present body are from all sources in previous time. The sources of these atoms may come from the atoms of the grasses of yesterday, breath-out air of a child last two days, the saliva of the wife last week, the meat last week, the baby urine last month, the food of the cow last three months, the feces on the road last year, the dusts last year, the death soldiers of World War, the victims of the wars, the sperm of the wild ox last century, the tears of sacrificed virgin girl last century, the bomb last decade, the river last century, and the chairs of religious leaders the last two centuries, the exploding stars trillion years ago, and countless phenomena before us. How can we create a time machine to move all present atoms back to yesterday, last month or last year, last decade, last century? The phenomena are constant and we can never change it in the past time. But we can control the quality of illumination of countless phenomena by creating the wanted phenomena with time. We do not control time, but we can control our behaviors to create results when others phenomena are moving and changing. Time management can be seen as behaviors management to create the wanted phenomena to lead to wanted results. Travelling with the speed near the speed of light can reduce the speed of the electrons orbiting in the atoms of the atomic clock. And make the human atomic clock slow down but not time. The astronauts travel near the speed of light can slow down their metabolism so that when they come back the Earth, they may look younger than their grandchildren but not smarter. The author Julian Barbour in his book *The End of Time*, argues that quantum equations of the universe take their true form when expressed in the timeless realm containing every possible now or momentary configuration of the universe. We are thinking and communicating with the definitions and assumptions formed long before we were born. These definitions and the experience help us understand the world. To understand the vital role of definitions, assumptions with the process of thinking, let do this imaginative exercises. What are your thinking, feelings, and responses when you see?

· A two-year-old boy is being beaten by a forty-year-old man.

· Your two-year-old son is beaten by a forty-year-old man.

- Your two-year-old son is being beaten by your forty-year-old spouse.
- Your forty-year-old spouse is being beaten by your two-year-old son.
- Your forty-year-old spouse is being beaten by your twenty-year-old son.
- A nearby twenty-year-old girl, lame, is passing a crowded road.
- A nearby twenty-year-old boy, lame, is passing a crowded road.
- A nearby seventy-year-old woman, lame, is passing a crowded road.

What do you think if your five-year-old son insists that he has seen a one hundred- year - old man driving his school bus? Your mind understands the value of time so you will hardly believe it. Time is nothing special but a relative definition help human beings understand the changing world based on the moving of an electron around its atom. In the changing world, things are interdependent and constantly interacting with each other. To understand the kind of interaction in the interdependent changing world, humankind created the chronology, calendar, days and time, which are have relation with the moving of an electron around the atom. Then the events and interactions of the world are put chronologically. Time is the same as other relative definitions like adjectives, nouns, verbs, adverbs, and so on used to describe the world. Buddha and Lao Tzu are the enlightened ones, who understood the vital role and the characters of mind. By mindfulness and meditation, Buddha understood that the world is spaceless and timeless; the world is interchangeable and interdependent. There is is no ego; there is no separate self in the world. The mind and its products create a distinction and definitions to help people think and communicate better with other people. The world is interchangeable and constant changing so that any attachments to the nothingness or ego are the wrong assumptions; the wrong assumption leads to wrong thinking, wrong acting, and misery. World are interchangeable and interdependent so that "one in all", "all in one", "part in the whole" and "the whole in the parts". There are some basic vital conditions to help the interchangeable world illuminate. These conditions may call golden rules, basic principles, the art of livings, and values in religions; which taught by enlightened ones, religious leaders and great philosophers of humankind. Enlightened ones also warn that wrong understanding, wrong assumption, wrong attachment, and violating the life principles will lead to dying and extinction.

References:

Astronomical unit. (n.d.). In Wikipedia. Retrieved July 17, 2017, from http://en. wikipedia.org /wiki/Astronomical_unit\

Atom. (n.d.). In Wikipedia. Retrieved July 17, 2017, from http://en.wikipedia.org/wiki /Atom Atomic clock. (n.d.). In Wikipedia. Retrieved July 17, 2017, from https://en.wikipedia. org/wiki/Atomic_clock

Barbour, Julian. (1999). The End of Time: The Next Revolution in Our Understanding of the Universe. Weidenfeld & Nicolson. Cell biology by the number. (n.d.). Retrieved July 19, 2017, from http://book.bionumbers. org/how-quickly-do-different-cells-in-the-body-replace-themselves/

Choi, Q. Charles. (2015, March 27). Quantum Record! 3,000 Atoms Entangled in Bizarre State. Retrieved July 19, 2017, from https://www.livescience.com/50280-record-3000-atoms-entangled.html

Earth mass. (n.d.). In Wikipedia. Retrieved July 17, 2017, from http://en.wikipedia.org /wiki/Earth_mass

Earth. (n.d.). In Wikipedia. Retrieved July 17, 2017, from http://en.wikipedia .org/wiki/Earth Hoyer, Stephan. (2012, December 19).

Electrons: how fast is an electron traveling around the nucleus?. Retrieved July 19, 2017, from http://www.quora.com /Electrons-How-fast-is-an-electron-travelling-around-the-nucleus

International System of Units. (n.d.). In Wikipedia. Retrieved July 17, 2017, from https://en.wikipedia.org/wiki/International_System_of_Units

Johnston, Hamish. (2015, March 25). How to entangle nearly 3000 atoms using a single photon. Retrieved July 19, 2017, from http://physicsworld.com/cws/article/news /2015/mar/25/how-to-entangle-nearly-3000-atoms-using-a-single-photon

Learning Astronomy. (n.d.). Solar System vs. Galaxy vs. Universe. Retrieved July 19, 2017, from http://www.learningastronomy.com/solarsystem_galaxy_universe.html

Milky Way. (n.d.). In Wikipedia. Retrieved July 17, 2017, from http://en.wikipedia.org /wiki/Milky_Way

Planetary mass. (n.d.). In Wikipedia. Retrieved July 17, 2017, from http://en. wikipedia.org /wiki/Planetary_mass

Quantum entanglement. (n.d.). In Wikipedia. Retrieved July 17, 2017, from https://en. wikipedia.org/wiki/ Quantum_entanglement Quark. (n.d.). In Wikipedia. Retrieved July 17, 2017, from http://en.wikipedia.org /wiki/Quark

Reece, T. Margaret. (n.d.). Physiology of self-renewal. Retrieved July 19, 2017, from http://www.medicalsciencenavigator.com/physiology-of-self-renewal/ Scientific American. (n.d.).

How fast is the earth moving?. Retrieved July 19, 2017, from http://www.scientificamerican.com/article/how-fast-is-the-earth-mov/ Sharp, Tim. (2012, September 17).

How big is Earth?. Retrieved July 19, 2017, from http://www.space.com/17638-how-big-is-earth.html

Solar mass. (n.d.). In Wikipedia. Retrieved July 17, 2017, from http://en.wikipedia. org/wiki/Solar_mass

Solar system. (n.d.). In Wikipedia. Retrieved July 17, 2017, from http://en.wikipedia.org /wiki/Solar_System

The size of atoms. (n.d.). Retrieved July 19, 2017, from http://hyperphysics.phy-astr.gsu.edu/hbase/Particles/atomsiz.html

The Week Staff. (2012, October 23). Six cases of children being raised by animals. Retrieved July 19, 2017, from http://theweek.com/articles/471164/6-cases-children-being-raised-by-animals

Time. (n.d.). In Wikipedia. Retrieved July 17, 2017, from https://en.wikipedia.org/wiki /Time

Walker, Jim. (2004, November). Atoms. Retrieved July 19, 2017, from http://www .nobeliefs.com/atom.htm

Chapter 24: Hysteria and conditioned responses

Hysteria and mass hysteria is the phenomena of infectious frightening; which are the results of wrong imaginations, wrong perceptions about fearful things or things conflict with people's strong beliefs. The unconscious misinterpretation and misperception about the environment, that people do not consciously know, cause a frightened and extremely stressed state in people. The fear, stress, and misperception about the environment make people so much stressed that they may become panic. The overactive of the autonomic central nervous system not only make their bodies filled with stress chemicals but also creating the vicious process of arousing in mind and brain. People mostly have symptoms like the symptoms caused by excessive stress chemicals: cortisone, adrenalin, and noradrenaline. Excessive of these stress chemicals with extreme fear can cause panic and the physical symptoms that are similar to hysteria. Hysteria has a variety of symptoms, including anxiety, shortness of breath, fainting, insomnia, irritability, nervousness, as well as sexually forward behavior. These symptoms mimic symptoms of other more definable diseases and create a case for arguing against the validity of hysteria as an actual disease, and it is often implied that it is an umbrella term, used to describe an indefinable illness. In sociology and psychology, mass hysteria, also known as collective hysteria, group hysteria, or collective obsessional behavior, is a phenomenon that transmits collective illusions of threats, whether real or imaginary, through a population in society is the result of rumors and fear. In medicine, the term is used to describe the spontaneous manifestation, or production of chemicals in the body, of the same or similar hysterical physical symptoms by more than one person. In horror films, when the crowd sees some of their members suddenly become panic, act in anxious ways, or bearing the mysterious pain, all of the other members in that crowd will have the signs of frightening and stress in their face. The fear in the film can also make the audiences in cinema screaming when seeing the sudden attack in a stressful situation. The infecting with fear of relating people is so complicated that we hardly know about by conscious mind. The sophistication of translating fear is the result of countless phenomena from the environment interacting with the mind. Can you create the minor hysteria in your family? Imagine that one of your family members comes late in the evening. If that member falls before the door and lying in the unconscious state, there are some bloody spots and some tearing on clothes, and little signs of fear on the face. I think that many people in this situation will suddenly have a feeling of fear or frightening. The fear is the product of the stimulating mind. In this state, even hearing the big noise of closing the door, the barking of the dogs or the running of mice on the ceiling can cause extreme stress in these people. Do you think that that the family members are the victim of hysteria? At the dinner table, if the father of the family has feelings of fear, anxiety because of the problems and pressure from work, even he does not speak about his problem; I think all other members will be infected with the feeling of fear and anxiety just by looking the way of the action of the father. They will have a little feeling of fear and anxiety and may overreact to minor problems, despite the fact that they do not know what is happening with the father. The human brain can catch many subliminal messages that people do not consciously know and create the corresponding emotion and preparation. Perhaps members of the family may suffer the mind hysteria if one member of the family has negative emotion like fear, anxiety, pain, and misery. Watching horror films, we will understand about hysteria, the transmitting of negative emotion, the anxiety, fear, and the suffering of people. These negative emotions are highest when the relating people only have seen the suffering but do not know the causes, so the mind is in the alert state to protect them from any threat. People suffering hysteria are the victims of not only the excessive stress chemicals like cortisol, epinephrine, and norepinephrine run throughout the body that create the symptoms of stress chemicals described in table two: "the most symptoms of stress that we can find in many patients", they but also become the victims of the endless circulation of frightening inside the mind. Curiosity help people find out the answer to the causes of the problems they met, especially the negative problems. After understanding the causes of the phenomena and problems around them, the mind may feel safe and calm down. In the previous time of human being, the sophisticated phenomena, the disaster, the powerful natural phenomena, people has to use the power of God and the Holy Spirit to explain for these. To some extent, the belief in God and the Holy Spirit have created all unknown phenomena help people feel safe and certainty for thousands of years. Unfortunately, these old beliefs had prevented the researchers and works of many scientists. The religious leaders had experienced feelings of fear and anxiety when seeing the scientists did the researchers that went against their religious beliefs. Reading the history of any sciences, we will find the difficulties that the religious beliefs and old beliefs had created for the development of science. I think the relating people in the past may suffer the hysteria with the feeling of fear, anxiety, and panic when they did the things that against their highest beliefs. A lot of severe punishments had been taken place to prevent any actions against the highest beliefs of groups. People are so afraid that they misinterpreted any disasters, epidemics, and difficulties they suffered were the punishment of God, Devil or Satan. Countless myths, rumors, legends, and heroes created by our ancestors in an attempt to explain the existence of countless strange phenomena they met. Regional festivals and rituals, taboos also were formed with these myths, legends, and heroes; following these things, people in communities will feel safe and protected; doing against any these things, people in communities will feel unsafe, frightened, fearful and panics. I think these are the sources of mass hysteria. Mass hysteria occurs when a group of people believes that they are suffering from a similar disease or ailment, sometimes referred to as massive psychogenic illness or epidemic hysteria. Below are some cases of hysteria recorded in human history.

June bug epidemic, USA 1962, In 1962, a mysterious disease broke out in a dressmaking department of a US textile factory.

The symptoms included numbness, nausea, dizziness, and vomiting. Word of a bug in the factory that would bite its victims and develop the above symptoms quickly spread. Soon sixty-two employees developed this mysterious illness. Researches by scientists showed that the case was one of mass hysteria. No evidence was ever found for a bug, which could cause the above flu-like symptoms, nor did all workers demonstrate bites.

Soap Opera Hysteria, Portugal 2006 "Strawberries with sugar" is a popular teen girl's show, aiming to depict the adventures of typical Portuguese youths. In May 2006, an outbreak of the "Strawberries with sugar virus" was reported in Portuguese schools. Three hundred or more students reported similar symptoms to those experienced by the characters in a recent episode. The symptoms included rashes, difficulty breathing, and dizziness. The Portuguese National Institute for Medical Emergency dismissed the illness as mass hysteria. This hysteria makes us have a better understanding of the influence of media.

Mount Pleasant, Mississippi 1976 School officials suspected drug use after fifteen students fell to the ground writhing, but no drugs were found. At one point, three hundred students of school's nine hundred students stayed home for fear of being "hexed"

West Bank fainting epidemic, 1983 The 1983 West Bank fainting epidemic was a series of incidents in March 1983 in which 943 Palestinian teenage girls, mostly school-girls, and a small number of Israeli Defense Forces women soldiers fainted or complained of feeling nauseous in the West Bank. Officers of both sides have accused that the other side has employed a toxic substance. No evidence has been found on both sides to prove the assumption of using the toxic substance. Investigators concluded the wave of complaints was ultimately a product of mass hysteria.

US Navy, San Diego, 1988 The US Navy evacuated six hundred men from barracks; one hundred and nineteen men were sent to San Diego hospitals with complaints of breathing difficulty. No evidence of toxins, food poisoning, or any other cause was found.

North Carolina, 2002, Ten girls developed seizures and other symptoms at a rural high school in North Carolina. Symptoms persisted for five months across various grade levels. Incidents tended to happen around lunch hour. No evidence of toxins, food poisoning was found.

Mexico City, 2007 In 2007 near Chalco, a working-class suburb of Mexico City, mass hysteria resulted in a massive outbreak of unusual symptoms suffered by nearly six hundred adolescent female students at Children's Village School. The afflicted students had difficulty walking and were feverish and nauseated. No evidence of toxins, food poisoning was found.

Afghanistan, 2009, Starting around 2009, a spate of apparent poisonings at girls' schools across Afghanistan began to be reported, symptoms included dizziness, fainting, and vomiting. The United Nations, World Health Organization, and NATO's International Security Assistance Force carried out investigations of the incidents over multiple years but never found any evidence of toxins or poisoning in the hundreds of blood, urine, and water samples they tested. The conclusion of the investigators was that the girls were suffering from massive psychogenic illness or mass hysteria.

Brunei, 2010 and 2014 In April and May 2010, incidents of mass hysteria occurred at all girls in secondary schools in Brunei. The most recent notable event happened on the 24th of April 2014 in a public secondary school. The phenomenon caused a wave of panic among many parents, educators, and members of the community. Some of the students affected by the phenomenon claimed to have been possessed by spirits, or jinn, displaying histrionic symptoms such as screaming, shaking, fainting, and crying.

Sri Lanka, 2012 From November fifteenth to twentieth, 2012, more than 1900 schoolchildren of fifteen schools in Sri Lanka and five teachers were treated for a range of symptoms that included skin rashes, vomiting, vertigo, and cough due to allergic reactions believed to be mass hysteria.

Charlie Charlie Panic, Colombia, 2015 Four teens in Tunja, Colombia were hospitalized, and several in the Dominican Republic were considered "possessed by Satan" after playing the Charlie Charlie Challenge viral game. After scientists have a deep understanding of hysteria, coupled with the many outbreaks of recent mental diseases, social events, social problems, and health problems, which are substantially increasing the number of patients, we will understand the real cause of all these problems. Most of them come from the mind. I just want to put quotes to prove the power of the mind.

> "If you tell a big enough lie and tell it frequently enough, it will be believed." **Adolf Hitler**

Do we eat, wear, buy, and do based on the essential values to satisfy basic needs? Or do we eat, wear, buy, and do based on emotion, temptation and greed? The answer to the question above will determine the quality of the behaviors. The problems are not the objects; the problems are our mind, our thinking. The best way is changing the thinking and mindset. The pattern caused one problem of a man will still linger in his mind, his thought, his actions, his behaviors, and his breathing. Moreover, this pattern of thinking will influence and appear in his teaching, breeding, raising children, studying, using medicine, working, achieving, eating, and injecting vaccine, and all his other behaviors. That is why the best way to have a happy life is to repair our thinking, changing attitude, changing the pattern of perception by self-training, mental therapist, practice meditation, and contemplation. With the weak man, small problem, small changes from the environment can create big stress, pain, and misery. With powerful man, small changes of environment do not deserve his attention; big solvable problems make him excited to deal; the unsolvable problems or the facts of life make him courageous to accept. Owning for personal development, nothing can cause a powerful man to feel sad, stressed, painful, or miserable. The most effective way of creating change is the change should start from inside and by oneself.

- Can you imagine the responses of your body when you are eating food but other people told that is dirty food, dangerous food?
- Can you imagine the responses of your children's body and your body when you feed your children the food that you think it is poisonous or dirty?
- Can you imagine the responses of your body and your child when your child get the vaccination but all of your minds are obsessed with negative thinking, negative consequences, negative expectation and with the feeling of fear, doubt, and anxiety?
- Before vaccine injection: Can you imagine the subliminal message you communicate to your child and your husband if you are frightened of the thinking that bad things may happen if your child gets vaccine injection?
- Can you guess the consequences of any activities or social phenomena, which all relating people have negative thinking, negative expectation; they are all stressed, fearful, doubtful, anxious, and panic?

Getting the right answers to these questions you will understand hysteria and all social phenomena have relation with the mind.

References:

Acocella, Joan. (1999). Creating hysteria in women and multiple personality disorder. Retrieved July 19, 2017, from http://www.nytimes.com/books/first/a/acocella-hysteria.html

Frater, Jamie. (2009, March 16). Top ten bizarre cases of mass hysteria. Retrieved July 19, 2017, from http://listverse.com/2009/03/16/top-10-bizarre-cases-of-mass-hysteria/

Hysteria. (n.d.). In Wikipedia. Retrieved July 17, 2017, from https://en.wikipedia.org/wiki/Hysteria

Kleinfield N. R. (1992, September 29). Fear and fiction: The furor at P.S. 3 -A special report; lead threat exposes and engulfs a school. Retrieved July 19, 2017, fromhttp://www.nytimes.com/1992/09/29/nyregion/fear-fiction-furor-ps-3-special-report-lead-threat-exposes-engulfs-school.html?pagewanted=all

Mass hysteria. (n.d.). In Wikipedia. Retrieved July 17, 2017, from https://en.wikipedia.org/wiki/Mass_hysteria

Pooley, Jefferson and Socolow J. Michael. (2013, October 28). The myth of the War of the Worlds Panic. Retrieved July 19, 2017, from http://www.slate.com/articles/arts/history/2013/10/orson_welles_war_of_the_worlds_panic_myth_the_infamous_radio_broadcast_did.html

Chapter 25: The relation between mental problems, environment, and conditioned responses

The children and patients with mental disorders, who usually have bad behaviors, bad emotion, bad feelings, fear, anxiety, panic, and overreacting to the small changes of environment, are the victims of living conditions. The signs or symptoms, to some extent, are the conditioned responses with the unwanted stimulations. The fact is the stimulations have many phenomena defined as patterns, varieties, and frequencies; which are caught by the subconscious mind and known or unknown by the conscious mind. Moreover, in a panic state, the mind may make many wrong conclusions about phenomena and emotions it has. Because of the unknown about the complexity of stimulation and the wrong conclusions of the mind, patients may overreact to mild stimulation. If making statistics about the spiritual life of these patients, we will find that these children and patients have experienced threatening, punishing, beating, and ignoring. They may have suffered a stressed and painful of the living environment during childhood or the previous time. The condition of living has created a lot of stress and pressure on them that lot of bad responses, bad behaviors formed as the conditioned responses to the stimulating. The neocortex and limbic system of the brain remember all the varieties and frequencies of the condition, which have created stress on them. Under stress condition, the limbic system may mismatch and misinterpret the normal condition into the stress condition. The conditioned responses, dysfunction of the brain and of limbic systems, and stressed state are the best explanation for the overreaction of these children and patients before mild stimulation from the environment. In return, their overreaction may make them much more stressed if they do not receive help from the beloved ones and the environment. The vicious circles of stress may form and make them get severe mental illness. Unfortunately, the medicine to treat mental diseases does not reduce stress for them if they still live under the stress condition. Let review the definitions and characters of mental disorders to understand the assumed relation.

Definition and understanding of mental disorders

> A mental disorder is a behavioral or mental pattern that may cause suffering or a poor ability to function in life. Such features may be persistent, relapsing and remitting, or occur as a single episode. Mental disorders are usually defined by a combination of how a person behaves, feels, perceives, or thinks. We may all know that behaves, feels, perceives, and thinks can be conditioned by the living conditions. In 2013, the American Psychiatric Association redefined mental disorders as "a syndrome characterized by a clinically significant disturbance in an individual's cognition, emotion regulation, or behavior that reflects a dysfunction in the psychological, biological, or developmental processes underlying mental functioning."

The unconscious mind can remember the pattern of stressful information; next time, if there is something similar, the unconscious mind can detect signals very quickly and call out the conditioned responses long before the conscious mind know what is happening. The unconscious mind silently activates the stress chemicals and activates the autonomic nervous systems independently with the cognitive mind. The activation of the stress system can be subsidized if we pay attention to the emotion and feelings when it is weak. If a lack of mindfulness, the activation of stress may overwhelm the mind, then mobilize all the conscious mind and subconscious for stress or strong emotion. The living environment conditions the conditioned responses in all people. After conditioning, only seeing, hearing or visualizing the stimulations can make people have the same state of mind as the previous time. In an experiment with the dog, researchers put the dog in a cage, created electrical shock simultaneously with the ringing of a bell. After several times of shocking and ringing bell, researchers have created the conditioned response to stress in the dog. After conditioning, just hearing the bell ringing, the dog trembled with fear as if there was a real electrical shock. It means that the dog has conditioned response to stress just by hearing the ringing bell. The dogs can catch the strange smell of other strange animals, people or objects in the air so that they may bark loudly. The owners of the dogs cannot catch any strange signals in the air does not mean that the strange signals in the air are not present. Many animals can catch the signals or phenomena below the sensory threshold of human beings. In fact, our autonomic nervous systems can catch the signals under the sensory threshold and creating necessary changes - as conditioned responses for survival. Most of the time, we do not know anything about the process and we cannot control the process. Only the mind outliers like meditation practitioners can control the functions of the mind. With vigorous practicing of mindfulness, close observing mind, body, and emotions, they creating countless connections, immeasurable changing in qualities of the brain. Their brain has up to a new level so their brain can understand the appearing and be disappearing of emotion, of the activation of autonomic nervous systems, and of any small changes in the body. Moreover, they can control responses of the autonomic nervous system as normal people use cognitive mind. These above describing perhaps are so tiny about the complication, sophistication, and potentials of the human brain. The brain can help people have unlimited potential in a good state. Unfortunately, the brain can create the massive destruction of the self and human beings if the brain is in a bad state. All mysterious phenomena and destructive phenomena available in human history are the results of the human potential brain.

How living environment and adult people can create changes in children?

Environment and adults consciously or unconsciously condition the conditioned response to the kids with the reward and punishment mechanism. With the reward and punishment, children easily direct to the specific behaviors that parents want. Children are so weak that they have to adapt to the environment; if adapt the environment or follow the order well, they will get the rewards, and get the feeling of joy and safety. On the other hand, if go against the environment or disobey the orders from parents, they will get punished and get the feeling of pain, hurt and non-safety. They are so weak that they cannot bear the pain from the punishment. Moreover, they are so immature that they do not know how to reduce the pain from punishment. They are in a stressed state. they start to learn to act whatever as long as the action will bring safety for them. Repeating with the conditions, the feelings, the rewards, and punishments, the kids have conditioned with conditioned responses. After conditioning, next time, just by seeing, hearing or sensing a part of the previous condition, the kids will have the sense of joy or fear, happiness or sadness, and feeling of warm or feeling of worry inside. Kids are so smart, they will spend the time to learn the way responses bring for them feelings of happiness, warmth, joy. The conditioned responses repeated gradually become habits and characters that help the kid feel safe with the least of energy. Gradually, the conditioned responses are so deep in mind that when kids become adolescents, adults, or elderly people, if they see the pictures have a lot of familiarity with the living environment during childhood they will relive the previous feeling in the body. During childhood, if children are joyful during playing, swimming, running in paddy fields, when becoming adults they will relive the same feelings just by catching the pattern of the living condition of the childhood. Some adults just hearing the sound of children playing, all their childhood memories and happy feelings flush to the mind as if they are living back of the moment of childhood. Many adults in Vietnam have these memories and joy when seeing the picture of children playing in paddy fields, riding buffaloes, dancing in the rain, swimming in the river. These are the memories of their childhood, all the feelings appear as conditioned responses of the mind just by seeing, hearing or reading the events. The westerners also have the joy and happiness when reading "The Adventures of Tom Sawyer" by Mark Twain or many other stories, fictions books. We ourselves all condition the corresponding responses, which go well with the living conditions. Some people have the feeling of missing home and countryside very much when living far away from home because they have formed the patterns of the deepest emotion, the happiest feelings inside their mind with some special occasion in childhood, these feeling will suddenly pop out just by seeing or hearing the familiar things. How about the children who live in the unhappy environment with a lot of fighting, shouting, killing, crying, beating, negative thinking, blaming or cheating; these kids are also conditioned negative responses with these conditions. The conditioned responses are deep in the mind by the repeat of conditioning. After conditioning, the kids may become frightened, trembled, or unsafe when they meet part of the pattern of the condition. If the kids were beating a lot during childhood, when becoming older, they may still have the feeling frightened or anxious with the staring of strangers, the screaming, or the sound of breaking. If make a deep investigation, we may find out that they have heard these sound or images when being beaten. The children from an unhappy environment can be obsessed with many normal things; afraid many normal things or normal sound; and they may have strange responses to these things. In fact, they have the responsibility of stress with these normal things. The normal stimulation can make them stress, can make them feel unsafe; can make them lose enthusiasm with studying, working, and afraid of joining with the crowd; in reverse, these responses make their problems gradually become worse. The conditions of living that create the feeling of getting rewards or punishments are so much complicated with countless events and phenomena happening. We may never have a thorough understanding of these conditions. We may never know what are the exact perceptions in the mind of the victims lived in the crucial environment. Practicing in the healthcare sector, I have seen many people get the feeling of pain like a headache, the aches in parts of the body before the changing of the weather. This experience is the best explanation for the assumption that our brain can senses many small changes in the living environment then create some specific chemicals that creating changes inside our body long before we consciously have the awareness of changes in the environment. These specific chemicals are the products of conditioned responses of the mind to the changes of living environment; these chemicals may create tensions of muscle cells and blood vessel cells in the head, neck, and intestine; and countless changes inside the body that we do not consciously know. We only notice that these changes inside the body when these changes created the perceivable symptoms. In fact, many animals can understand the changes in the living environment then they have the corresponding responses to make them safe. My grandparents taught me to watch the way that dragonflies fly to know that the weather will rain or sun. If the dragonflies fly at high altitudes, the weather will sun; if fly at low altitudes the weather will rain; if flying at middle altitudes, the weather will shady. Some people are conditioned responses the specific emotions and feelings with many others things like richness, poverty, the young, the old, the illness, the pain, the failures, the money, the fame, the property, and so on. They may be conditioned by the actions or feelings of joy and happiness, pain and disgusting, respect and gratefulness, or disrespect and ungratefulness with each of these factors. Furthermore, these conditioned responses will go along with them, affect many later decisions, and affect the quality of their living. The information put in the subconscious mind of children can affect their lives when they grow up. In the function of the mind, the researcher assumes that the capacity of mind mainly belongs to the subconscious mind, and they do not know how much information, how many patterns of responses, and how many phenomena that stored in the mind and brain of human beings. With the theory of hologram, the human brain can store countless unknown information that controls the activity of thinking, acting and the functioning of the autonomic nervous system. Many trainers use NLP techniques (Neuro-Linguistic Programming) to condition the good responses to the people. Trainers can condition the joy and happy feelings inside the participants as the responses with pain, failure, taking action, denials, losses or even the death. After conditioning, they can have the feeling of joy, pride in the failure; they may have feelings of happiness with the losses, the good feelings with their defects, disadvantages, or weakness. These good feelings are the best source of the energy to push them to countless actions for success. Good thinking not making the result, but the good acting is. The focus of mind by good principles helps to create good feelings that lead to actions, thinking, and corrections. Many accumulate of good actions will create a good life. This is part of motivational and educational programs. These programs may create wanting changes. Unfortunately, the wrong conditioning of the mind can be like the following, the participants live in an environment that has a strong influence on them. The group leaders may use the psychological technique, the art of persuasion, the art of conditioning, the art of using NLP. The participants are conditioned with the responses like the feeling of joy, and pride in the bad behaviors like beating, kicking, breaking, destroying or killing. Even the participants may have noble feelings, the feeling of highest fulfillment, and the divine feelings when they taking action of killing or sacrificing. In fact, many people sacrificing themselves to kill other people without any hesitation of the feeling of guilt. The examples from all around the world help us understand how powerful our mind is. The good conditioning is the best preparation for the good life, for the miracles of life. On the other hand, bad conditioning is the worst preparation for the bad life, for problems and miracles in life. We are nothing except the beliefs, thoughts, opinions, and philosophy we keep in mind. Blindly keeping can make us become the slaves of these ideas then we consciously and unconsciously destroy ourselves. It is very helpful for the patients, the injuring people, and the miserable people to meet with the good trainers; the trainer will help them to adopt the good responses, the good habits of thinking to make them have a good life. If would be tragic for the men if they adopt accidentally or intentionally the wrong responses, the wrong habits which lead to failures. Observing the people around, we can see that the men with many defects and diseases adopting the right responses, the right mindset, they are even living in poverty or difficulty can achieve far more than the handsome, healthy men adopting with wrong responses, wrong mindset living in abundance. Understand the mind, the conditioned responses, the power of the brain and the psychology of achievement, people can understand many paradoxes of life and can create many miracles in life. Television and media, videos, programs, and films can stimulate high emotion in viewers, with vivid pictures and sounds and many techniques in psychology. Understanding about the human being, the producers mix many arts and techniques to make the watchers have the feeling of pain, joy, hurt, delight, sorrow and sadness as real as the actors do. In the brain of watchers, the pattern of activating the brain cells are the same as the pattern of activating brain cells in the actors and actress. The mirror neurons in the human brain make people have feelings as vivid as they experience it in real life. The mirror neurons help watchers' brain imitate the activities of actors' brain that creates the acting. It means, to some extent, the patterns of activities in movies have left some tracks inside the brain of watchers. With the transient emotions from real life and from watching the film, the watcher may be conditioned some responses after watching the film, these conditioned responses are the most obvious if the conditioned responses bring the good feeling in watchers. Looking around you will see the kids are easy conditioned the responses of their heroes. They may have acts the same as the act of their heroes. This is the reason why television and media can condition the conditioned responses in viewers; media can be effective tools for the coders to code the mind of viewers. Anything from the environment can arouse the high emotion, with reward and punishment can leave some tracks in the mind of individuals. The patterns of the reaction of individuals in the future can foresee from the habits of feeding the mind from the past and the present. The hours of watching negative media, reading bad news, wasting time on meaningless films, to some extent, can affect the behavior and the life of the individual. Just looking at the expanding of useless media, the resources and time consumed for negative media, many researchers and trainers can have the sense of gut feeling how devastating the negative media is; and how tremendously helpful if people can take advantage of television and good media.

Debating ideas about the relation between autism, ADHD and depression

It is not the masking of autistic symptoms or advantages of diagnosing. We are talking about the abilities or disabilities of the individuals to get lifelong support from society or not! Then the chance of work, act, learn and operate all machines in the communities. It is not advanced diagnosing!

When we view autism as poor abilities to master social skills, speaking, giving a speech, communication skills. The small advantages of the lifestyle of past and present, of the countryside and city, and the advantages in the instinct of girl vs boy; all character of autism will be easy to understand.

What if in the past, playing together, in nature, with trees, fishes, and animals, the kids have all these experiences and unconsciously applied all these therapies?

It is the skills: who diagnosis for autism? I know the one who helps autistic kids are just bachelor = normal people with specific skills of interacting (no medicine, no drug, no special therapies) to help the kids have skills. And when we do realize that it is the skills, parents can realize since the kids small with several months old and have the earliest effective interventions. And just with small teaching for these parents, they can become the best special teachers for their kids and can help their kids 24/7 with love and patience.

When it is the skills, parents can sense something wrong since the kids of 2 months old, or 3 months old or 4, 5, 6, 7, 8, 9, 10, 11, 12, 13, 14, 15, 16, 17, 18, 19 months old. They can feel the early signs of poor social skills via everyday activities, every talk, every interaction. And they can help/cure the kids by massive interaction (this is also the advice of all specialists). All these kids can only get official diagnosing from 10 to 30 months later. It is too late when the golden time of forming the immature brain is finished. On the skills, by nature, parents can sense something not normal on time and have a natural intervention on time, they can save their kids. They can have normal healthy kids and millions of other parents!

Are autism, depression, obesity, mastery, outliers, talent, ADHD, poor learning, stress, abilities, seizures, drugs, violence, PTSD born or created by a continuous and stoppable process? What is the role of the environment?

If it is the process, the problems have to grow from small to impossible. So what if we can sense the problems since it was small. Stop before it is impossible: the problems will not appear, we need not try hard to make it disappear!

If it is born, we should not touch or say about it. If it is created, we should help them vigorously to master the process as early as possible because the time of forming the immature mind is rare and precious and hard to reverse it back to normal

Because:

Most therapists, psychologists still think that it is born, even their work of consultations seems effective.

And

What if stress & pressure made adults depressed put on infants and babies? What are symptoms in growth, eat, sleep, learning & behaviors?

Language is the product of a living environment which is formed well from the combination of the quantity of time and the quality of mind- as your native language and my native language, we speak it naturally without thinking at all. We are not born with our native language, so I doubt the connection kids with autism or delayed speech to their living environment and their feeling that they cannot learn well the native language and the metaphors. You can test them with Aesop fables, pretending game, funny game, role-playing games. You will realize that they are not good at understanding, interacting, communicating or persuading as normal kids.

"You like your child want to eat organic food, why?"

"And why you force your child to play in the boring artificial environment: shopping center, box home, clean pavement, fake-plastic fruit, cotton dogs, plastic fish."

"These expensive fake, plastic or cotton toys with shape of dog, cat, chicken, robot, apple may tackle fully in the corner of the room and your kids do not pay any attention much. But just 2-penny fish, crab, turtle, your kids may be excited to play with them all day, when."

References:

Mental disorder. (n.d.). In Wikipedia. Retrieved July 17, 2017, from http://en.wikipedia.org/wiki /Mental_disorder

Awaken you wonderful we

Part VI: Belief System, Obsessed Desires, and the Work of Potential Brain

Chapter 26: Coding the mind, the role of practicing in learning skills

Let see the function of the brain in an example of a new driver with the first driving. In driving car, the first time people learn to drive taking lots of courage to step in car, a lot of focus to memorize where to put hands, feet, when to use hand, when to use feet, how to look at mirror, how to understand the signs, the signals from nearby cars. The mind is conditioned with the orders like "if... then...", then the mind controls the body. Drivers have to concentrate with as much effort and concentration as possible and as little nervousness as possible during the first drive. After many times of practice, the mind has formed well the corresponding responses with the signals from the environment. The conscious mind gradually works effectively with the coming signals and things happening on the road. The mind decodes the signals and the conditions into the patterns then sends the patterns of signals to unconscious mind to remember. After decoding the receiving patterns, the unconscious mind can understand all the strange things happening during the drive. The process of learning, practicing, and thinking is like the process of putting the dots of knowledge in the conscious mind and unconscious mind. Series of dots put into the subconscious mind sent by conscious mind during the practice of driving. The dots or patterns or knowledge can be understood like: if see the turn left signal then turn left; if go to crossroad then slow the speed; if want to turn left then slow speed, see around, see mirrors, turn on the light to let other vehicles know then turn left.... A series of coding these dots are taken place in mind; it takes time. The mind has conditioned the responses with the driving. Any new action needs to practice for the first time like driving, reading road-signs, swimming, eating, walking... needs a lot of focus and consciousness. The new drivers consciously remember the things need to do and consciously take action with hands and foot.

Conditioned driving

> Learning driving is like the process of condition response to the mind with the orders of if... then...
>
> If seeing the turn left signal then turn left;
>
> If going to crossroad then slow the speed;
>
> If wanting to turn left then slow speed, look around, look mirrors, turn on the turn-left light to let other vehicles know then turn left.

After months, years of training, and practicing, we master the driving, the subconscious mind knows exactly these dots, and it can call out the exact information or responses that match with the environment that we do not consciously know. After many time of practicing, the mind is conditioned so well with the responses that when practicing any needed responses, the drivers do it unconsciously and tirelessly. If drivers drive well, the process of calling out the dots of information in the subconscious mind, do by the subconscious mind, is silent and unrecognizable, but very effective that the drivers do not notice anything at all when on road.

You can pay attention to your next driving: you drive your car unconsciously; you do not pay any attention when you turn your car at the corner, you do not pay any attention to control the hands to make change the land on road, or slightly turn your car to avoid the small rock or small obstacles on the road. Sometimes I was astonished by the perfect function of my mind and my hand when avoiding an obstacle on road. The process of avoiding obstacles may include seeing the object, finding the direction to go, just moving the hand a little to twist the steering wheel a little enough to direct the car to a new lane. The process of turning the car is the same. With you or skillful drivers, it is very easy. But with people do not know how to drive, with the people have not seen the car before, it is not an easy process. How about train drivers, pilots, and truck drivers? I think with each people, they so are familiar with the process of their driving that they do not notice at all. To try to understand this, you can try to drive a truck, or operate any new machines, you will see how difficult to operate these new machines. However, with the people have conditioned well the responses with these machines by operating these machines for three, five, or ten years, their answer about the difficulty of operating these machines is as easy as the driver drives a car.

Skillful drivers can play CD, talk with children, listen to audios, or think in advance to prepare for the work simultaneously with driving the car. The drivers do not mind or pay much attention to driving on the familiar path. Driving skill now become automatic responses. The skillful drivers drive the car in the mountain road so effortlessly and effectively than other people who first met them may think they have a genius for driving. Skillful drivers drive automatically with less energy, less stressful and more effective than the first time of driving; driving now is much easier than their assumption before taking the driving test. After drive for one three years, the drivers have mastered the skill so well that if let them retake the test for the driving license. In fact, the test for driving license is still the same as before and still is a big problem for the people who take the driving test.

The more of driving, the more of thinking, the more dots of knowledge about driving put in subconscious mind, the more drivers can drive safely, quickly and effectively. During driving, the subconscious mind scans the environment to detect any signals then creating the corresponding responses. During the driving, conscious mind does not have to work hard to control the drive; any strange signals are caught by subconscious mind first then create responses. If people or the mind does not understand the strange signals, subconscious mind slightly stimulates the stress system to prepare for dealing with strange signals. The stress can be calm down if the conscious mind has time and concentration to understand the strange signals; with understanding, the conscious mind can calm down the stress inside the body. If the driver drives in the forest, a small branch of tree fall on the top of the car with big noise, it can create some corresponding changes inside the driver's body like sweating, short breath, fearing, palpitation and a little of stress. These changes only happen with the unskilled driver or non-experienced driver. During driving in forest, the first or second branch of tree can make driving a little stressful, to the third branch, fourth branch or eighth branch fall on the top car does not make driver any signal of stress at all; because the diver knows that is branches of tree, they are not dangerous to him. We can make the mind and emotion calm down by good training; the training makes the mind become familiar with the environment, and understand the environment. The understanding of the signals helps the subconscious mind and conscious mind to create corresponding responses to signals. A good driver can understand and solve all problems on the road so he can create a feeling of safety so the mind does not activate the stress system.

Driving is one of the skills that modern people need to master. It is the same as any other skill, the more you practice, the more you master. To an accountant, the skillful work of doctors can make them hard to understand. To a technician, the brave, confidence and determination of a leader or a manager make him astonished. Most foreigners astonish with the motor driving skill of Vietnamese people when they come to Vietnam, some of them are so afraid of the complexity of motor driving on the roads. Some of my female friends also feel afraid of driving motor in Vietnam only after some years of living abroad.

An assumption of a car accident happened by an unskilled driver. The new drivers do not have much knowledge about driving. So that the mind has to do a lot of things during the first drive, the conscious mind tries to remember the knowledge of driving skills, the way of moving hands, moving legs, see the rear mirrors, see the signals from nearby cars. The subconscious mind does not understand information and signals it received during the first drive, it activated the stress system constantly for any receiving signals it does not understand - the strange signals. Even small, non-dangerous signals can misunderstand as threatening and stimulate the subconscious mind. Pedestrians far away, the road signs with three instructions, crossroad, a loud voice of nearby vehicles and foggy day can make the driver stressful; they can misunderstand as a thread for safety because of not understanding. The subconscious mind arouses vigorously, disturb the focus of the conscious mind to make the driving is a more stressful task. The subconscious mind can recall any stored information in mind then create a conditioned response. Stories of self-talk during the first drive may be like the table below:

Negative self-talk

> "A pedestrian walk far away on road, I can crash over him - this is true because I have ever seen, read or heard about this situation, it has the same pattern like this".
>
> "That car drive too fast, I have read the news of this fast-moving car cause accident with the nearby car".
>
> "Do not move too close to my cars, we can crash each other".

Serious things happen with new drivers are moody and negative drivers. The first drive, conscious and unconscious mind does not understand well the receiving signals on road; the subconscious mind will pull out a lot of unrelated outcomes from the receiving signals; sometimes, it irrationally pull out the serious outcomes, many negative stories pop out in the mind. With arousing mind, the receiving signals from driving misinterpreted into the threatening to the safety of the driver. The unconscious mind sends arousing messages like "watch out" or "danger". It simultaneously activates the stress system; stress chemicals flush to the entire body as the conditioned response to make the driver prepares for the coming attack. It can make new driver has signed: freezing, trembling, sweating, changing the volume of voice, increase heartbeat, palpitation and many other symptoms in table three: the most symptoms of stress that we can find in many patients. Arousing mind makes the driver so stressful and exhausted that he cannot drive long hours for the first time. If the subconscious mind continues to arouse, it creates a series of the endless circle of stresses and outcomes. Arousing distracts the focus of driver, it makes the driver feel overwhelming with driving. To the point of over-stimulated, the new driver falls into extreme stress, the conscious mind cannot calm the mind and the emotion. He loses control of the mind and body. The signs of over-stress are so much obvious; he is in a mad, crazy state; he shouts at nearby drivers; easily losing temper; he cannot control himself. He drives like crazy; he presses gear unconsciously, turns the car suddenly. Serious car accidence may happen unless someone stops him. If looking into the cases of car accidents, we can see many cases have the same pattern of causes like because of losing control or lacking awareness of the driver.

The responsibility of system one, or unconscious mind, is to detect any harm to our obsessed needs. If system one sense anything is not right, anything can destroy our desired things. The mind may misinterpret it as attacking signals. It means that it may be dangerous or harmful. The stress system slightly activated as a conditioned response. The drip of stress chemicals appears in our bodies. It makes us have some of the transient signs in table 6: the most symptoms of stress that we can find in many patients. When people know exactly what they need, or the things they obsessed, the mind will focus on scanning to find out any bad things to these needs. Only the most experienced people and the most obsessed people have the ability of quick scanning environment to find out the good things and the best things to their obsessed desires. They are so obsessed with the desires that their ability of scanning now becomes part of their instinct. Making ability becomes part of the instinct takes lots of time to form so only outliers can thin slice the situation in the blink of an eye to having gut feelings. They can sense something strange and then create some changes inside the body, but they cannot consciously explain exactly what it is. This is also true with the professional athletes, the motor-racing drivers, and the Olympic athletes. They have practiced so hard that they can create the exact corresponding responses to any obstacles during the games in a blink; perhaps these skills are part of the instinct. The fact is our ancestors did not know anything about these skills one hundred years ago.

If the mind can detect the wanted or desired things, we will have feelings of gaining and happiness. The things that satisfy the individuals' desires will slightly activate the happy chemicals in the individuals' body so that the individuals have the transient sense of joy, happiness or safety; these happiness chemicals will create some changes in the appearance of the body. Malcolm Gladwell explained a lot of critical situations with gut feelings in his book "Blink: The power of thinking without thinking". Reading Blink, we can understand how marvelous our brain is. Experienced people can have the first impression comes from gut feelings about the situation or people; if investigating deeper about the situation and people, most of the time they will see that the first impression is right.

This is the potential of our brain. Someone can have the first impression and transient gut feelings from the work of the subconscious mind. Someone has to train a lot to have a good first impression, to have the power of thinking without thinking. Malcolm Gladwell suggests that it must take up to ten thousand hours of hard work to become outliers, who possess the ability to thin slicing situation with gut feelings.

Out of perceivable message means the massages with no perceivable image, no perceivable voice, no perceivable sound but the mind can perceive the message is the way of subliminal programs in CDs, DVDs or programs to create changes in the participants. The technique Neuro-linguistic programming (NLP) is mainly coding the mind with the wanted responses with specific stimulations in order to change participants' behaviors, which used by some trainers. Trainers insert the subliminal messages below the conscious mind's ability to detect sound and image in the program. The participants cannot recognize it consciously so conscious mind cannot judge it right or wrong to reject it; however, the unconscious mind can catch the message and accept the message unconditionally, then the unconscious mind will create a reaction inside the body which is correspondent to the subliminal message. The subliminal message can go direct to the subconscious mind and create the wanted changes. If that subliminal message is caught by the conscious or perceivable, the conscious mind will judge the message; most of the time, the subliminal message will be rejected by the conscious mind and cannot create any wanted change in the participants.

If the subliminal message in the program is negative like danger, killing or watch out, the subconscious mind will active the stress state as the conditioned response with danger, stress chemicals will circulate in the brain and body of receivers. With high technology machines, researchers can detect the small changes in heartbeat, brainwave, muscle tension, sweating in the participants' body. If receiving the negative subliminal message, the receiver can become tired, slightly stressed and have a nightmare when sleep. If continuous receiving the negatives subliminal message for a long time, the receiver can be extremely stressed. On the other hand, with people receive the positive subliminal message; they have nothing changes in the indicators of the heartbeat, brainwave, muscle tension, sweating. Furthermore, they will have a good dream when sleep, this can be the effects of happy chemicals.

The using of subliminal message popular in many training programs is proof of the potential of the human mind. The responding to the subliminal message is the proof the ability of subconscious mind with the catching the unheard, unseen, untouched message from the condition, and the ability of subconscious mind in creating the corresponding response as the conditioned response of the mind with the condition. The subconscious mind does the scanning environment and stimulating the corresponding state in the body with the perceived message long before the conscious mind know what is happening. Experts have exact gut feelings in the critical situation long before they consciously know what is really happening.

Researchers can do experiments to prove these abilities of the mind. The experiments on mice, animals and social data can prove these characters of the mind. The effects of chemical creating happiness and stress state can easily prove by some experiment. To this point, we all agree to the potential of the mind, the characters of the mind and the role of chemicals in the state of mind. We can move to the next interesting section of the book.

Chapter 27: The brain with obsessed desires

The limbic system controls the emotion, short-term memory, and autonomic nervous system. The cerebral cortex forms the function of the mind as an executive, cognitive, thinking with logic and imagination, control kinesthetic, hearing, and visualization. The cerebral cortex stores long-term memory and conscious behaviors. Human beings have a potential brain with unlimited power. The problem is why we get severely stressed and be the victims of chronic stress in spite of the fact that we are very smart and successful.

Human beings have been evolving a lot from our ancestors; we not only have the need of survival but also we have many other needs; we not only obsessed with the need of survival but also we obsess with many other needs. Some groups of people have only basic needs; other groups of people have many needs. To some extent, the needs are expanding substantially in many groups of people with the advancement of living standard. The needs to push and motivate people to work harder, longer and more persistently. Owning for the needs, human beings have created many great advancements and developments for themselves and human kinds. On the one hand, people are the masters of the needs, they create many miracles with the noble deeds of noble need, the selfless needs. On the other hand, people may be the victims of vicious needs, the selfish needs.

Human needs to be explained by Abraham Maslow:
Abraham Maslow had taken researchers about human's needs and described the needs of human beings in "Maslow's hierarchy of needs":

The first needs are physiological needs, to do with the maintenance of the human body. If we are unwell, then little else matters until we recover.

The second needs are safety needs, about putting a roof over our heads and keeping us from harm.

The third needs are social belonging needs, about satisfying our tribal nature. If we are helpful and kind to others, they will want us as friends.

Fourth needs are esteem needs, for a higher position within a group. If people respect us, we have greater power.

Fifth needs are self-actualization needs, to 'become what we are capable of becoming', which would our greatest achievement.

Human needs explained by Tony Robbins

Recently, Tony Robbins has explained these needs of modern people in a much more understandable way. According to Tony Robbins, people have six basic needs:

The first needs are needs of certainty - the need for safety, security, comfort, order, predictability, and control.

The Second needs are needs of uncertainty or excitement. We need variety, surprise, challenges, excitement, difference, adventure, and change. People hate boring things.

The third needs are needs of connection and love. As the human being, we all need to connect with others, and we all need love from others. The need come from communication, unified, approval, to feel connected with human beings, intimate and loved by members of the family and other human beings.

Fourth needs are needs of significance. Every people like to be significant. People need to have meaning, special, pride, needed, wanted, sense of importance and worthy of love. They do all things to get and protect their significance. Most of the luxury products made to make people feel of significance.

Fifth needs are the needs of development. People need constant emotional, intellectual and spiritual development. This need drives us to study more and do harder to make us develop.

Sixth needs are needs of contribution, the need to give beyond ourselves, give, care, protect and serve others, to leave a legacy.

What do these human needs mean?

Most people have their own set of needs. With specific individuals, receiving rewards means that they receive tangible and intangible things that satisfy their needs. Receiving rewards will make people feel safe, happy, joyful, inspired and motivated; receiving rewards make people filled with happy chemicals.

On the other hand, with some individuals, punishing these individuals means they will suffer the losses of tangible things or intangible things, which are the things they need to satisfy their needs. Being Punishment means bearing the losses. People perceive the actions of other people as punishments if the actions make them have the feeling of losses and the feelings of reducing their need satisfaction. Punishing make people have the feeling of reducing their certainty, their excitement, their connection and love, their significance, their development, and their contribution. These actions of punishment will make people feel unsafe, disappointed, annoyed, angry, sad, and extremely stressful.

At some stage of life, they have one or some needs stronger than other needs. With some groups of people, these needs are increasing. They need more and more. To satisfy these expanding needs they have to accumulate and possess thousand precious things. If outside conditions meet our needs, it means these needs are satisfied, the happy system activated, chemicals of happiness appear in brain and body make us have good feelings. As a human creature, we want to have more happy feelings. The actions of animals are to satisfy the need for survival; on the other hand, human beings act to make them have a feeling of happiness. The drive of thoughts, behaviors of human beings is feelings - happy feelings. Collecting, accumulating, achieving, receiving, wearing only make people feel happy; they are happy when these things are satisfied with individuals' needs. All actions are to find joy from hunting, training, studying, kickboxing, playing, beating, killing, breaking, or suicide. People have a sophisticated brain than people can imagine, with memory, intelligence, and imagination, people do not find joy directly from the actions. They find joy in every action based on their perception of the actions. Memory and imagination make their perceptions have private meaning. These are two kinds of joy: short-term joy and long-term joy, or short-term gain and long-term gain. All animals' behavior is to have immediate satisfaction; they do not have the much ability to think in long term. All worthwhile achievements in the world are the result of long-term gain, the mind of human beings makes them direct the action to the long-term gain. The potential of the brain helps them accept short-term pain gracefully and joyfully on the way to accomplish worthwhile results.

Unfortunately, from times to times, some people have many more other selfish needs. To satisfy these needs, hundreds or thousands of specific things they want to own to satisfy our needs, to have a happy feeling. For examples, they need to have more money, houses, status, position, fame, successful business, have more land, more cars, wealthy for family members. The specific desires are different from individual to individual; To some extent, these desires are the core of the individual's belief. If these needs are satisfied, people will feel happy; if the needs are not satisfied, people will feel pain, miserable or stressful. In the modern world, the brain of people not only has the responsibility of helping people to survive but also the brain has the responsibility to make people have the feeling of joy, happiness. The potential brain works all day to satisfy the needs of their owners. Individuals with specific desirable needs, the unconscious mind has the responsibility of scanning the environment to see things outside can satisfy their needs or damage their needs. With the huge power, the unconscious mind of individuals can scan the environment in a blink of an eye according to the obsessed needs; the scanning is so slightly and quickly that the individuals do not have any conscious idea about the scanning and the finding of the unconscious mind. After getting the conclusion, the subconscious mind will send out the signals by forming the chemicals like happy chemicals and stress chemical; and the electrical signals inside the brain. Well-trained individuals will have clear gut feelings from the inside and the outside environment.

For example, with the mother, she obsesses with the need for protecting her child so strong that she can have the gut feelings of what happened to her child when the child crying. These gut feelings are much better than the child's father, even if the father is a very successful man. The lawyers have good gut feelings when scanning a dozen pages of contract than the ordinary people do. The doctors have a better gut feeling about patients than ordinary people do. The power and sensitivity of gut feelings depend on the power of desires and the mastery of people in the area. These gut feelings are the abilities of the unconscious mind of the experts and experienced people, who obsess with ideas or goals.

Our brains have two systems: fast thinking and slow thinking described well in the book "Think fast and slow" of Daniel Kahneman. According to the author, two systems combining into the way people think. The system one is fast, intuitive, and emotional; the system two is slower, more deliberative and logical. According to Sigmund Freud, the human mind has a conscious mind and subconscious mind. The conscious mind works slowly and logically in analyzing information; it takes lots of energy for functions, and it needs concentration to function well. The unconscious accept the information as the dots of knowledge send from a conscious mind; it stores the dots of knowledge for future actions. The subconscious mind works fast, intuitively, automatically and emotionally; it works in a blink that individuals did not even realize of its working; it works base on the memorized information send from the conscious mind. The subconscious mind only accepts and memorizes the receiving information without denying. When getting new information or new signals, the conscious mind tries to understand signals; it requires time, energy and focus. After getting the pattern of signals, the meaning of information, the conscious mind sends the pattern to the subconscious mind to store it for future use. This process can be like sending many dots of information to the subconscious mind. The more dots the subconscious mind has, the more the mind can functions well with less effort. The conscious mind does its job well when people are in happiness, peace and total concentration. People who have little chance of taking action, little time of thinking, no curiosity, no safe, and often in stress; their conscious mind does not function well; so that they have very few dots of knowledge in their unconscious mind. This is the reason that un-experienced people have functions of the brain are worse than experienced people do, and the trainees do not work well as the seniors.

According to Howard Gardner, there are seven types of intelligence. Each individual has talent in specific areas. Working in strength areas makes the brain function very well. The joy and smooth of working in strength makes people healthier and happier. When individuals do the work they love, the working stimulates the mind creating happy chemicals; they happily work with curiosity, imaginations, deep immersion into work, lacking the sense of timing; these are the characters of people reach to the state of flow in work. Working in a happy state help them understand quicker, more exactly than people working in a stress state. When people work in a happy state, they work much more well, no tired, no pain. Moreover, they find joy, happiness, and excitement in working. Working in strength areas makes people happier than sitting idle; gradually they love the work, and working is the vital parts of their happiness. They work in spite of getting old or getting no payment. Their faces radiate happiness, joy, and excitement during working time.

> "Success follows doing what you want to do. There is no other way to be successful." **Malcolm Forbes**

> "When you are courting a nice girl an hour seems like a second. When you sit on a red-hot cinder a second seems like an hour. That is relativity." ***Albert Einstein***.

There is the relativity of thinking that makes big difference in the feelings of people in a stress state and people in a happy state. Feelings create the relativity of time. If individuals experience the happiness state for one hour and in stress state for ten seconds, they will know the relativity of time. All of you can do the test when you are courting a nice, beautiful girl an hour seems like a second. When you are courting with an ugly, selfish girl an hour seems like a year. Moreover, the outcome of the courting and chatting may remain for weeks or months after that event. The first kiss of a couple is the sweetest kiss ever because it is the fruit of countless previous happy events; they may think they cannot live without another. But the kiss of a frustrated couple with lots of yelling, beating, screaming is the frightened, contemptuous kiss because it is the fruit of countless sad events; they may think it is better to get the divorce. That is the perception of relativity or thinking of relativity.

> The first kiss of a couple is the sweetest kiss ever because it is the fruit of countless previous happy events; they may think they cannot live without another. But the kiss of a frustrated couple with lots of yelling, beating, screaming is the frightened, contemptuous kiss because it is the fruit of countless sad events; they may think it is better to get the divorce.

The relativity of time also happens when people work in their weakness and work in their strength. In doing in weakness, there are countless things that the subconscious mind does not understand, it is very difficult for the mind and body to function well, the focus of conscious mind always be irritated by the subconscious mind with a small of stress chemicals. There are very little dots of knowledge in weakness areas; moreover, deep in the mind, there is the hatred with the work relating to the weakness, so that it is very tired to work in weakness for both conscious mind and subconscious mind. To the people working in weakness or the hatred are so terrible they experience pain, stress and miserable even they gain many material rewards from the work. Moreover, people work in weakness can adopt the bad conclusion or bad belief about their ability, which will leave tracks in their future. People work in their weakness or hatreds may experience the early symptoms of stress like a headache, migraine, nausea, upset stomach, insomnia. For more detail of symptoms they experience, let look at table two: the most symptoms of stress that we can find in many patients.

> "The important thing is not to stop questioning. Curiosity has its own reason for existing."
>
> **Albert Einstein**

Curiosity and imagination can only appear when people are in the safe and happy state, in stillness and peace of mind. Looking a little boy in the peaceful and happy state, observers can see the happiness radiating from the way he acts, runs, curiously questions, talks, plays, jumps up and down to every corner of the room; the little boy in happiness can run, talk, play endlessly and without any tired. People watching this little boy can sense the abundance flow of energy inside of him and radiates from him. He is like a small tree with high vitality.

Working in strength areas, the mind works in a happy state, the mind works very efficiently to analyze, collect, accumulate, and combine the knowledge. Moreover, the unconscious mind of people accumulates the abundance of knowledge. With these abundances of true knowledge, subconscious mind functions so accurately and silently to get the job done in a blink of an eye that they do not recognize. With the stillness and clearness of mind, we can have gut feelings about the good or bad indicators of the situation. This is the talent of the outliers.

The mind cannot have curiosity and imagination in a stressful state. The subconscious mind in stress only scans the environment to see the threatening from the environment. Stress chemicals running throughout the body and brain, interrupting the focus of the mind, arousing the mind constantly, making people have the feeling of the feeling of the cold. People in the high position in career, which they hate or find no meaning, usually experience tired, stressful and unsatisfied at work; even worse they feel extreme stressful with many feeling like the symptoms of the cold. It is liked they are wearing a burden on the successful career. This is why it is very difficult to succeed and get peace in doing with weakness. When people work in weakness, conscious mind has a lot of things to do; when the job is done, they do not really feel joyful, excited or happy; there are no happiness chemicals in the brain so that they very quickly get tired in the doing. One hour of work in weakness seems like ten hours - this is perceptional relativity. The perception of the phenomena may make people feel stressed or feel happy. It is not the same for every people.

Chapter 28: What influence the belief system of individuals?

These are the wrong beliefs that people or children may adopt from environment unintentionally or intentionally. The misunderstanding of human needs and wrongly using the reward and punishment techniques by parents and adults may create ill beliefs for their children. Children may adopt the wrong belief as the conditioned response to find safety in the environment. Each wrong concept and belief seems like a splint to splint the thinking and acting of children. Children have a wrong belief system are under the seamless web of splints that splint the hands, legs, and mind of the children. If these children do not get help or do not grow big enough to break the wrong belief system, they will be the victims of the living environment.

The wrong opinions of a child may become the child's belief

> "You cannot do it."
>
> "You are too weak to do it."
>
> "Look at the way you work, I think you will be a failure in life."
>
> "Fuck you! Prison is the best place for you."
>
> "You have to do farming like this unless I will beat you."
>
> "Do you know who you are? Luxury places are not for you."
>
> "Dumb, stupid, stubborn, lazy boy. I do not think you will be the success."
>
> "Study hard, find a stable job, you will have a stable

> life, this is our dream, you know? My son"
>
> "Getting a stable job is the dream of us; you should not leave it, my son."
>
> "You are so stupid that you cannot do the demanding job."
>
> "No one in our district can ever do that job, so please sit down and stay in that safe place, my son"
>
> "Follow my advice I will happy to help you. Otherwise, get out of our house and do the things you like."
>
> "I love you; I want to do good for you. So do not deny our pieces of advice and help."
>
> "Do you love your parents? If yes, let follow their wishes to make them happy."
>
> "When the thing goes wrong, find someone to blame;"
>
> "Alcohol is a good drink make me feel comfortable in stress situation;"
>
> "Study is for big dummy head, I am smarter than most of them, so no need for me to study anymore;"
>
> "The rich are selfish people; they are dump heads with luck"
>
> "I want to get rich without doing anything"
>
> "Beating is a good way to solve any conflict"
>
> "He dare to look at me with that way, I have to teach him a lesson."

On the other hand, there are many good opinions, beliefs may become the beliefs of the kids owning for the understanding basic human needs and understanding the art of using reward and punishment by parents and adults. Parents who master the art of using reward and punishment based on the understanding of human needs will make their children feel safe, motivated and inspired before any hard works, obstacles, and challenges. This is the art of conditioning the mind. When kids feel safe, inspired and motivated; they will do more, learn more and try more. These are the ways to help kids may find out the good knowledge and beliefs for themselves. Adopting a good belief may be seen as placing the wings to uplift individuals to overcome difficulties and obstacles.

The good opinions of a child may become the child's belief

"You can do it"

"Nick Vujicic can do many things with no hand, no leg, so can you. His height is less than 1 meter, no hand, no foot, but when he goes, many young men with the height more than 1.7 meters want to work for him to make his moving easier and on time. When he talks, hundreds of young handsome men and beautiful, healthy girls want to listen to his talk? Is this the paradoxes of life? What is most important in life?"

"Disable is not in hand or leg, disable is in the mind, take control of your mind and you will control your life."

"If you think you can or cannot do, you are right."

"I am healthy, I am lucky, I am great. I can handle well any challenges."

"Challenges make me stronger, challenges make me smarter, and challenges make me better. I welcome challenges."

"Stable is failures, I have great potential, a giant sleeping within, wake the giant up with a dream and massive action"

"What the mind can conceive and believe, you can achieve."

"Success leaves track, find the right track, follow it, you will succeed"

"Many men born with defects, diseases but they have the best attitude, clear goals, serving heart and principles to create massive action. They are far more success than many other healthy men. I trust in you that you will succeed; you can do that. You can feel safe that I will support you unconditionally."

> "Break and failure are the ladders to achievement. You cannot find any big achiever never break anything, or never making any failure. Break and failure give them tremendous opportunities. It is fine if you break anything or fail in the way of doing. I know it is the price of your success in the future. So make sure that I will support you, do not afraid of break and failure, keep moving on; my son."

These pieces of advice, opinions of parents and adults based on their understanding may become the self-talk inside the receiver's head. These adopted opinions may become the silent thoughts appear every single time. These opinions may become the receiver's belief. The belief system of a person is all the concepts, ideas that person thinks true or false. These concepts of the things, like should or should not to do, have or have not to do, are accepted by the conscious mind and stored deep into subconscious mind as the dots of knowledge. People live under the hologram of countless dots they put into the mind. The mind will call on these dots when it needs materials to judge an idea, information or a situation before taking responding actions.

Belief formed by what we feed the mind by reading, listening, thinking, doing; from the close friends talk to us, and the self - talk we do every day. During childhood, belief is formed mostly by parents, we memorize the concepts; from these concepts we take actions. The rewards or punishments we perceived from the environment when taking action will determine the meaning of the receiving information. People do things in a way to avoid pain and gain pleasure. The outside environment sends signals and information to the mind; the mind will analyze it by feeling it create the signals. If perceiving reward, the mind will memorize the condition. Next time, if we response based on the pattern of knowledge and we gain pleasure and reward, this knowledge will become part of our belief systems. Gradually, the mind may create conditioned feelings based on the patterns of information.

The young kids have easily conditioned the responses with the reward and punishment by parents and environment. The small children do not have their own idea, do not have their own concepts to reject information, they do not have a barrier to protect their mind, do not have enough strength to make them feel safe in case of go against the advice of parents. Small kids have to adapt to the environment, they memorize the pattern of receiving information and advice; if using pattern of information makes them safe and pleased, they tend to repeat this advice many times to gain pleasure. Gradually, the information and advice may become the children's belief.

On the other hand, they will memorize the pain condition to stay away. If encountering the condition makes them get pain or punishment, they will stay away from the condition. The subconscious mind will remember the pattern o the condition and the perceived negative emotion as the dot of knowledge. Gradually, these dots become part of the children's belief. The subconscious mind will use these dots very quickly and silently to create conditioned responses. The subconscious mind can sense the pleasure or happiness from the condition of the environment in a blink, long before the individual can understand what happens.

The subconscious mind will create conditioned responses with each of condition. The subconscious mind of the kid will send the gut feelings for the kids when it encounters with part of the condition. Encountering with the condition of stress, the subconscious mind will create the gut feeling of stress; and the children may have some obvious symptoms of stress. Encounter with the condition of happiness, the subconscious mind will create the gut feelings of happiness; and the children may have the obvious signs of happiness.

The pattern of knowledge, conditions, and corresponding responses will put in subconscious mind like the dots of knowledge. People may have the awareness of the patterns of information and responses they have if they pay attention to their responses to the environment; with the awareness, they may control and correct the beliefs they have. If people lack awareness, they may be the victims of the wrong beliefs they have. Just watching groups of people angrily arguing and fighting to protect their opinions, we will understand how powerful of different beliefs can make; and how sophisticatedly the beliefs can make people think they are the owners of their opinions, perceptions, and beliefs. Countless conditioned responses have created silently inside their mind to protect their opinions, perceptions, and beliefs that they do not know.

I have seen many examples of conditioning the responses of fear with small kids by adults. Small kids became stressful after making a mistake. A small girl trembled after breaking a dish. A small girl was very nervous and anxious about making a mistake because of the thinking that her parents would punish her. A good kid was so nervous and pitiful with the thought that her parents would disappointed with her disobeyed behaviors. A boy was happily playing and talking suddenly became frightening and trembling because of breaking an expensive toy. A boy became fearful and stressed with the staring of his father. A small boy was so afraid that he fearfully followed any orders of adults just by listening that he will be punished by his father he does not obey their orders. These are the most common examples that many people know or experience. Other adults may create many characters like ghost, devil, monster, demon, police, and a bad man to make the small child obey their orders. These feeling of stress, fear, and panic are the conditioned responses in the kids' mind to make kids obey any order from adults temporary. Unfortunately, these conditioned responses go along with the development of the kids; all of these negative feelings and experiences may form the bad hologram about life for kids. Constantly living under stress conditioned will make kids affected by rebelling responses, abnormal responses, and abnormal behaviors. The outside appearances, behaviors, health are the reflections of the state of mind.

Kids can make mistake, it is normal for the kids. Unfortunately, the overreacting of parents with the mistake of kid can make kids pain and hurt so much that kids are obsessed with the wrong patterns of behaving and responding. Kids have unintentionally conditioned the responses of stress and fear with any mistake. There are a series of events, objects, people, behaviors and countless phenomena relating to the time that kids fell into stressed, fearful and terrified. The mind of kids will remember all the perceivable phenomena and countless phenomena that are under the sensory threshold. In the terrified state, the mind may misinterpret all of these phenomena with painful experiences. After a crucial punishing, if seeing, making any parts of previous painful conditions, kids may fall to extreme stress. Experienced parents can easily see the signs of stress or fear in their kids, which are described in table two: "the most symptoms of stress that we can find in many patients" so that they can help the kids calm the stress down, sooth the fear in their kids.

Unfortunately, parents may fall to some traps of thinking that they not only ignore the fear and stress of the kids but also they unintentionally making the stress severer, creating the deep scars in the soul of their children. Parents unintentionally condition their kids with extremely stressed response to the minor stimulations. Sadly, the pattern in this paragraph appears every day, not only with the kids but also with all other people in society like workers, employees, employers, teachers, students. They are the receivers and the creators of the bad conditioned responses like fear, pain, stress, and panicking that they do not know if they do not practice compassion. In other words, we are the creators and receivers of stress in our community. We are the creators and receivers of misery in our family and community. We are not only the effects of the living environment but also we are the causes of our living conditions. We are the receivers and creators of any results we have. So in order to change the results we have in life, the best way is starting from inside, not start from the outside environment; start with the circles of influences. Why do we not know that we do involve in the problems we have? In the next parts, I will show you some of the traps in thinking that we do not know; and how to overcome the traps.

Chapter 29: The work of the potential mind

Our potential brain works day and night, twenty-four hours a day to scan the environment to find out things outside are safe or dangerous. Our ancestors used the potential of the brain to scan the environment to find out whether or not it was safe or dangerous. The human being in the modern day still has this ability of scanning environment; furthermore, the scanning ability may be more sophisticated. Because modern people have more needs, they obsess about these needs. Their brain not only scans the dangerous signals for their survival from the environment but also potentially the brain scans to see whether or not there are any attacks from the environment, which may harm their needs. The human mind is very sensitive to anything that harms their assets. There are some people so obsessed with their needs and assets that they have many assumptions in their mind like the table below. In their mind, they have to possess some specific things to satisfy their obsessed needs. Getting, possessing and dominating bring to these people the feeling of safety and happiness. Whatever they think they have to have, whatever they obsess with will be the focus of the mind, then from the mind, its control of the process of thinking, speaking and acting.

People with the need of more; want more, more, more and more things to make them feel happy. They are so obsessed with these needs and possession so much that these things will be the priority of the mind. Even some people so obsessed with these addicted feelings so that they forget or destroy the chance of satisfying the six basic needs described by Tony Robbins. Then the responsibility of the subconscious mind is to scan is there any things harm their assets; is there any things danger for our needs. If there are any signs of attacks to assets, the stress system will be activated, the person with need of more will overreacts vigorously; the pattern of their actions is same as a caveman saw a tiger. I have seen many crucial punishments, violent actions, the act of crimes arise from unwanted things happened.

The need for more

> "I need more money to have the feeling of safety."
>
> "I need five houses to prove my significance, to make sure I am rich."
>
> "I have to be rich to prove for my family that I am a good person."
>
> "I have to have the luxury bag to make me feel happy with the admiring eyes of friends."
>
> "I have to have ten luxury bags, ten Channel shoes to make have the feelings of importance and happiness"
>
> "I have to have ten supercars to show my status, people will admire me."
>
> "My dress makes me much more beautiful than teacher's dress."
>
> "I hate that guy because he did not praise my luxury bags."
>
> "I hate my friends because they do not thank me for my help. I have helped them with a large amount of money."
>
> "I get mad when seeing him makes my suit dirty."
>
> "If he scratches my luxury bag, I will kill him."

Last year, I had the bad impression when seeing a car driver beating a motorbike driver crazily until the motor driver bleeding and falling down. The crucial beating started just because of a small scratch the motorbike driver created in the car. How crazy when people are driven by greed. The car driver was so obsessed with his car that he cannot bear anything happening to the car, he acted crucially without any compassion for the pain that the motorbike driver had to suffer from him. If any bad thing happens to his car or anything he loves, he may get mad and react wildly and crucially without paying attention to the result. He is the victim of negative emotion and the creator of tragedy for himself and his society.

Greedy people are usually disappointed; they cannot be satisfied with the condition of living, even in the abundance of living. Their greed changes constantly that they never know what their good condition of living is. All fairy tales and stories have the figures of the greedy man and good man; one of these stories is The "Tale of the Fisherman and the Fish". The greedy people usually get disappointed, angry at every activity. They always find lacking instead of abundance from the environment. They are obsessed with many luxury and expensive things. Once they get these things, they immediately feel bored with them very quickly. Because of the desires and the focusing of the mind, the people with the need for more always feel angry, disappointed and unsafe. Each time of feeling of danger, anger, and disappointment, their subconscious mind usually activates the stress system with the stress chemicals. The constant activating of the stress system makes them fall to extreme stress. Observe closely we will see that they are the victims of stress with many symptoms in table two: the most symptoms of stress that we can find in many patients. The greedy people can feel stressed, unhappy and miserable even when they live in a villa in Beverly hill, driving supercars, wearing luxury accessories. These expensive things cannot make them happy for a long time. Living in luxury building, they still are stressed and have want of jumping out from the windows. They take every action like giving, eating, taking, serving, studying, and doing with negative feelings, the feelings of pain and losses. Experienced people can see the negative pattern of pain and loses in their thinking, talking, and acting. Physicians can detect the stress symptoms in their bodies; the symptoms described in table two: the most symptoms of stress that we can find in many patients. There are many teachings from great men about how to have a happy living.

The right understanding of adjectives

Adjectives used to describe the character, traits of object: brave - cowardly, calm - windy, cruel - kind, courteous - discourteous, rude; discourage - encourage, dreary - cheerful, generous - stingy, gentle - rough, clean - dirty, nice-nasty, polite-rude, honest - dishonest, justice - injustice, mad - happy, major - minor, real - fake, straight - crooked, transparent - nontransparent, and true-false.

Some adjective describes positive traits of people: accessible, active, adaptable, admirable, compassionate, empathetic, energetic, enthusiastic, humorous, imaginative, and impressive.

Some adjective describes negative traits of people: angry, anxious, cautious, charmless, conceited, cowardly, critical, crude, cruel, discontented, discouraging, discourteous, frightening, greedy, hateful, miserable, and reactive.

Let see the countless information an adjective can describe. When we first meet a new man, we want to know more about him by stories and descriptions of characters in the adjective. What is the right to understanding the traits of men? A trait of a man will tell that when things happened to the man, he will have the adjectively conditioned responses to the events. The quality of responses of the individual is described by the adjective trait of the individual. The responses are the combination of all conditioned responses in the whole body: face, cells, brain, chemical, hair, muscles cells, thinking, self-talking, nonverbal message, words, energy, behaviors, and so on. Countless parts of his body seem to conspire to make him have the trait of characters.

For example, he is a humorous man means that he will have humorous conditioned responses to whatever happened to him. In other words he responses humorously.

He is a cruel man means that he will have cruel conditioned responses to unwanted thing happened to him no matter how rich, how powerful and how healthy he is.

He is a corrupt man means that he corruptly response to most of the things happen to him, or all of his body will conspire to create corruptive conditioned responses in the most situation no matter how intelligent, how powerful, and how rich he is.

He is a good man, but the environment makes him corrupt small from things cost $1 to $5 things. He has unconsciously conditioned his mind in the corrupt trait. Gradually he becomes a corrupt man. He tends to act corruptively to whatever happened to him. His richness, intelligence, wealthy, and power fail to make him good. These advantages are only the levers, which multiply the bad causes he made. For example, the power and intelligence can make a corrupt politician success in stealing one million $ in building the 4 billion $ dump to protect the capital and make electricity; the intelligence of scientists can make him successfully get the profit of ten thousand $ by removing some screw in building a spaceship. With people in society: farmers, workers, entrepreneurs, leaders, engineers, teachers, and religious leaders, what characters do you want they have?

> The core or majority of a man is traits, character, not intelligence, or standard of living. Virtue men do not need the enforcement of the law to make good, but the corrupt men use his intelligence to take profit successfully by violating human law legally.

Traits of a person used to describe the pattern of conditioned responses of that person to the environment. Someone have conditioned responses consciously or unconsciously by the living environment. To know what conditioned responses and characters someone has, they need to live mindfully to understand what is happening inside his body and outside the body. People who understand their characters can make changes in characters if needed by conditioning the mind with visualization of the wanted responses.

The teaching of great men about the misery that needs may bring

> "To live a pure unselfish life, one must count nothing as one's own in the midst of abundance." **Buddha**
>
> "A crust eaten in peace is better than a banquet partaken in anxiety." **Aesop**
>
> "Content makes poor men rich; discontent makes rich men poor." **Benjamin Franklin**
>
> "Who is wise? He who learns from everyone. Who is powerful? He that governs his passions. Who is rich? He that is content. Who is that? Nobody." **Benjamin Franklin**
>
> "It is the eye of other people that ruin us. If I were blind I would want, neither fine clothes, or fine houses or fine furniture." **Benjamin Franklin**
>
> "The discontented man finds no easy chair." **Benjamin Franklin**

What is the exact meaning of contentment? What is the character of people with the contented mind? The one who has content mind have surely will have conditioned positive attitude and conditioned good feeling whatever bad things happened to them. They will happy and grateful to focus their mind to find the answers to the problem they have. Fortunately for them, happy feeling and grateful thinking will make their mind in a good state to focus on solving the problem. Most of the time, contented men have positive thinking, solution-oriented thinking, positive views point, and happy feeling despite what happens to them. They welcome events happened to them without any greedy expectation. Contented men choose a positive attitude and happiness despite the events and environment; they choose based on their understanding of life." Contented men will rejoice because thorn bushes have roses."

Unfortunately, discontented men suffer negative feelings and stress all day whatever good things come to them. They have conditioned anger, conditioned negative attitude, and conditioned stress to whatever seemingly insignificant unwanted thing in abundant good things happen to them. They have unconsciously conditioned the negative thinking, feeling to whatever unwanted things happen to them. Discontented men are the slave of greed, anger, ignorance, and changing sensual feelings. Look at the pattern of reaction to the event, people will know that a man is contented or discontented. Sadly, they are the slaves and the victims of their imbalanced mind that they do not know to change it. More surprisingly, discontent men always think their conditioned greedy thinking, their conditioned angry emotion, their conditioned negative responses are right, they even dare to fight to protect their opinions, thinking, feeling, and responding." Discontented men will complain because rose bushes have thorns."

Rare people are wise, rare people are powerful and rare people are actually as rich as they usually think. Most people live in self-centered, discontented mood, anger, and envy. They count everything is on their own. They feed their ego to grow big enough to swallow them. In the constantly changing society, they have to run, work, and chase to a lot of things to get more, have more to satisfy their needs, to make them feel happy and joyful. Unfortunately, their happiness in possessing things do not last much; they easily feel discontent with new things and start to want more. Greedy people never get real happy with the things they have. They cling to the changing things in society. Much of clinging lead to disappointment, they fall in anger and anxiety in the abundance of living. Each time they feel anger, their body is flushed with little stress hormones.

People in modern society have a lot of desires that need to be satisfied, they will fall into stress constantly if they get unwanted things. Their bodies may always be filled with stress hormones. Because of stress, they tend to overreact to small things, stay away from the crowd and like to stay alone in order to find their safety. People become stress because their obsessed desires are not satisfied; so that they like to do something to help them relieve stress. With stressed people, smoking, playing, eating, shopping, drinking wine, using the drug, quitting school, playing with friends, rebelling, shouting, running, self-injuring, fighting, breaking objects and playing the game are the activities that may reduce the stress. Unfortunately, their needs of more are increasing by the influence of the environment, surrounding crowd and adopted bad habits. Each moment of stress, the bad habits help them a lot in relieving stress, so that they rarely listen to their own voice of conscience and gut feelings, which remind them to stay away from bad habits. The unconscious mind of the greedy individual always detects the unsatisfied things, it misinterprets the unwanted things as threat or dangers, then constantly sends the signals creating stress state to cope with unwanted things. Greedy people get stress or anger long before they consciously know what is happening. If they lack mindfulness, if they do not pay attention to the small changes in the body, the anger and stress may become too big that they cannot consciously control anymore. They have many symptoms in table two "the most symptoms of stress that we can find in many patients", and their overreaction and their anger can make people so afraid that they want to stay away from them.

Their anger and overreaction can make their relatives hurt or anger; even worse, their relatives get mad or angry with them. Gradually, stress and anger make people stay away from them. They lack a deep connection with their relatives. The anger can destroy the relationship very quickly, and may leave the wound in the soul of everyone. Gradually, the six basic needs of the human being like certainty, uncertainty, connection and love, significance, development, and contribution are not satisfied because of the anger and stress. The anger and stress create vicious circles affecting life, if not stopped properly, the people with anger and stress can become the creators and victims simultaneously in life.

For example, when a manager with a need is not satisfied, he becomes anger and stress. Every staff around him can sense there is something wrong with him and they should stay away from him. The unconscious mind of staff is alert; the unconscious mind may misinterpret normal signals into the danger, the mind lacks focus on work. The whole office is in a stressful state because of the manager's anger. Everybody filled with hormones of stress. Staffs have to "work to safe". The even small normal thing happens like the ring of the fall, the big noise outside, a call of someone's name, and the sounds of close the door may see as threatening signals. Staffs are so much stress that they are transiently sweating, chill in the neck, chill in the back, trembling, over-alerting, shaking and over caution. All staffs want to stay away from the manager. The six basic needs of staffs are not satisfied with a stressful environment. The staffs become more anxious and stress because of the stress of the manager. The staffs get more symptoms of stress like cold symptoms than next-door staffs. Working in the stress state, staffs will have no safety, no curiosity, no creativity, no fun, no need for contribution and development; they only work to find the safety at work. Because of the wrong behaviors of manager, the staffs feel so unsafe that they do not want to try new ideas, do not make innovation, do not want to take the challenges; all they want is to do is do things that brings safety. The work in a stressful environment is so hard for staffs that eight hours of work seem like the year of work; they are exhausted; they experience the relativity of time. Gradually, working in a stressful environment makes staffs hate the work. The reason that they do not quit the works because in making the decision of taking the work, they count the cost and benefit of working; in staffs' perception, they still feel the benefit is more than the cost. Because the benefit from the work can satisfy some of the staffs' needs so that they can bear the cost of the work they hate.

On the other hand, staffs work in a happy environment, the basic needs are satisfied, staffs happy, have more energy to work. They are "safe to work"; they do a good job. They work in a happy state; people are safe, funny, happy and joyful with the work. They are rarely stressful at work; they feel that the 8 hours of work pass very quickly. Gradually, they love the work. The love and joy at work can create may extraordinary things for the company and society.

Emotion and energy of working places can be the difference makers to the effectiveness of the work. Furthermore, when workers return home, the emotion they have at work also affects the emotion they have at home. To some extent, the emotion and energy someone has in differences places are interdependent with each other. The difference in the quality of emotion between people compounds over time can create a big difference in the quality of life.

The obsessed needs and obsessed desires of greedy people make them easily become stress. They are so busy to chase to changing things that they forget the real needs of themselves and others. Mother Teresa has sensed the hunger of modern people. The hunger only is satisfied by the love, connection and caring of surrounding people.

> "Being unwanted, unloved, uncared for, forgotten by everybody, I think that is a much greater hunger, a much greater poverty than the person who has nothing to eat."
>
> **Mother Teresa**

These are the different expressions the need or want, the need for love, the need of care for, the need for significance and the need for significance. Being unwanted, unloved, uncared for, forgotten by everybody is the tragedy of our modern life. These unsatisfied needs will create misery for all relating people. The fact is with the development of technology gadgets, the hunger of these needs are getting worse and its effects seem to be out of control. More and more people being stressful in abundance life; get depression even in the success of career; the number of people with mental problems is soaring, the number of people with modern diseases is soaring also; which go against with the development of the quality of physical living. Mother Teresa sensed the pain, misery because of the hunger of modern people "being unwanted, unloved, uncared for, forgotten by everybody, is a much greater hunger, much greater poverty than the person who has nothing to eat." These are the six basic needs of human being. If someone hunger for these needs, they may fall into extreme anger, sadness or extreme stress. They will do useless actions, careless actions; make useless things in the hope of satisfying the hunger. People suffering from hunger can have the symptoms in table three: "the most symptoms of stress that we can find in many patients." By looking at table three, physicians and experts will realize that most people with health problems and social problems have these symptoms earlier long before they get the problems in health and society. Most of the mental diseases are the serious side effects of stress chemicals. Temporary, most scientists cannot explain correctly the reason why people diagnosed with mental problems are soaring. Some experts even think of the improvement in diagnosis to explain this. It is not the right answer. The right answer appears if we pay attention to the mental life and spiritual health. In my mind, the development of technology that creating technological gadgets makes the hunger and poverty of modern people become more serious. The technology devices have helped people connect with faraway people and disconnect with the near-by people simultaneously; the devices has worsened the quality of the relationship; destroy the connection and love with the near-by people. The development of technology devices is the best explanation for the soaring number of people with health problems and social problems. And worst of all is the ill philosophy dominating the mind of people make them think they have a self, ego and constant, and the philosophy putting money first not love, connection, characters, and attitude first have made modern people more greedy, more angry with any mild unwanted things. Greed and anger are the powerful invisible forces not only prevent people from coming closer but also push people away. Greed and anger also make people create more solid covers to make them safe. Every people: adults, students, engineers, doctors, nurses, employees, employers, soldiers, politicians, managers, kids, children, and pets are the hunger for love, connection, and compassion. They would be touched, moved, and cried by the touching of mother Teresa or their beloved ones.

Most of the intelligence mind will not understand the bare words of fact, to understand the hunger of love, please watch these series videos on youtube.com to know the hunger our children and beloved ones.

Table 24: The videos on youtube.com help people understand the needs of human beings.

	Name of videos on youtube.com	Craving and inside changes
1	Babies' Reaction When Daddy Comes Home Compilation	With the deepest hunger, no one can hide the strongest emotion. They love each other, but they have to stay away for a long time. The baby boys, baby girls cannot hide the happiest feelings inside. The sudden attack of massive happy chemicals make the mind cannot control their body; they are astounded, startled for a while then hugging, screaming, kissing, running, crying, the tears of happiness of the meeting people. No words can express their happiness. Achieving goals, money, and getting promotion will not make them happy like this.

Having seen some dogs are so excited, so happy that they are startled then urinate incontinently when seeing their owner after a long time no see. |
2	Dogs Welcoming Soldiers Home Compilation (2012)	
3	Father Surprises Cheerleader	
4	Homecoming Heroes	
5	Little Girl's Priceless Reaction To Dad's Homecoming Will Leave You In Tears!	
6	Marine Surprises his sister on her wedding day	
7	Military Surprises	
8	Most Emotional Soldiers Coming	

	Home Compilation	
9	Navy Dad Surprises Daughter for Valentine's Day at Westosha H.S. - The World Surprise	
10	Soldier Dad Surprises Daughters At School And Their Reaction Will Melt Your Heart	
11	Soldier Surprises Daughter at Manchester Schools	

Our children, kids, adults and loved ones have the same need for hugging, embracing, and kissing.

12	Animals Hug to their Friends Humans its Emotional	Our children, kids have the same need of hugging, embracing, and kissing. Our beloved, adults ones also crave for this. Sadly, a lot of rules, fame, procedure, fear, pressures from life, and old paradigms have made the adults forced to hide their craving needs. They forget that life is funny, life is love and life has to be filled with smiling,
13	Baby Elephants love to cuddle	
14	Because hugs are the best therapy (people and animals hugs)	

15	Cats begging for Hugs	craving illogical mind. Einstein understood is the enlightened one understood this.
16	Cute Baby Goats - A Cute And Funny Baby Goats Compilation	
17	Humans Hugging Other Animals	
18	People And Animal Hugging Each Other With Love (heartwarming and touching video)	
19	Love All Animals - A Compassionate World Begins with You	

Reading the top ten diseases of United State of America and other developed countries, I think these diseases are the effects of stress. The diseases are direct proof of the effect of stress in modern society. Researchers can create stress on animals; serious and chronic stress, they will get the same problems in animals that people have. I have heard many stories about the abnormal behaviors of the pets like dogs, cats when they left alone, with the feelings of unloved, unwanted and uncared for. For a long time, these pets can have problems the same as modern people have. The statisticians can make the calculation to see the relation of stress with health problems and social problems in society. They can make the statistics to see the relation of time of using technology devices, time of exposing to the technology devices and the number of people diagnosed with the health problems and social problems; they will have the relationship between these trends. Moreover, using the questionnaires with the symptoms of table three, "the most symptoms of stress that we can find in many patients", to ask the people having problems, we will get astonishing results. Reviewing the statistics from the CDC, the top ten leading cause of America,

The top ten leading cause of America

1st Heart disease
2nd Cancer
3rd Chronic lower respiratory diseases
4th Accidents (unintentional injuries)
5th Stroke (cerebrovascular diseases)
6th Alzheimer's disease
7th Diabetes
8th Influenza and pneumonia
9th Nephritis, nephrotic syndrome, and nephrosis
10th Intentional self-harm (suicide)

Source: http://www.cdc.gov/nchs/fastats/leading-causes-of-death.htm

From the National Institute of Mental Health, the top global mental and behavioral disorders that cause the global years lived with disability (YLDs) 2010 are:

1st Major depressive disorder
2nd Anxiety disorders
3rd Drug use disorders
4th Schizophrenia
5th Alcohol use disorders
6th Bipolar disorder
7th Dysthymia
8th Autism and Asperger's disorder
9th ADHD and conduct disorder
10th Eating disorders
11th Other mental and behavioral disorders
12th Idiopathic intellectual disability

Sources: http://www.nimh.nih.gov/health/statistics/

References

National Institute of Mental Health. (n.d.). Global YLDs contributed by mental and behavioral disorders as a percent of total global YLDs (2010). Retrieved July 19, 2017, from http://www.nimh.nih.gov/health/statistics/

CDC National Center for Health Statistics. (2017, March 17). Leading causes of death. Retrieved July 19, 2017, from http://www.cdc.gov/nchs/fastats/leading-causes-of-death.htm

Part VII: Real Hunger in Abundance Living and Countless Problems

Chapter 30: The real hunger of modern people and its consequences

"The greatest disease in the West today is not tuberculosis or leprosy; it is being unwanted, unloved, and uncared for. We can cure physical diseases with medicine, but the only cure for loneliness, despair, and hopelessness is love. There are many people in the world who are dying for a piece of bread but there are much more dying for a little love. The poverty in the West is a different kind of poverty - it is not only the poverty of loneliness but also of spirituality. There's a hunger for love, as there is a hunger for God."

Mother Teresa

*** *** ***

Most diseases in modern society are the results of stressed state: chronic, even serious stressed. There are four causes of creating a stressed state, which leads to mental diseases, health problems, and social problems. These causes are lack of connection, lack of love, stressful environment and lack of ability of the individuals.

These four causes are interdependent. Combination of these four causes can create extreme stress in the individuals; in return, the stress worsens these four causes. The development of technology devices reduces significantly the quality of connection and quality of love between people. Especially, the love and connection parents give to their children.

Table 25: The four causes of human problems

The four causes of human problems	
1. Lack of connection	Human beings are the creatures of nature and society. So their basic need is the connection to the natural environment and social environment. They need to connect to all beings: parents, people, adults, kids, brothers, nature, trees, animals, and natural living environment; technology devices make this lacking worsen.
2. Lack of love	Unconditional love, unconditional support, and love come from understanding. Most of the love they received are angry love, blind love, ignorant love, greedy love, selfish love, and conditioned love; receiving these love making them more painful and stressful.
3. Stressful environment	Stress from family and the living society: parents, sibling, and adults, schools, teachers, friends, subject, and tests; environment: all things they see as the threatening. They do not get enough love, connection, ability and

	understanding to overcome the mild unwanted problems. And people also stressed because of unsatisfied basic needs.
4. Lack of suitable difficulties or challenges which lead to poor skills, poor ability, poor knowledge, or ignorance	Lack of suitable difficulties or challenges leads to a lack of essential skills and ability make them left behind. Conditional love, lack of connection and many threatening make them do not feel safe enough to learn more, do more, try more, ask more and play more to gain real powers, strength, and abilities. They misunderstand many essential things, and conflicts in human society as threatening. They are not understood by adults that the real things they need are unconditional love, connection, close contact, and supportive environment to feel safe to gain essential skills to understand and deal well with the problems they meet.

The best combination of love, connection, and good understanding creates an individual's ability. Love, connection, and understanding of the environment create inspiration, motivation, and safety for children to learn more, do more and risk more. These lead to strong abilities of the children. The best combination of love, connection, and understanding helps ordinary children become geniuses; and help them achieve far more success in life than ordinary people can imagine. On the other hand, the worst combination may create pain, fear, sadness, disappointment, hurt, wound, depression, and anxiety for the children. The smart children may affect extremely stressed if they live under the worst combination of these four factors. The lack of love, lack of connection, lack of understanding, stressful problems, and stressed state of mind interact with each other form a circle of cause and effect or a dot of cause and effect. Gradually, countless vicious circles are formed. The connection of these circles creates a downward spiral or downward life. The circle of cause and effect leave mark on thought, belief, brain structure, emotional life, spiritual life, cognitive thinking, gene, physical body, metabolism, skills, talent, ability, cognitive behaviors, and habits of the children. Gradually, children may affect some mental diseases, social problems, health problems, and bad characters.

On the bright side, we live in a society where there are talented people, genius, the saints, great men, and successful people; all of them grew up with naked small children. On the contrary, there also are the criminals, the slaughters, the poor, the disabled, the ill, and many miserable people in our society; all of them also grew up from naked small children. Some people are the sufferers of the living environment; in other words, they are the creators of their destiny.

What is the best combination of these four factors, what is the worst combination of these four factors? There is no exact answer, the combination is not only the science of achievement but also is the art of living well. Parents and leaders have to use the head and the heart to get the understanding; then they need to use the head and heart in serving and using the art of reward and punishment.

> "If your actions inspire others to dream more, learn more, do more, and become more, you are a leader."
>
> **John Quincy Adams**

I will prove the assumption in table fourteen "The four main causes cause most of the problems" by the theory and the knowledge that I know. I hope that researchers and statisticians will quantify these causes, and carry out the treatment to the needed people.

First, I will use mental disorders with the known symptoms of the disorders but do not fully know the causes. The mental disorder is increasing substantially in our modern society. Most concerns are autism, depression, and ADHD happening to many healthy children without any previous indicators. Especially, autism causes most of the worry in parents. Even worse, these problems happening to small children seem out of control, it creates stress and worries for many parents. I chose autism as an example because autism has some characters that are not understandable for the researchers, physicians, and scientists. On the other hand, the autistic characters easily explained by the assumption of the four causes in table eight.

The signs of Autism, from National Autism Association with my explanation in brackets and italics

Autism is a neurodevelopmental disorder characterized by:

- Social impairments (*"Lack of interacting skill or social skill, these skills needed a lot of effort to study and master"*).

-Cognitive impairments (*"Lack of cognitive thinking, this skill is very hard to form and master"*)

-Communication difficulties (*"How hard if you have to learn a new language or to live in a new country where there is only has danger? It is harder for the autistic children to learn to speak and read other emotion if the children have no joy or no safety in learning"*)

-Repetitive behaviors (*"The signs of the children have very little skill or learn just a few behaviors, they tend to repeat a few behaviors they learned"*)

Early Signs: a person child ASD (Autism spectrum disorder) might:

-Not respond to their name (*"They do not have much impressed with their name, they do not have the feeling of joy or happiness when hearing their name"*).

-Not point at objects or things of interest ("*Lack of interest in things. What is your interested when you are fearful, tired and stressed*")

-Not play "pretend" games ("*This game need a lot of cognitive thinking and imaginative thinking, the ability belong to emotional thinking. How hard to play pretend game with police officers, technical engineers or serious people? How easy it is to play a pretending game with healthy children who have a highly imaginative mind, irrational thinking, and little of prejudices!*")

-Avoid eye contact ("*Autistic children do not know to read information from the eye as normal children do*")

-Want to be alone ("*Lack of all vital social skills so the best way is to stay away from the crowd. They have suffered enough how painful when they contact with other. Sadly, this pain may come from the beloved ones*")

-Have difficulty understanding, or showing understanding, or other people's feelings or their own. ("*Autistic children lack the emotional intelligence so that they lack understand others and understand themselves*")

-Have no speech or delayed speech ("*How hard for children to learn to talk? Lack of love, connection, understanding, and a lot of stressful problems make children afraid to learn to talk. The slower start of speech makes them more stressed than healthy children also*")

-Repeat words or phrases over and over ("*It is very hard to learn, so when they learn anything, especially learning with joy, they tend to repeat that words: let observe the emotion or feeling when the autistic children repeating words*")

-Give unrelated answers to questions. ("*They do not have the cognitive thinking or intelligence to understand the questions and words of questions. They may give unrelated answers. Unfortunately, if autistic children get pain from answering, they may be so much more fearful with the learning that they choose to withdraw from learning*")

-Get upset by minor changes. ("*Living under the constant stressed state caused by living environment, they will be in response or upset with minor changes: minor changes can stimulate the fight or flight in autistic children. You can understand this when you are stressed or angry because of fear, overwork or in a stressful situation. How much love, connection, and understanding you need from your beloved ones?"*)

-Have obsessive interests. ("*Autistic children only know very little things, like or love very little things, and these things may bring joy for them, so that they may have these interests."*)

-Flap their hands, rock their body or spin in circles. ("*Perhaps they learn these behaviors by mimic the behaviors of characters in the shows on television*")

-Have unusual reactions (over or under-sensitivity) to the way things sound, smell, taste, look or feel. ("*The things with sound, smell, taste, look or feel may have some similarity with the stressed situation they have suffered. The familiar sound, smell, taste, look, and feel may appear in the situation that caused negative events in their family. Their unusual reactions are just the conditioned responses*")

-Have low to no social skills ("*Social skills are the hard skills learned from the environment. The autistic children are so much stressed that they learn very little or no social skills, on the other hand, the healthy children have enough joy, love, and connection to learning these social skills*").

-Avoid or resist physical contact (*"Physical contact creates many emotional signals; they will avoid and resist if they do not feel joyful, happy, and peaceful with physical contact. Quick-tempered parents usually make their children do not feel safe with any of their behaviors. Unfortunately, if they do not get enough physical contact, they may be indifferent with other people"*).

-Demonstrate little safety or danger of awareness. *("The show of lacking abilities")*

-Reverse pronouns (e.g., says "you" instead of "I")

People with autism may also:

-Have unusual interests and behaviors. (*"This is because of lacking skills and poor learning abilities"*)

-Have extreme anxiety and phobias, as well as unusual phobias (*"Any normal things in the living environment that created or related to their previous the stressed state will become their phobias. New Office workers may fear many things during their first day at work; they may have a lot of phobias. Experienced workers are less fearful than new workers are. Phobias come from not understand, misunderstand or previous experience"*)

-Line up toys or other objects. (*"Perhaps this is the mark of logical intelligence and spatial intelligence the autistic boys have"*).

-Play with toys the same way every time. (*"They learn only a few ways to play with toys"*)

-Like parts of objects (e.g., wheels)

-Become upset by minor changes. (*"Minor changes can be interpreted into big threats with stressed people"*).

Other Symptoms:

- Hyperactivity (*"A way of reducing the stress that they suffered in unusual ways; Moreover, constant acting help release enormous energy in small children"*)

- Impulsivity (*"Acting without thinking, they lack emotional intelligence, lack of compassion so that when they are irritated, they usually act with little thinking"*)

- Short attention span (*"The stressed state in mind and stress chemicals in the body make them lack of concentration."*)

- Aggression (*"Another word of expressing the overreact of hurting people"*)

- Cause self-injury. (*"To some extent, the self-injury activities may help them relief with pain in their brain and body. Who likes tattooing? Who like hurting themselves and others? Do you have any experience that you are so stressed that you want to hurt yourself?"*)

- Meltdowns (*"The tension in mind, thinking, and brain will lead to exhaustion very quickly"*)

- Unusual eating and sleeping habits (*"Eating and sleeping are affected by the feeling they have. Unusual feelings lead to unusual eating and unusual sleeping habits. Autistic children normally eat in fear, eat in sorrow and sleep with fear"*)

- Unusual mood or emotional reactions (*"This is the results from stress and hurt that they have suffered"*)

- Lack of fear or more fear than expected. (*"This comes from lack of understanding of the environment."*)

When I read these symptoms of autism, I got a chill. I visualized that these autistic kids had been gone through serious stress. Moreover, they are still being so stressful that they upset by minor changes. Observers can easily see and feel the stressed state through their actions, their reactions to the environment, and their reactions to stimulations of the environment. They can sense the stress chemicals available to autistic children. The effects of adrenaline, norepinephrine, and cortisone in table three: "the most symptoms of stress that we can find in many patients" may found in every autistic child.

I want to find out what are the real causes of autism, I cannot satisfy with the presumed causes by some researchers: A genetic basis to autism, environmental pollution, or the Valproic acid - a medicine for seizures. If one of these causes is true, they can create autistic mice in the laboratory. In fact, mice with autism have not yet successfully created; some researchers believe that the mice injected with Valproic acid have some autistic symptoms are not autistic mice. Moreover, if one of the above causes is true, so how can we explain the ratio between the numbers of autistic boys and autistic girls. Most of the living areas of autistic children are in cities, the very rare case of autistic children in the countryside, or rural areas. The fact there is all the above assumptions are wrong because these assumptions fail to prove the character of autism.

I think the real causes must belong to the lifestyle of family members (love), the caring for autistic children (connection), the energy in their families (peace - stress) and the ability of children; these are the four causes combine each other and create the effects on children.

The first health problem individuals possibly affect at the early stage of life is autism. If the infants' needs for connection and love are not satisfied, the infants may become irritation, anger, and stress. Even worse, the stressful atmosphere in their family caused by parents can make the stress of children more severe. Close observation can easily realize the stressful atmosphere in the families of autistic children. Their parents may be stressful with work, society, financial problem; lack of love and support from a partner or tired of the boring partner. Parents become stressed, make a lot of crying, a lot of blame, a lot of fucking, shouting; a lot of ruling of "have to", a lot of contempt signals. Many parents also get the symptoms of stress in table three: the most symptoms of stress that we can find in many patients. One of my vivid moments was about my first child three months ago, in the morning, he woke up, making some fun activities, but when he saw my wife suffering pain because of scram in her leg, he nearly burst into a tear. We had to hug him and calm him down. This has triggered in me with the thinking of what happening with children in a stressful family. I have read a lot of many mothers got depression after giving birth. The depression of the mothers comes from the stressful atmosphere in families that many readers and people have seen. How about the small children and the infants in those families, what suffering they have to bear; finding out the effects of stressful environment on small children are my main concerns. Some people in Vietnam said that the mother and father with over 30 or 35 years old are too old for giving birth and their children may get the defects and problems. This is just the people's assumption because the Westerners do not think that and they do not find the scientific proof for the assumption. After searching I found out that the habits, thinking, lifestyle, and emotion of the parents over 35 years old are too rigid, too tidy, too boring and too stressful for the forming and developing of fetus and children. The main concerns for the development of the children are the lifestyle and energy of living environment, it is not the number of years old of parents.

Lacking love, lacking connection combining with the endless stress can create health problems in young kids. Depending on the varieties of stressful environment, of lacking love, of lacking connection, the infants can get a different degree of stressed state. The fact is the effects of stress on the physical ability and mental ability of children varies so much that scientists have to use the term of Autism spectrum disorders (ASD) to describe the variety of autism.

Children affect which symptoms in the list of symptoms depend on the degree of stress that they have to suffer from the environment. The ability of an individual depends on the stage of life, gender, characters, instinct, strengths, and weaknesses. The ability of individuals, the lack of love, the lack of connection, the degree of the stressful environment and the intervention of physicians will determine the variety of the autistic symptoms. The above combination varies so much that the symptoms and progression of autistic children have so many varieties, scientists have to use Autism spectrum disorder (ASD) to describe autism.

The basic symptoms of autism, illustrated by the table below, are often accompanied by other medical conditions. These symptoms are the results of the constant stressed state that the autistic children have suffered. The varieties of each symptom depend on the environment and the abilities of children. Each specific group of symptoms with a right degree can create a specific definition of illness in medical care.

Table 26: Basic symptoms of autism accompanied by other medical conditions

Core autism symptoms	Associated neurological issues	Associated systemic issues	Related disorders
Social deficits	Sleep deficits	Immune dysfunction	Sleep disorders
Language impairment	Mood disorders	GI disorders	Mood disorders
Repetitive behaviors	Anxiety		Anxiety disorders
	Hyperactivities		Attention deficit hyperactivity disorder
	Lack of attention		Obsessive-compulsive disorder
	Seizures		

Sources: www.autismspeaks.org/what-autism/symptoms

The autism and other health problems in young boys and young girls are the serious side effects of excessive stress chemicals; these excessive stress chemicals come from the bearing of extreme stress in life.

Infants and kids are afraid of big noises, aggressive environment, beating, shouting, unsafe environment. Most of all they are afraid of a beating, comparing with others by their angry parents. They are afraid of the activities that harm the six needs of human beings. They are so weak and fragile that they need love, connection, peaceful environment to grow. Unfortunately, in modern society, there are plenty of technology devices, which attract the attention of children and family members; it means that these devices take away the connection and love of small children. Parents lost a large amount of time to connect with their children and other members. Children do not get enough love and connection they feel uncomfortable with some symptoms of stress. If not handle well, they may be stressed and make some bad behaviors like crying, shouting, and screaming. Making bad behaviors, children may receive back the anger of their parents and adults; which may make children more hurting and stressed. Their discomfort makes their unconscious mind misinterprets many unsatisfied things as threatens from the environment. It activates the stress system in children's bodies. Each time of stress, the stress hormones pump into the body and brain by themselves. If stress continues, it compounds into severe stress with many complications.

The complication at the first few years of life is autism; autistic children often have the stomach problem, which is the result of stress chemicals described in table three. Stomach disease usually occurs when people are worried, anxious and stressed. In the hospital, experienced doctors often prescribe psychotic medications with gastric medication for patients with acute stomach ulcer after some severe incidence. Patients with serious trauma in the hospital usually prescribed the gastric medication to protect the stomach because the stress from trauma may upset the stomach. In fact, people experienced serious stress usually got acute gastroenteritis. Worry and stress are some of the main factors cause stomach pain or intestine problems. The autistic children usually have digestive problems is proof that autistic children have been experiencing severe stress.

Why have the autistic children been gone through severe stress? During infant time, children are soft and weak. They need the love and connection of parents to feel protected, safe and happy. Children are extremely afraid of their parents to abandon them. Scientists have done a study to show how much love, how much connection animals need. In the documental film: "Emotional intelligence" of Daniel Gilbert has a short video to record this test. Researchers confined a baby monkey in a separate cage, left him very hungry. When the door of the cage opened to free the baby monkey to run in a room, where there are milk and a sample model of mother monkey. The model of mother monkey and the bottle of milk were parallel, separated by a panel. The little monkey rushed to the model of mother monkey; he twisted, hugged and played joyfully with the monkey model even he was very hungry. This video set a deep impression on me about the obsessed need of love and connection that small babies need. It creates a chill in me when I hear or see some parents punish their children crucially. The crucial punishment may relieve the anger for parents and make the children so afraid to obey the orders, but crucial punishment also leaves a big scar on children's soul. Their ignorance and ego of parents are so big enough that parents do not know they are creating bad karma for their children and society.

In some distressful families, parents always argue, blame, and shout at each other. They do not make enough love action, they do not care much for others to satisfy each other's needs. Parents' basic needs are not satisfied, it creates stress in the family. This is the beginning of the tragedy for their small children. To some extent, the financial situation makes them worried, along with lack of love, lack of support and lack of connection that make parents sad, angry and anxious. If the sadness, anger, and worry are not calmed down, parents may get severe stress. Some mothers even get depressed after giving birth. Because of being busy at work, spending time with technology equipment, parents spend very little time with their infants. This time is not enough to satisfy the need for love and connection of the infants. Even worse, not only lacking the number of time parents spend with their children, but also is the quality of time they spend with their children is terrible. They hug their children in anger, sadness and contempt mood. Even worse, there are some breastfeeding mothers feed the child while they are sad and crying because of the stress and loneliness. These sources of milk are poisonous for their children's physical and mental development. The infants lack love and live in the stressful environment with big noise, big cursing, big cry, less of hugging and kissing, lack of talking face to face. The subconscious of children is alerted and sensible to detect unwanted things and threatening signals. Moreover, they are too weak, too fragile; they do not have the ability and receive enough support to calm the arousing mind. These lead to over stimulate the mind, create an extremely stressed state, even worse, some children fall into seizures and panic state at the early stage of life. Full of chemical stress circulate around the young bodies. Repeated many times, children may be conditioned by the stress responses to the environment. After conditioning, children easily become stress as the responses to mild stimulations.

Some watchful mothers can read these early abnormal signs. Children may have the early symptoms of overload adrenalin and norepinephrine and cortisone-like sweating, nausea and vomiting, crying, pale skin, feeling shortness of breath, dizziness, weakness or tremors, headache, feeling nervous or anxious, a lot of crying, screaming, and sudden awake at night. These are the signs of stressed children. These symptoms may have long before the symptoms of autism. These symptoms listed in table three: the most symptoms of stress that we can find in many patients. The children start to cry a lot and or have some abnormal actions. If parents can intervene in time, they can save their children. They can calm the children with their love by hugs, time of contact, time of talking, and with a peaceful state of their mind.

Autistic children do not have the ability to read the emotional signals, so they misinterpret and cannot understand well with the emotional signals they receive. To join in community, the most important skill is reading and understanding the thinking and feelings of opposite people by the emotional signals. Lack of connection and lack of love at the early stage of life, autistic children do not understand these signals and tend to afraid of these signals. People usually afraid of or overreact to things they do not understand.

"In this world, there is always danger for those who are afraid of it". **George Bernard Shaw**

Autistic children are not able to interact with and understand the other person's ideas. It means they lack emotional intelligence. Emotional intelligence is the ability to understand human emotions, which formed in the early stage of human life. The infants have the premature brain, the brain is in process of developing to mature brain during several first years of their life. Children crave for human affection, love, and human connection to feel protected, safe and happy. The happy state during early childhood is the best condition for the perfection of the immature brain. On the other hand, the stress state during early childhood is the worst condition for the perfection of the immature brain. It is very dangerous if bad thing interferes with the perfection of the immature brain. The bad intervention can leave the defect in brain structures and brain functions.

The role of connection and love to the development of newborn baby may found in the living of children in orphanages. During the early stages of life in the orphanage, the infant babies receive caring well; they have enough support for physical development. Children in orphanages do not have to live in a stressful environment like autistic babies. Unfortunately, they do have enough love and do not have enough connection with the human being to form social skills in critical time. The lack of love and connection can abnormalities in the orphans' mind and brain and create a little stress on them. The effects of abnormalities and mild stress are obvious after they adopted by their parents; some adopted children have a lot of difficulties to join in communities, new family, and classes. These adopted children lack the critical skills to survive in human society. Joining in everyday activities in society is much easy with normal children, but it is very difficult and stressful for children from orphanages. At the early stage of life, children in orphanages lack love and connection with human being in the most important period of developing of the brain. The lack of love and connection during the development of the brain leads to the lacking of vital social skills. To some extent, the autistic children also lack these vital social skills as the children in orphanages because they lack love, lack of connection, lack of vital skills and living in a stressful environment. Fortunately, the children in orphanages do not have to live in a stressful environment like autistic children, so that they have different problems with the autistic children.

Why these autistic children lack social skills but some autistic children have good abilities in logic and learning other skills. Most Autistic children like to look at cubic things and moving objects. They do not pay much attention to the emotion signals from the faces and eyes of people. Perhaps they lack emotional skill; they are not good at emotional intelligence so that they cannot understand the importance of eyes and faces in expressing information. Lacking the ability to understand messages, emotions, or feelings in people's eyes and faces make them not interested in seeing it. Not seeing the face makes them miss many chances of learning, interacting to improve emotional intelligence. As a human being, interaction skill is the most important skill for good living in a human society where people mainly communicate with emotional signals. Lacking social skill, autistic children find it is hard to integrate into the community. Early first signs, the children are indifferent, not concentrated, slow language and aggression, making strange behaviors, doing things unnaturally. These are the indicators that the children are under stress and have emotional disorders. Autistic children cannot read other people's emotions in the environment so they are afraid of interacting with people. They chose to stay away from the crowd to protect them from the harm.

Most autistic children are in the cities, in industrial zones, rarely in rural villages. Because in cities autistic children have less time connecting with nature and other human beings, less time of playing freely, less time to play with other kids than the children live in rural areas. They only play with toys, televisions, phones in artificial spaces, these things only make interested for short time. These spaces have no vitality, no energy, no fun and nothing that stimulates and creates curiosity in children. The young children need the space of living, which is funny, freely, naturally and rich in energy to create more energy in children. The energy of children and environment exchanges in many ways we do not know. Therefore, there is little energy in artificial places of living. You see how tasteless when watching artificial flowers with closed, clean spaces versus how joyful for children plant a rose in the garden, watering it and watch its growing with blooming flowers. The difference between the energy in the countryside and the energy in the home of autistic children may be the same as the difference between the energy in kindergarten and the energy with nursing homes. I have worked with two Singaporean doctors; they made me rethink the role of the natural environment. One doctor shows very interested in a mantis in his flowers pot; he took a lot of pictures of the mantis and post on his Facebook account with excitement. I was astonished by his behaviors because, in the countryside of Vietnam, we see a lot of mantises on the trees. The other Singaporean doctor told that he is very like to live in Vietnam because after working hours, he can go to see hundreds of ducks swimming, birds singing, cows and buffalos on fields. You can sense that energy of joy by seeing the happiness in the eyes and actions of children; as a father, just seeing or remembering these kinds of actions of my child help me understand how important to give space for the children to playing freely with full energy.

If kids are not satisfied with their deep need and have to live with the boring environment, they gradually lose interest, lack of vital skills and dull their instinct. Lacking energy from environment make kids uncomfortable, lose the interest in things, in life, lose the enthusiasm to read environment, do not feel happy, and do not feel energetic in living; they become indifferent with life. These are the signs of losing the vital fuel of life, lacking the active energy. If paying attention to the behaviors, the emotions and the reactions of the children, parents can have a better understanding of their children, their energy, and emotions they have. If there are any abnormities in the behaviors and emotions of children, parents need to solve those abnormities as soon as possible. Parents should care for the fluidity and the natural manner in behaviors of young children; even parents should try hard to encourage their children to speak funny words, silly words, playing freely. Most importantly is making children smile; parents should make stressed children smile as much as possible. Because smiling is in action shows that children feel safe, secured, protected and extremely joyful. Parents should take precaution to unnatural signals every time like rigidity and stiffness in actions, lack of emotion in actions, lack of energy and enthusiasm in playing of young children; these signals are against nature, it means that children may feel unsafe. Parents have to get a real understanding and make their children feel safe.

In the rigid environment, children's needs are not satisfied, they may feel uncomfortable; their unconscious mind activates the chemical of stress in case of need for their safety. Live in a closed, rigid environment, children may lose all chances of forming some vital skills to deal with problems in real life, especially in a stressful situation. Small children in the countryside are more likely to play with nature, to play with one another, with friends of the same age; they have tremendous opportunities to learn, think, negotiate, play, and interact with other human beings; these activities sharpen their vital social skills. Gradually, owning for the supportive environment children can increase their intelligence; the intelligence may be the combination of emotional intelligent (EQ), adaptive intelligent (AQ), spiritual intelligence (SQ), social intelligence (SQ), and intelligent quotient (IQ). In my opinions, if the environment supports well for the children, they can develop these multiple intelligences astonishingly. Children in rural areas can gain some good skills from playing in nature that helps them adapt well to the changes and pressures from the environment. The disadvantage of children in rural areas is they lack a good education, lack of time and resources for studying. To some extent, the difference in living environments has helped the children in rural areas overcome the family stress better than autistic children in the city.

> "Look deep into nature, and then you will understand everything better." **Albert Einstein**

Children in the city have less chance to interact with others; they spend most of the time on television, smartphones and playing toys. Time for parents in city play with children is very little. Most of the time children in Vietnam spend time with the domestic helpers who have little connection, compassion and little love for children; they only for care physiological needs. Most of the domestic helpers rarely talk, embrace and hug children with love like their parents do. These domestic helpers without emotion are like robots. The first important stage of life of autistic children in the city, they have far less time spent on direct contact, direct communication, close connecting and close interacting with other people than normal children do. If paying attention, parents can read the early signs of stress and indifference in their children. Can you imagine the scenario: "parents and adults in city arguing loudly, a lot of shouting and crying, beating and skipping meals, meanwhile their small children lie in bed with frailty, scare, intense, tremble and indifference, you will know what they want." They are in extreme stress state with a lot of stress chemicals run throughout the body. Early visible problem is stomach upset with a lot of vomiting and excessive acid. Each stress, cortisone, adrenalin, and nor-epinephrine pumped into the body. Children activate the stress system as if they are in a dangerous environment; all functions reduced, just putting all the effort in stress state like "fight or flight". Unfortunately, they cannot fight and they cannot fly except crying and screaming. Stressed children may turn away, have feelings of insecure, indifferent to many things and do not look at their parents' eyes. Because of fear and stress, when parents hug them, they resist with the stiffness in muscle, do not put their head on their parent's shoulder comfortably; they cry more often, sudden awake during sleep. These are the signals that children are in problems. When there is stress in the family, the autistic children are the weakest member of the family, bearing the most consequences of the stress, conflict and negative emotions in the family. They have signals of stress with more watchful, awake and unsafe at home as if they are in the new environment. They need the love and connection of parents to calm negative feelings down. If parents misread the behaviors of children, they not only miss the opportunity for their children to gain the materials to support the development of emotional intelligence in the previous phase of life but also, they worsen the stress that their children have to bear. Observing children in safe, we will see they are stretching arms, playing freely and naturally;

talking and singing endlessly, smiling all day, making many funny and silly actions; hugging comfortably and sleep comfortably on the shoulder of parents.

Why is the earlier stage of life the precious time? Precious time relates to the development of the brain. Infant's brain lack lots of normal functions; infant babies cannot see, cannot hear; they just feel the emotions and energy from the surrounding. The first stage of life is the period of the rapid perfection of the brain. It will be very dangerous when the first phase of this life is interrupted, especially caused by panic or stress. If we look at the living conditions of autistic children, there is a lot of pressure and negative energy, which is harsh and stressful for the immature brain of the children.

If we make statistics of direct interaction time between parents with autistic children and parents with normal children, we will see the relation. Epidemiology of autism also shows that when parents are older, their children are more likely to have autism. For me, this is evidence of poor energy in interaction and less connection and the bad lifestyle of living. The old people often prefer more silence, serious in action, strict in order and neatness than the young parents do. This also reduces the chance of playing for children and creates additional psychological pressure on the children.

Why the number of autistic boys higher than the number of autistic girls, which is four times higher in the United States and eight times higher in Vietnam. This is the evidence of the advantage in individual ability; here is the instinctive advantage of gender. From ancient time, women were often at home, doing agriculture works, caring for and protecting their children from danger. Thus, they created a high degree of emotional intuition; quick understand the child feelings; and a comprehensive scanning the intention of strangers. Mothers have to have good judgment of stranger's intention standing behind their children in a blink of an eye. Just listening to the crying of their babies, mothers can understand what the babies need, are they in danger or not. This ability is perfect for the instinct of mothers because it is formed from the early stages of life. With them, emotional skills and social skills are the most prioritized. Baby girls prioritize develop emotional and social skills earlier than baby boys do. With good interaction intelligence, baby girls tend to care for others, smile, make fun, talk and affection behaviors more than baby boys at the same age. In Vietnam, cute girls usually get more hugging, cuddling, loving action, kissing on cheeks and talking than baby boys do. In characters relate to gender, girls are familiar with adjective "cute" which belongs to emotional intelligence and boys are familiar with adjective "smart" which belong to logical intelligence. Baby girls usually like to play the game with emotions like playing with dolls, playing drama, when becoming older they like the work of caring for people. These are the reasons that the emotional intelligence of girls formed earlier than boys do.

On the other hand, boys are different. In the ancient environment: men hunted, built houses and fought. Therefore, men need broad coverage, fast and accurate action with strength. The intelligence optimal for men roles and functions is logical and spacing, and reasoning intelligence. Most boys form IQ, logic, reasoning earlier than girls do. The most favorite games of boys are matching, fixing, repairing and playing number games, which require logical thinking. This is the reason why modern scientists, engineers, IT, mathematicians are mostly men. In boys, the development of logical thinking during the first year of childhood is the most prioritized. Emotional intelligence is not optimal for the roles of men so that emotional intelligence can develop later.

A team of researchers led by psychologist Stuart Ritchie, a date of an ongoing, long-term biomedical study of people living in the United Kingdom with 500,000 enrollees. Researchers found that women tended to have significantly thicker cortices than men have. Thicker cortices have been associated with higher scores on a variety of cognitive and general intelligence tests. Meanwhile, men had higher brain volumes than women in every subcortical region they looked at, including the hippocampus (which plays broad roles in memory and spatial awareness), the amygdala (emotions, memory, and decision-making), striatum (learning, inhibition, and reward processing), and thalamus (processing and relaying sensory information to other parts of the brain).

The problem begins to happen to the small young boys, who have logical intelligence, spatial intelligence and do not have emotional intelligence, live in stressful condition. These young boys lack love, lack of connection and have to bear the stress, conflict of the environment in the early stages of life. Because of sexual instinct, girls have the opportunity to develop emotional intelligence earlier than boys do, so they have the ability to resolve the conflict, calm stress so that, to some extent, stress or conflict does not harm them at the earlier stage of life. Otherwise, the earlier development of logical intelligence and spatial intelligence does not help much the baby boys in dealing with stress; in a stressful environment, boys tend to fall into extreme stress. Owning for the difference in the instinct of gender, girls do not fall into the state of severe stress as most boys do. Only a small difference, formed earlier, have helped girls become more prominent than boys in combating autism.

The habit of autistic children perhaps is the evidence that boys have formed the intelligence of space and logic before affecting autism. This logic and space intelligence have been showed when autistic children play; many autistic boys turn his gaze on cubic things; they like to put, match cubic things in stack or sequences. I wonder if the intelligence of the baby boys has any relation with the intelligence of their parents.

The difference created by emotional intelligence between boys and girls in dealing with stress may obviously found in the two situations of conversation. If given a task for a female comedian to ask her professor for letting her retakes the exam because of the bad result. Simultaneously, if giving a task for a male engineer to ask his professor for letting him retakes the exam because of the bad result. We will see many of the differences on their faces, the atmosphere of conversation, and the quality of conversations. The female comedian is more open-minded, more flexible than the male engineer is. The first conversation is flexible with full of smiling, cheerfulness, and relaxation; the conversation is very interesting. In reverse, the second conversation is rigid with full of anxiety, rigidity, stress, a lot of mumbling; the second conversation is so stressful boring. The first conversation both people are relaxed, the unconscious mind detect the signal of safe and happy; the happy state is activated, so both people are happy, more open to talking. The positive energy of the first conversation creates a good result that satisfies both people in a natural way. On the other hand, the male engineer's behaviors are so rigid that the conversation may make him have the feeling of stress, anxiety, boring and misery during the second conversation. These signals are caught by the subconscious mind of the professor so that it makes the professor in the state of alert; these alert signals also be caught by the engineer man. Both men in the state of a little stress, people can feel reserved and closed signals. The answer engineer man gets tend to fit with the atmosphere of conversation. The difference in EQ in both intelligent individuals can make different results in social life. Perhaps, these differences accumulating with time is the most contribution to create outliers.

If look close to autistic children or children with other mental problems, we can see they are nervous, panic, startled, frightened and paralyzed and apathetic to many things in the environment. The nervous system of autistic children is not fully developed. First few years of life is a precious time for children to complete the brain and nervous system. They need emotional materials from the interaction, from love, from the adoring eyes of loved ones, from cuddling, patting, from the warmth of hugs and many social behaviors to perfect the development of the immature brain. Moreover, there is always tensions and stress in the stage of developing the immature brain. That leads to the formation of the brain with many dysfunctional functions. Researchers have seen individuals with autism tend to use different areas of the brain to perform mobility tasks compared to normal groups.

There are no same specific signals and symptoms in every autistic child. Autism is a disorder of the whole body system, evolving over time and constantly interacting with many factors from the environment. As a result, people use a rainbow ring as a symbol to describe the diversity of autism.

How about the young babies left in the jungle, adopted by animals? These babies lack connection with human beings, lack of support for physical development, lack of love from parents so they lack social human skills. To some extent, they get a close connection, love, and care for wild animals. Through the imitation and the influence of the living condition, these children have learned some survival skills, which help them overcome the problems in wildlife. Living with the wild animals, these children have conditioned with the responses of these wild animals. The repeated responses in babies by the influence of the environment of living created the animal habits in the babies adopted by animals. From the adopted habits, repeated many times, the individuals will have specific adopted animal characters. These animal characters make them very difficult to live with other human beings.

By experimental in mice, we can see these effects of lacking love, connection and excessive stress on the development of animals during the early stage of life. If the mouse is isolated and put in the over-stressful state by shocking at an early stage of life, we will get an autistic mouse. If the mouse is not isolated and being over-stressful, we will get a mouse with some of the side effect symptoms of stress described in table three. If the mouse is isolated from the early stage of life and not being stressful, it will be very difficult for the mouse to join in the normal activity with others mice because of lacking the interaction skills. These are also the problem with the animals in the zoo, the tamed animals; if we free these mature animals into the jungle, they will die soon because of lacking vital skills for survival and connection with other animals. If my guessing is right, this will be evidence of real problems in our modern society. Infants and young babies are the first victims of the problems.

This can be a curse to our future generation who belongs too much to machines, artificially intelligence and robots, technology devices and living in the environment with lack of love, lack intimate action and lack human connection and lack of support. The new conditions of living from now on will entirely different to any conditions in the previous history. The new condition has conditioned the new responses, new skills for our future generations. Unfortunately, these new responses are not helpful for us to cope with stress. In fact, the conditioned responses children adopted from the condition of living make them more stress with the stressful environment and diminish the ability to learn new vital skills. Lacking vitals skills lead them to be more stressful; in return, the stress worsens the ability to learn vital skills. Gradually, the combination of stressful environment and lacking social skills create many problems for personal, family and society.

To this point, we can see autistic children have lost their emotions and defect in brains. Most autistic children have a less emotional expression, no attention to the emotions of the opposite person when interacting. So the brain affected, losing the function of the normal brain. If late in realizing the problems with children, it will be very difficult to help autistic children because the brain has already completed the basic development. The brain of autistic children lacks normal structures, the normal connection between the parts of the brain compared to the normal brain. Treatment by a specialist is very difficult, expensive and not much effective if not taking the roots of problems. Many accompanying symptoms in autistic children are treatable with some medicines. The most effective way is parents and adults can check themselves and their kids with the symptoms of overstress chemicals described in table three: "the most symptoms of stress that we can find in many patients". If yes, they can make the intervention as quickly as possible with these real causes.

I have taken time to practice compassion with the feelings of any children I met who are punished severely by their children. Especially the children when their parents are quarreling. Sometimes I cannot stand the ten minutes in places of those children with the pain, fear, and injury they are bearing. Their parents dive into personal anger and stress so blindly that they do not pay any attention to their children who are extremely fearful and stressful. Furthermore, the conflicts make them less talking, less chatting, less making love action, less caring, less direct talking, and less interacting to soothe the stress of the child. The stress and pain they are bearing lead them to lack of interesting in studying, lack of supporting and lack of vital skills. These are the first step in endless circles of stress that they have to bear.

In my mind, the overreacting, rebelling, indifferent responding, screaming and shouting with the anger of some children are not the intentional behaviors; they are the conditioned action as the responses to the stressful condition.

They fall into the stressed state because of their wrong perceiving thoughts, their wrong perceiving opinions from the environment; and their overreactions to the environment. These kids are the individuals that need the love, connection, compassion, understanding and patience from their parents the most. Please do not hurt them anymore.

Remember the moment you have the feeling of insecurity, anxiety, and fear when you are in a strange environment, difficult situations, and dangerous situations. How much love, how much support and how much caring, do you need in those situations? The autistic children have badly experienced the insecurity, anxiety, fear and extreme stress in early-stage life. The feeling of pain and insecure make children not only lost the enthusiasm, and refuse to learn new skills; but also make the results of learning is terrible. The children getting severe stress in the early stage of life lack a lot of essential skills for social interaction. The lacking of vital social skills makes them afraid of coming to a new crowd, new environment, and new places. The autistic children mostly separated from nature and human interaction by the inadvertent or deliberate blind love of their parents; the isolation makes the children have less chance and less enthusiasm for learning social skills which leads to abnormalities in the mind and brain of the autistic children. The children lack some vital skills for social interaction. The lacking makes the child hesitate, afraid to interact with strangers, afraid the crowd; feel unsafe, unprotected in the condition need interacting. They seek security, safety by living alone.

Sometimes, when kids hunger for love, for being cared for, for being wanted, they act in different or abnormal ways to satisfy the hunger. Parents and adults usually misinterpret these abnormal behaviors as the behaviors of spoilt children. They may disappointed and angry; even worse, parents may use violence to punish their children violently. The punishment of parents can make children so afraid that they stop the abnormal behaviors; but the hunger, cause of unwanted behaviors, is still in the children, furthermore, the punishment of parents can lead to severe stress for their children. I have heard many stories of naughty children transformed into good and talent ones by the love, the care for of parents or teachers; who have the empathy with the children and since the deepen need of children. They use loving and caring action, compassion, patience, and respect to nurture the hidden talents of naughty children.

Medications can relieve the symptoms, but cannot cure autism. Some researchers have figured out some ways to help to relieve the symptoms:

Some researchers have injected autistic mice with oxytocin, and they found oxytocin has some good effects on autistic mice. They think of carrying out more research to find a way to apply oxytocin to treat autistic children in the future. As we know, oxytocin is a natural hormone appears when people make close contact: make love, have sex, kiss, hug, playing with parents and children, and breastfeeding. These intimacy activities help create oxytocin in both parents and autistic children; which helps them feel more inspired and happy to overcome the stress. When the mothers give birth, oxytocin released at the highest peak. If mothers do not have much close contact with the children; do not make love and get affection from fathers, all parents and their children will be lack of oxytocin, this leads to lack of joy and happiness in family life and makes stress for all members. Some mothers are so stressful after giving birth that they may get depressed. Mothers and children in the family are the early victim of stress in the family. If test them with the question of the symptoms in table three, we will know how much stress they are.

Some experts found that pets: dogs, cats, parrots can relieve symptoms in autistic kids. In fact, dogs, cats, parrots are emotional animal. I think pets create a little feeling of being loved, being cared for, being wanted for autistic children so that they can relieve the symptoms in autistic kids. In fact, these feelings so little compare to the feeling that parents can give to them.

> "All that I am, or hope to be, I owe to my angel mother."
>
> **Abraham Lincoln**

These may be the sharing of most successful people who have a happy childhood, their mother or father may not have a college education, but they may have their Ph.D. in parenting.

These are the evidence show that the most effective way to help autistic children is eliminating the stress in children by the unconditional love, the connection, the caring of parents and family members. Infants, especially autistic children need much more love and connection by more hug, more intimacy talk, more talk eye to eye, more kiss, more skin contact, more caring, affection actions, more contact with other people. Parents can massage children more regular; help children exposing to nature more often, and make children happy by creating a peaceful and happy environment of living.

When the children become older, if they may be more stressful because the four causes lack love, lack of connection, lack of vital skills for interaction and live in the stressful environment; they will get many other health problems or diseases. The seriousness of problems depends on the seriousness of stress, the lack of connection, the lack of love and the lack of social skills. They may get the diseases in the category of top ten diseases or the top ten causes of death in every country in the world.

Think out of the boxes:

Are abilities, geniuses, outliers, failures, autism, ADHD, depression, seizures, anxiety disorder or talented caused by a single factor or by a continuous process that can slow down, stopped or reversed? And how can we master it?

1. All autistic kids have delayed speech or poor communication skills or poor social skills; these problems can be predicted and prevented well by parents very soon during the early months old of the kids. So can we prevent autism by preventing delayed speech and preventing poor social and emotional skills for kids?

2. Best for kids: accept we may wrong to create more chances for kids grow. Socrates smart because he said he did not know anything. I feel cramp of gut feelings when seeing the parents of kids with lots of problems said they know all things and start to blame all things except themselves for their problems.

3. By observing and reading the body language, eye contact, and interaction skills, do you think we can predict early signs of autism, ADHD since 2,4,6 or 8 months old or long before the official diagnosing?

4. By observing, reading the body language, making eye contact, do you think that we can predict early signs of autism, ADHD since 2, 4, 6 or 8 months old?

5. Do successful cases of intervention for autism and difficult speaking overthrow the ideas of the cause is by genes and brain structure?

6. Do successful cases of intervention for autism overthrow the ideas that fixed genes and brain structure is the cause?

7. Group of autistic kids is included in the group of delayed speech kids, because most of the autistic kids have delayed speech, and none of the autistic kids can communicate and manage emotion well, so autistic kids are included in delayed speech kids, right? Then can we prevent autism by predicting and curing delayed speech, poor social skills, and poor emotional skills in the small kids? I know that all are learnable skills and can be done well by all parents.

8. I awaken when a parent told me about the obvious symptoms of autistic kids: 1. No social smiling, 2. Lack of eye contact, 3. Not responding to their name, 4. No social anticipation or Peek-A-Boo, 5. Poor visual tracking, 6. Lack of social babbling, 7. Fixation on unusual objects. I see that these are just signs of learnable social skills.

9. If kids with are taught to speak, communicate and master emotion well, do they still have autism? I see none of the autistic

kids can communicate well and master emotion well in special schools? So I doubt the temporary ideas about autism and think that there are always simple ways to teach angel kids all of these skills!

10. Is there any autistic kids do not have delayed speech, is there any autistic kids communicate well, is there any autistic kids manage emotion well? What exactly the percent and the number of the kids? Does the answer give you any clues?

11. Kids with autism, ADHD have poor communication, poor languages and strange react; do you think parents can predict the problems by observing since 2, 4 or 6 months old?

12. Million angels: "They may live in stress, eating in fear, sleeping in anxiety, playing in the boring safe side, wearing luxury clothes in discontentment, studying with pressure, getting lifesaving vaccination hysterically, and sexing with contempt. They never find real joy and happiness. Stress chemicals: Adrenalin, noradrenalin, and cortisone can create countless side effects on patients, which listed in any medical book."

13. Nature of learning is learning without stress, learn just with joy, enthusiasm, with love, endless energy, and participate in all intelligence. The environment just supplies Unconditioned Love, Connection – Understanding, Encourage Environment, and Chances of Building Abilities.

14. Never do I see the high percent of autistic kids have same problems of delayed speech and poor social skills or poor EQ like this, the percent may be more than 80% or 90% of autistic kids. So I doubt that this is the big clues in dealing with the problems that we forget in dealing with the problems.

15. Playing is learning, watching is learning, sleeping is learning, and doing is learning... Kids may experience "Flow" from the early stage of life. Kids' most powerful tools are the weakness, beloved, cute, enthusiasm, pay attention, curiosity, asking, imagining, and learn, try, fail, think, learn, try, fail, think, learn, try, fail, think with joy and safety. Think about that before each

time of intervention.

16. Sorry, Is autism a single event or a continuous process? What does rainbow tell us, and what is the mechanism of special education?

17. Sorry, what if autism, ADHD can be predicted, prevented or relieved effectively by family members as the special teachers do?

18. Walking, thinking, speaking native languages, studying countless skills, one-year-old kids, two-year-old kids, three-year-old kids never have to sit at a table to learn. But that time kids can learn more than anybody can imagine. Think about that before any blind intervention.

19. What if parents know the way to eradicate delayed speech for all kids, and make kids have high EQ, will the autism be eradicated too? I see there is no autistic kids can communicate well or have good social skills!

20. You do not teach healthy kids to learn the languages: English, Japanese, Chinese, and Vietnamese... but kids can make it become their instinct. That is the nature of learning without learning, Kid under three years old never have to sit at the table to learn, but they learn every time with joy.

References:

Autism Speaks. (n.d).Symptoms. Retrieved July 19, 2017, from http://www.autismspeaks.org/what-autism/symptoms

National Autism Association. (n.d.) Signs of Autism. Retrieved July 19, 2017, from http://nationalautismassociation.org/resources/signs-of-utism/

Price, Michael. (2017, April 11). Study finds some significant differences in brains of men and women. Retrieved July 19, 2017, from http://www.sciencemag.org/news/2017/04/study-finds-significant-differences-brains-men-and-women

Chapter 31: The real cause of mental problems and social problems in older kids

When people become anger or stress, they will have the symptoms of stress described in table two: some of the symptoms like shortness of breath, palpitation, cramped muscles, fearfulness, pale skin, scare of big noise, insomnia, susceptibility, tiredness, chilliness. These people with stress usually go to the hospital for health check more often than happy people do. Chronic stress can make people become sick, exhausted, and get flu symptoms; some children even suffered gastric and intestinal problems. The children go through the stressful state because so many unwanted things or hurtful things happened to them but they do not know how to reduce stress. Gradually, disease appears during childhood or adolescent, they may have other problems, such as depression, anxiety, eating disorders, mental disorder, intestine disorders, addict drug, addict smoke, ADHD and so on; these are also the kinds of physical disorders, cognitive disorders, and mental disorders happen to children in our society. These problems are the products stress on the development of children. The increasing trends of these problems recently are also the reflection of increasing stress in our society. In a stressed state, children easily become anger, they express with screaming and crying to attract the attention of their parents, to get the love, help, connection and paying attention from their parents. Unfortunately, if these bad behaviors repeat gradually, children may get bad habits that annoy their parents. Because of stress, children may get some bad habits. To cope with bad actions from children, most parents and adults give their children high tech gadgets like smartphone and computer, where there is game with sound, pictures, flash of light to attract the attention of children; other time, they may use violence or pressure to force the children to get rid of the bad habits. All of these ways can make children become more obey the order of adults but these ways also the causes of severer stress in children life. If parents use the negative way like violence, and pressure on stressed children, they will make their children suffer more stress with hurt, pain, and fear; in other words, parents may unconsciously enlarge the wound in the soul of their children. The more stressed children are, the worse habits children may get. Stress, wanting, and bad habits are the causes of misery for all members of family and society. So that the most effective way to help children in stress is by understanding, making them feel significance, love, connection, compassion, and patience.

Children like to react in stress situation with rebelling, shouting, screaming, doing unusual things, drinking alcohol, using drugs, eating, smoking because these things have the mechanism to relieve the stress that they have to suffer. Understanding the mechanism of stress and reducing stress can help adults understand that become naughty children is one way of stressed children to reduce the stress they have to bear.

What happens with the obedient children? On the one hand, they have to bear the stress and conflict of the family. On the other hand, they are so obedient that they do not do anything against the orders of their parents, they do not want to make any naughty actions; even doing these may help them reduce stress. This is the reason why good children in the family are the ones who suffer stress the most. Furthermore, male kids like to take action, like to run, play or use motion in studying because of their instincts; the female kids like to ruminate the negative emotions and feeling that they have in a stress situation. This perhaps is the reason to explain the problem that stressed kids will have. In fact, there is a big difference between the genders in the problems of ADHD and depression in kids. According to healthline.com "Males are almost three times more likely to be diagnosed with ADHD than females." According to "Teen depression statistics & facts" from teenhelp.com:

"17.3% of adolescents that had a major depressive episode in 2014 were female."

"5.7% of adolescents that had a major depressive episode in 2014 were male."

> The naughty child likes rebelling to reduce stress. Good child bears the stress without any rebelling because of their goodness and responsibility. That is why the good child gets more stressed than a naughty child get. Gradually, the good child may get mental health problems because of their goodness, responsibility, consideration, and helplessness.

Moreover, the stressed state and the massive of stress hormones to prepare for "fight and flight", but the male children cannot fight or flight. They have to stay still in the environment of stress with the disability of acting and bearing all the stress and stress hormones. It means male children have to bear the severe destruction of massive stress chemicals in the body than female children so that male kid usually has the atonic symptoms with other diseases; the male kids may be the victims of physical stress. The female children usually ruminate the negative thinking, negative emotion, and negative feeling, so that the female kids will have psychical symptoms with other diseases; the female kids may be the victims of psychical stress or emotional stress. We can easily see different the pattern of symptoms: atonic symptoms, atonic symptoms and psychic symptoms in many other health problems in small boys and small girls. For example, the disease like epilepsy, the disease also has the big difference between the patterns of symptoms in the young boys and young girls.

The vital roles of male and female to the survivals of human beings had made women evolved toward mastering the vitals skills for giving birth and caring for children and had made men evolved toward mastering the vitals skills for hunting and protecting. So that men and women have different strengths and weakness; they are complete each other; they are fit to each other, but they never same to each other. Because of the difference between the strengths and weakness between men and women, they have the different pattern of acting in dealing with stress. The different patterns of responding with stress have left the different tracks in health problems in men and women. Men and women may have the same health problem but the varieties of symptoms in the problems between men and women are not the same. Under stress situation, men are more likely to become the victims of physical stress, and women are more likely to become the victims of mental stress.

Let see some facts done by scientists to show the difference of dealing with stressful situations between men and women. From Uspharmacist.com, in stress situation:

Men more likely increase sleep but women decrease sleep. Men more likely increase appetite but women decreased appetite. Women more likely to decrease the consumption of energy but men do not. To fight and flight well, men need to prepare enough energy and restore energy quickly. The fear and anxiety that women have may harm their children so that they cannot sleep, cannot eat.

Men and women more likely to decrease the concentration.

Women more likely increase interpersonal sensitivity but men do not. This difference may come from the vital roles in human spices: men with fighting and protecting and women, women with giving birth and caring. You cannot kill an animal when having high interpersonal sensitivity, but you cannot care for children without interpersonal sensitivity. In a stress situation, men and women still keep their instincts, and these instincts may make the stress and anger become worse.

Men have more suicidal ideation but women do not. This may be the results of so many responsibilities put on men. Failure, losing and breaking is very terrible with men, especially when he bears a lot of responsibilities in family, community, and country; perhaps this is true with Japanese men. The compound of these things can make the man have more of suicidal action.

Eating, sleeping, and acting makes a man do not suffer physical problem like leaden paralysis. On the other hand, women eat less, sleepless, and usually ruminate more the thoughts and feelings that make women so much more tired than men are. Women more likely to increase leaden paralysis.

The statistic from Australian social trends 1998, "Health experiences of men and women", men have higher death rates at all ages and report more serious conditions than women. Women report the less serious conditions more often than men report and assess their own health more negatively. Moreover, the two leading causes of death were cancer and ischemic heart disease, together accounting for 50% of all deaths. Male to female ratios for these causes of death were 1.7 and 1.9 respectively. The greatest disparities were for accidents and suicide, male to female ratios of 2.6 and 4.2 respectively, which together accounted for only 6% of all deaths despite their prominence in the younger age groups.

Because of many unwanted things happened, parents may become stressed, their body is in the state of highly alerted, even a normal noise can make them startle and overreact. Adults or older children in tension are easily fallen into anger and panic with normal stimulations. Older children and adults with chronic stress may lead to many health problems like depression, decreased immune function, irritability, worry and insomnia, cardiovascular diseases and metabolic diseases. All of these stressed people should be a test of the symptoms of stress chemicals to have the early intervention.

If we make statistics show the trends over the years of the causes such as divorce, family stress, domestic violence, the number of quarrels, the closeness to nature; time of parents completely at home, communication between family members, spending time for others; and the time spent on TV, smartphones, online games, technology devices, social web. Other statistics show the trends over the year of problems like mental problems: depression, personality disorders, autism, suicide, harassment, dropouts, disruptions, schizophrenia and addictions; and social problems, personal problems. We will easily figure out the relations between these trends. The first group of charts is to measure the quality of interaction, the quality of the relationship between people. The second group of charts is to show the results of interaction, results of spiritual life. The quality of interaction can feel in the love people put in action, attitudes in behaviors, the individual's zeal in action and the nature of the action, which are the energy of action that the dumb, the deaf or the blind can sense the vitality of actions. These elements are invisible and sensible; it is difficult to evaluate and only feel by heart. These are some of the indicators for the love, connection, ability and stress relating to individuals.

> "Love begins at home, and it is not how much we do... but how much love we put in that action."
>
> **Mother Teresa**

In fact, the monks, living in the mountains, no electricity, no tap water, no modern facilities, no money, only them with nature and meditation, experience the highest of happiness. Visitors and entrepreneurs visit these monks also feel happy and relaxed because of the energy radiating from the monks. Zen masters have reached the highest states of love, connection, understanding and peace of mind. People can know the state of mind of Zen masters by the gut feelings they have when hearing the words, watching their actions and perceiving the energy radiate from them. There are many people have reached to the high quality of living, they reach the state of the highest happiness, peace of mind, enlightenment, they have found the way of creating heaven on earth. Luckily, they have left their tracks for us to follow.

Up to now, I am waiting for the statisticians ignoring a series of meaningless lists of vague causes of mental disorder, social problems and many other problems in modern society. I hope statisticians start to measure the frequency of mental disorders, social disorders with the quality of mental and spiritual health. There are strong bonds between mental health, physical health, spiritual health, the living environment and the responses of individuals. People with mental or emotional problems often have worse physical health than those without. In fact, mental problems, emotional problems, and physical problems are the visible faces that have strong relationships with the state of the mind. Mental problems, emotional problems, and physical problems go together; they are the appearances of the inner state of mind. Mental problems, emotional problems, physical problems, and the state of the mind can summarize in sentences:

"As within, so without

As if Yin and Yang

Interdependent and interchangeable"

With man, within is the state of mind, it is the hologram of countless phenomena. These countless phenomena come from countless actions taken place before and after the forming of the fetus. Countless phenomena that his ancestors, parents, relatives do. Countless anger, stress, sadness, joy, happiness, fighting, and wars have been created by him and human kinds. Countless temperate actions, and rebelling actions, countless thought, thinking, reading, watching, eating, doing and cognitive thinking he has done each moment. So that the last evening he became angry and beaten his child unintentionally. The anger and the beating may have the image of the failure of his child, the actions of his child, his mother, his father, his ancestors, his holy spirits, his wife… and so on. His anger and his beating are in the seamless web of countless phenomena. In return, his anger and his punishment also create countless seamless webs of countless phenomena. Specific things as human beings perceive and die for are the illuminating of countless effects and the beginning of countless causes also. There is no begin, there is no end, there is no I, there is no you. We are the illuminating of countless phenomena, and we can give hand to create some more phenomena that make the process of dissolving faster.

People can live to 80 years old, quite long, but that number compare the thirteen billion years of the universe is just like a life of lightning to them, I mean a second to 80 years. Some scientists have proved that dinosaurs have lived on earth 180 million years. Human beings only have had languages and many other ways of communication and modern cognitive thinking for six thousand years. We formed conscious thinking, cognitive thinking, and so on… all things called mind and consciousness. Owing to conceptions, definitions, words, ideas, contracts, and belief system, currency, banks human beings have taken the giant leap in the scale of evolution. The ability of thinking has become much easier than our ancestors did; we can consume a large amount of knowledge about countless phenomena with just several words, definitions, and assumptions. The laws, the principles, and systems set out to help countless phenomena go back and forth in the world, the more of moving, the faster of moving, the better of creating. We have created far more achievements than we and other creatures could imagine, and yet we have not yet tapped into the small part of our potential.

Unfortunately, during the time on earth, modern human beings have become victims of mind and cognitive thinking. Money, possession, thinking of my and yours... and countless terms and definitions in Wikipedia which have helped the human being taken advancement now become the dangerous destruction of all humankind. No one can clearly define money, but all need it, work for it, and sacrificed for it. The fact is the money notes of some countries one time had the value equal to a buffalo, a big car now become the paper used to clean the shoes or cover the pieces of bread because of inflation. Inflation comes from lack of trust because of countless distrust behaviors.

Lacking trust and bond in society, people have weakened themselves. They do not feel safe so that they do countless destructive behaviors: they buy bombs instead of food, they buy cruise missiles instead of schools, and they spend money on military instead of on social security. The ignorance, the feeling of danger and the negative emotion like anger make them blind with the massive destruction of the wars in human history. Lacking trust, precious paper money becomes useless. In history, one truck of paper money of Nazi Germany only traded for one loaf of bread after World War II.

Because money sticks to so many tempting things, the greedy people become its slaves. People can sacrifice and destroy themselves and others to protect the products of thinking: ideas, concepts, possession, currency, money. People cut tree, pollute the air, the ocean for money; their ignorance makes them feel well with their destructive behaviors. They go hunting not because of the need but because of the greed. Ignorance makes them feel the destructive phenomena they created are the right things to do. "One in all and all in one" is the best explanation for all problems human being have now. I highly recommend parents should listen to the song:

    - Listen to "Color of the wind" by Vanessa Williams to understand people's mind and their ignorance.

    - Listen to "Because of you" of Kelly Clarkson to under the misery and the fear our children have. How parents will think about their stupid behavior when listening to the message of their children in the song. Hopeful they will aware of their behaviors. The chorus of the song with meaning "Because of you: I never stray too far from the sidewalk. I learned to play on the safe side so I do not get hurt. I find it hard to trust not only me but everyone around me. I am afraid. I am afraid. I am afraid because of you"

    - Listen to "No love" by No Love Eminem, Lil Wayne will make adults understand the difficulties and miseries children may meet in school. Please do not hurt them.

    - Listen to "Hall of fame" by The Script ft. Will.I.Am will make us understand the potential of our people. Please do treat them as heroes, do not treat as a stupid one, and do not treat them as a burden.

Listening to these songs, you may have compassion for surrounding people and our children. Please do make them feel safe, do make them feel understood, do soothe their pain with a connection, and do form the strength for them.

> "As within so without
>
> As above so below
>
> Defects within are compensated
>
> By unnecessary compensations of without
>
> Poor within are covered
>
> By unnecessary covers of without"

Within or without is just the separation of human thinking. Within and without is to talk about the sides of phenomena that we choose to look at. They are one, no separation. Within and without is the name of the nameless phenomena. To have better understand, let answer: do you stay still or moving? Are you changing or staying still? Are you in the north or the south of the sun? Are you more beautiful than the tree in your garden? Are you a good person or a bad person? Are you above or below the center of galaxy Milky Way? Are you living or dying?

Without and without is one. Within and with are changing as Yin and Yang. Within and without are mental health, emotional health, and physical health. Scientists and physicians have a glossary of terms to describe mental health, emotional health, and physical health. These are the same scientist used these glossaries to describe the people's problem.

The problems for scientists is how to know within. How do they measure the within to prove the relationship between within and without? As we know that within is the state of mind, within fluctuates from the happy state to the stressful state. Happy state goes with happy chemicals and stressful state goes with the stress chemicals. The effect of happy chemicals and stress chemicals appear entire the body. We can know how happy or how stress people are with the questionnaire about the quality of the thoughts, feelings, words, actions, and reactions. The state of mind will determine the kind of thoughts, feelings, words, and actions and the energy of thoughts, feelings, words, and actions. People only have one state of mind at one time; either they are the stressed or happy state. The effects of stress chemical on the body are more obvious than the effects of happy chemicals on the body. The stress chemicals create changes in the body describes in table three. With the development of technology, people can use machine detect and quantify some obvious changes in the body caused by stress chemicals. People also answer the questionnaire about the symptoms described in table three. Combine the obvious changes catch by machine with the answer in the questionnaire; we can know how stressed people are. The effects of happy chemicals on the body are easily be seen by the experienced people but have not yet quantified by the machine.

We can know how happy people are by observing and questioning the manner of thoughts, the manner of words and the manner of behaviors. By observing, questioning and using the machine to detect some obvious symptoms, scientists and physicians can know how the state of the individuals is. Defining of the within and defining the without, researchers can prove for the relation between within and without the individuals. They will see the relation between mental health, emotional health, and physical health; they are going together and are the expression of the state of mind of individuals.

Deeply communal, family oriented, friendly, kept these people healthy

There will be an astoundingly low number of individuals suffering from mental problems living in the United and happy society. In the introduction of book Outliers, Malcolm Gladwell told the story of a small and isolated Pennsylvania town called Roseto in the late 1800s. Roseto was an outlier in terms of health - death rates in this small village, populated by immigrants from the same small town in Italy, were unusually low. Doctors and scientists looked tirelessly for an explanation of the phenomena of the health of these people. They thought there must be something about the diet, exercise routines, genes or environment of the Rosetans to explain their unusually good health, but all of these hypotheses led to dead ends. Finally, Stewart Wolf, a physician, suggested that the very culture of Roseto, deeply communal, family oriented, friendly, kept these people healthy. The finding of Wolf always stimulates my thinking about the quality of the living environment: supporting, connecting, helping, love and the principles of actions will determine the state of mind, then determine the health of people.

Combine teaching of Buddha, the knowledge of all sciences, we will understand: it is in the quantity and quality of interactions among family members, between the members in society determines the state of mind, which expresses in the mental health, the emotional health, and the physical health. All the mental, emotional and physical problems of our modern society come from the selfish culture, where people not only reduce the interaction with other people but also, the quality of interaction is very poor. The shortage of quality and quantity of human-human interaction create a number of implications for the state of mind, which create mental problems, emotional problems, and physical problems. In fact, the case of autistic children is increasing is the proof that the poor quality of human-human interaction; the poor within lead to the poor without. So if statisticians make statistics about disorders like mental problems, physical problems, emotional problems, and social problems, they will see there are increasing trends of these problems at the approximately same rate, despite the standard of living is increasing.

The "Mental Health Trends in America 2016" by Will King from with the statistics and explanations are the best proofs for the theory of stress. The states with the lowest prevalence of people with mental health conditions also had higher graduation rates for high school, while states with a higher prevalence of people with mental health conditions were shown to simultaneously have more homelessness, obesity, and poverty.

Key Finding of Mental Health in the United States

- 18.5% of Americans were found to be experiencing some form of mental health issue, which translates to roughly 43.7 million adults.

- Nearly 4% of adult Americans report having serious thoughts of suicide, which translates to roughly 9 million individuals.

- Roughly, 10% of young Americans ages 12-17 reported having at least one major depressive episode in the last 12 months.

- More young people across the nation were found to be experiencing depression.

Increase in Prevalence of Mental Health Issues

- Nationwide, 43.7 million adult Americans (18.5%) experience a mental health condition. The number of 2015 was 42.5 million, meaning 1.2 million more Americans now reportedly experience some form of mental health issue in just one year.

- The estimate for those with serious suicidal thoughts was approximately 9 million (3.89%) going into 2016. The report of 2015 estimated 8.8 million with serious suicidal thoughts.

Increase in Youth Depression

- The youth with a mental health condition was qualified by having at least one major depressive episode in the past 12 months, roughly 2.4 million young Americans, with 1.7 million experiencing severe depression.

- The report asserts major depression is marked by significant and pervasive feelings of sadness associated with suicidal thoughts. In 2015, a report estimated the number of youth in America experiencing at least one major depressive episode at 2.1 million.

The earlier intervention the better for people, the family therapist Shameela Keshavjee said:

- Without early intervention, these teens miss out on the opportunity to develop the skills necessary to manage their symptoms, which can set them up to struggle in relationships, work, and school environments.

- The longer they go without these skills, the more entrenched they become in the effects of their mental illness, which can prolong or complicate any treatment they seek as adults.

Identifying Risk Factors: let look at the kinds of problems that go together to have a big view of risk factors. The good outcome of mental health goes with many positive results. Failure in dealing with mental health goes along with many other problems. All the negative outcomes or positive outcomes are just the perceivable signs of the real problems the communities.

- In two of the top-ranked states Vermont and Minnesota for a low prevalence of mental health conditions, each was observed to have lower rates of violent crime and obesity. Other positive outcome factors include lower rates of child maltreatment, homelessness, and unemployment.

- States with a higher prevalence of mental health conditions, such as Louisiana and Nevada, each placed high for six of the nine negative outcomes, including more crime and a lower percentage of high school graduates. Other negative factors included states with high poverty, high toxic chemical release, and lower rates of high school graduation.

- For children with a mental health condition, the report highlights the importance of having solid relationships in a child's life to mitigate risks and factors external to the home.

Keshavjee explained because the changes in socialization due to technology and social media have disconnected young people from each other and from reality. And young people turn to the social web like Instagram, Facebook, and texts to communicate to find a sense of belonging, of importance which can lead to unrealistic expectations of happiness, a decrease in empathy, false presentations of self, and possibly isolation.

The accumulation of all factors creates the most destructive of society. All the numbers and opinions of author Keshavjee in Mental Health Trends in America 2016 are the strong proof of the influence of stress on people. It is the development of tech development of technology has separated the chance of direct contact with young people. The later intervention the less opportunity to develop skill the young have. Less skill leads to excessive stress for these young people. When people have stress, they tend to use cigarettes, wine, drugs, drop out of school, rebelling or shopping to relieve stress because of the unsatisfied need to make them discomfort. Any of these activities repeat over time can become bad habits. Police officers will exhaust if they chase to catch, punish, and educate people with bad habits.

Monks, happy people, and kind people are the outliers in combating the mental problems and physical problems and on the way of the pursuit of happiness. I hope scientists and statisticians will help to find out the real cause of our society.

> "Love begins at home, and it is not how much we do but how much love we put in that action."
>
> **Mother Teresa**

What makes difference to help our children, the reality is not too complicated, while waiting for the scientists and statisticians to do research to verify this cause. We can help our children and ourselves to have peace, happiness, and meaningful life. We need to increase our love, enthusiasm, attitude, caring, connecting to each other by selfless actions to help relatives, family members, friends, and all human kinds. Everybody has specific needs in Maslow's Hierarchy of Needs. Tony Robbins summarized and recorded in six basic needs. These needs always exist in every individual; the needs are the drives to push individuals to act to get things to satisfy their needs. If people get things to satisfy their needs, they will have happy feelings. If people do not get the things to satisfy their needs, they will suffer the pain with angry, disappointed and stressed feelings. All people actions intend to satisfy these needs to get happy feelings. For example:

If someone needs money to satisfy the need for safety for their family, they will focus on the activities to get money stronger than the activities to get the reputation or activities of entertaining.

A mother is obsessed with the need for protecting her child so that all her activities focus to protect her child; she does not care much about the activities of playing, eating or entertaining. Especially if her child is ill, she will prioritize all her activities to care for her child; she does not care about recreating activities. All of her potential minds focus on protecting her child. If she has to go to a party with coworkers, during the party, her mind arouses a lot with the thoughts about her child; she does not mind what she is eating.

If a man is obsessed with specific goals, all his activities focus on getting those goals to get the feeling of happiness. All the potential of her mind focuses on the direction of getting goals.

Each child and individuals have specific needs with the varieties of demand for satisfying the needs. Parents should understand their children so that they can make their children happy and do not accidentally make their children hurting and stressed. Leaders and managers also have to have an understanding of their staffs so that they can make their employees happy at work to get effective work. Understanding people's needs and satisfying these need is the art of how to influence friends and people.

> A vast number of published studies have suggested a link between job satisfaction levels and health. Researchers found that job satisfaction level is an important factor influencing the health of workers. Organizations should include the development of stress management policies to identify and eradicate work practices that cause most job dissatisfaction as part of an exercise aimed at improving employee health. Occupational health clinicians should consider counseling employees diagnosed as having psychological problems to critically evaluate their work—and help them to explore ways of gaining greater satisfaction from this important aspect of their life.

Mary Kay succeeded with her cosmetic: Mary Kay brand because of the ability to satisfy these needs of the customers. She taught staffs that everybody walks in the shop always have a board hang in front of her chest with a note

"make me feel important"

When individuals serve these basic needs of others with loving, caring, supporting and encouraging, they and receivers will have feelings of happiness, joy a, d peace. No need for scientists to prove these ideas, all religious leaders, philosophers, and great people teach these ideas. Best of all, you can make an experiment with yourself by observing the feeling inside with each of selfish actions and selfless actions. Go with happy people, people will feel positive energy radiating from happy people; our unconscious mind will detect signals of the safety and happiness then activate happy state in our body mysteriously that we rarely consciously know what is happening inside. This is the reason why when we close to or listen to monks, great men or happy people, we can sense of warm feeling from them; we feel moved and touched by them. We are more relaxed and peaceful when staying with them. We experience good feelings, good energy. These feelings are very precious for us; these feeling may heal some wounds inside. Furthermore, this energy will grow, develop like a flood, swept away the negative things in us. Great men bring new energy and excitement to where they come; to the people they contact. The energy of love and serving is invisible and powerful radiating from them, it is far happier than the expensive material things can bring. The value of spiritual interaction is far more valuable than anything else.

How about "we fake it then we make it". Some wealthy people try to fake to make others happy with lots of gift and precious things to their family. They want to wear another mask at home which is opposite with the mask at work, the mask in public. This is a bad way for us to fake anything. Because when we fake it, we did some things totally different from our own belief. Our subconscious mind detects that there is some wrong here when we do it. People can sense the unnatural things from our action. It sends a small signal for the body to prepare a little stress chemical for fight and flight. Experienced people or sophisticated machine can detect abnormal signals from everybody in a pretended situation. We have to use a conscious mind to calm the discomfort down. In fact, love is like a kind of energy that deaf and blind people can feel; people can sense it is real or fake unconsciously; our unconscious mind very sensitive to pretending behaviors that it silently send the gut feelings of discomfort and watch out. We do not feel the preparing of war in our body, but experienced people can sense the tension. Our family members can sense this, especially our children. They open the gift with little joy and tension, their subconscious mind senses something wrong the unnatural behaviors, and subconscious mind sends signals to create stress chemicals for all relating people. The whole family covers with little tension. Some family members can feel chills or cold with pretending action. In fact, individuals in a stressful family get more cold symptoms than the ones in a happy family. This tension can break out if anything unwanted happens; people in the tension of pretending behaviors may overact of many normal things. The things that we are hiding will show out soon. This is the reason that we should not follow the advice of non-experienced people. Do not follow the advice from talkative experts: they have knowledge but do not have experience; they do not know the art of using this kind of knowledge. We have to put our heart, consideration, patience into every love actions.

> "A crust eaten in peace is better than a banquet partaken in anxiety." **Aesop**

Follow your own heart, if you want to make other happy, changing action is not enough, you have to change your own belief. Start with understanding, then put heart into action, put love into words and actions. It can be the unskillful behaviors but receivers still sense warm and happy feeling. From changing of belief, perceptions about people then make kind, adorable and caring actions. If you fake but make it real then you can make it. This is the way to make love. If you do not change this way, do not fake it, wait until you change your basic first.

I heard enough the comments of the staffs about their bossy managers try to pretend to be kind and caring; they had the feeling of nausea, chill with beautiful words without love from bossy managers. The fact is, no matter how small of action, the matter is how much love you put in action. The love, consideration, compassion, and openness put into action can make big difference for all people.

There are individuals who are successful in their work, in business, in film, they may be the idol, but the quality of their personal lives is tragic and broken. Part of the tragedy is that they do not pay attention to the feelings they have every day. Some time they misunderstand that the success in work can compensate every defect inside and in other areas. They do not know that success in work only satisfies some of their needs, not all their needs. There are some deep needs inside are not satisfied, the unconscious mind sends the signals of discomfort to remind them. However, they are busy with many activities, do not spend the time to listen to gut feelings, do not spend the time to know the most important things to them. Sometimes they have to wear the mask to cover the discomfort inside their body. Dive into work, activities, they gain some joyful feelings. Suppress the discomfort inside the body, to the one day, the discomfort of unsatisfying the deepen needs are so strong; they become exhausted, bored with work, bored with life; they may become a depression or want to find the way to kill themselves. Some people were such stressed and depressed that they committed suicide even when they were in very success in career. If make a deep investigation, scientists will find that sad, stressed, and depressed people have the many signs of overstress, they have many symptoms described in table three.

Individuals succeed in their career are very strong, they overcome the outside challenges. This strength is not enough to overcome themselves and their big ego. They need real power to conquer themselves, by controlling the mind, emotion, and ego; by controlling temptation and desire, by changing the belief from demanding to serving to have a peaceful life. Then we put caring and understanding into every action.

References:
Australian Bureau of Statistics. (1998, June 03). Health status: health experiences of men and women. Retrieved July 19, 2017, from http://www.abs.gov.au...!OpenDocument
Brave The World. (2016, August 9). Fifty real differences between men and women. Retrieved July 19, 2017, from http://bravetheworld.com/2016/08/09/50-real-differences-men-women/

CDC. (2016, June 16). Women and heart disease fact sheet. Retrieved July 19, 2017, from http://www.cdc.gov/dhdsp/ data_statistics/fact_sheets/fs_women_heart.htm
CDC. (n.d.). Leading causes of death. Retrieved July 19, 2017, from http://www.cdc.gov/nchs /fastats/leading-causes-of-death.htm
Cooper CL. Can we live with the changing nature of work? Journal of Managerial Psychology1999;14:569–72.
Cooper CL.ed The theories of organizational stress. Oxford: Oxford University Press, 1999.
E B Faragher, M Cass, C L Cooper. The relationship between job satisfaction and health: a meta-analysis. Retrieved from http://oem.bmj.com/content/62/2/105
Gladwell, Malcolm (2008). Outliers. New York: Little, Brown & Co
Holland, Kimberly; Riley, Elsbeth; Bueno, Tonya, d Krucik T. George. ADHD by the numbers: facts, statistics, and you. (2014, September 4). Retrieved July 19, 2017, from http://www.healthline.com/health/adhd/facts-statistics-infographic
Iaffaldno MT, Muchinsky PM. Job satisfaction and job performance: a meta-analysis. Psychol Bull1985;97:251–73.
Jackson, A. Elizabeth. (2015, November 20). Gender in cardiovascular diseases. Retrieved July 19, 2017, from http://www.acc.org/latest-in-cardiology/ten-points-to-remember /2015 /11/19/23/53/gender-in-cardiovascular-diseases
Jantz, L. Gregory. (2014, February 27). Brain differences between genders. Retrieved July 19, 2017, from http://www.psychologytoday.com/blog/hope-relationships /201402/brain-differences-between-genders
Kenny DT, Carlson JG, McGuigan FJ, et al., eds. Stress and health: research and clinical applications. Amsterdam: Harwood Academic Publishers, 2000.
King, Will. (2016. January 11). Mental health trends in America in 2016. Retrieved July 19, 2017, from http://www.goodtherapy .org/blog/mental-health-trends-in-America-2016-0111161

Lyness, D'Arcy. (2016, August). Depression. Retrieved July 19, 2017, from http://www.kidshealth.org/en/parents/understanding-depression.html.

MedlinePlus. (n.d). Recognizing teen depression. Retrieved July 19, 2017, from https://medlineplus.gov/ency/patientinstructions/000648.htm

National Institute of Mental Health. (n.d.). Major depression among adolescents. Retrieved July 19, 2017, from http://www.nimh.nih.gov/health/statistics/prevalence/major-depression-among-adolescents.shtml

Nine differences between the male and female brain. (2017, April 23). Retrieved July 19, 2017, from http://www.brainfitnessforlife.com/differences-between-the-male-and-female-brain/

Office of the Surgeon General (OSG). (n.d.). Reports of the Surgeon General, U.S. Public Health Service. Retrieved July 19, 2017, from http://www.surgeongeneral.gov /library/reports/index.html.

Paoli P. First European Survey on the Work Environment 1991–1992. Dublin: European Foundation for the Improvement of Living and Working Conditions, 1992.

Prednisolone side effects. (2017, July 5). Retrieved July 19, 2017, from http://www.drugs.com /sfx/prednisolone-side-effects.html

Price, Michael. (2017, April 11). Study finds some significant differences in brains of men and women. Retrieved July 19, 2017, from http://www.sciencemag.org/news/2017/04/study-finds-significant-differences-brains-men-and-women

Public Health Agency of Canada. (2002, October 3). A report on mental illnesses in Canada - chapter two mood disorders. Retrieved July 19, 2017, from http://www.phac-aspc.gc.ca/publicat/miic-mmac/chap_2-eng.php

SAMHSA - Substance Abuse and Mental Health Services Administration, (2017, September 13). Retrieved September 15, 2017 from Http:// www.samhsa.gov/.

Smith, Thomas. (2013, September 18). Women and Depression: Does Gender Matter?. Retrieved July 19, 2017, from http://www.uspharmacist.com/article/women-and-depression-does-gender-matter-43010

Teen Help. (n.d.). Teen depression statistics & facts. Retrieved July 19, 2017, from http://www.teenhelp.com/teen-depression/teen-depression-statistics/

Chapter 32: Still ignoring? Autoimmune diseases and suicides are inevitable

One of the most fascinating is the residents of Roseto in the "Outlier" of Malcolm Gladwell, a small town in Pennsylvania. Early in the 1960s, this small town became well-known to the national medical community because the residents had a very low incidence of heart disease despite the fact that they ate a high-fat, high-cholesterol diet and drank alcohol on a regular basis. Researchers sought to discover the cause of this unusual phenomenon and concluded that the supportive, interactive, and close-knit nature of the town's primarily Italian American population created an immunity to heart disease. The protection from heart disease occurred because these immigrants still maintained an Italian lifestyle, including very strong familial and social ties. Lifestyle is the prominent different maker in studying heart disease community by community, organization by organization and nation by nation.

> PARETO IN HEALTH/MEDICINE
>
> Remember when working with the mind: irrational mind, the giant brain evolved for millions of years, illogical mind and Placebo effects, Neuro-plasticity, Mirror neurons, affirmation, self-talk, nocebo effects, T1/2 or half-life of all substances, taboos, rituals, religious belief, compound effects, conditioned responses, and magical adaptability, illusive mind, self-healing or self-destroying, irrational thinking, Subliminal message, marketing of luxury brand, benefit of expensive products, and Hysteria. Remember the question of the old: "what do we feed the mind of beings every day?"
>
> AND what if all of these lead to negativity or

> positivity? Maybe Outliers or Failures!

Most of us know that the severe and untreatable of autoimmune diseases. We all know stress weakens the immune system. The serious problems with the immune system are the immune system disorders, which are unknown the real causes even we have a thorough understanding of its symptoms. Immune system disorders cause abnormally low activity or overactivity of the immune system. In cases of the immune system overactivity, the body attacks and damages its own tissues - autoimmune diseases. Immune deficiency diseases decrease the body's ability to fight invaders, causing vulnerability to infections.

In response to an unknown trigger, the immune system may begin producing antibodies that instead of fighting infections, attack the body's own tissues. Treatment for autoimmune diseases generally focuses on reducing immune system activity.

We all know that the body controls all functions of autonomic nervous systems. Hormone system plays an important role in the control of all functions of the body. The organs that control the hormones in the body are hypothalamus, pineal gland, pituitary gland, thyroid gland, parathyroid glands, adrenal glands, pancreas, ovaries (female), and testes (male). If there is any change in the environment like increasing the temperature, the high brain centers will send neurohormones to the hypothalamus. From hypothalamus, it sends to pituitary. From pituitary, it creates some hypophyseal hormones to stimulate the target tissues like adrenal cortex, testes, ovaries, and thyroid. Then from the target tissues, many hormones created and pumped into the blood to the target organs, then create needed changes in the target organs. The changes inside the body make the body adapt well to the changes in the living environment. In the process of creating hormones, all organs, target tissues, and hormones participate to create hormones also participate to the send back the inhibition signals to other organs, target tissues to stop sending stimulations signals when the number of hormones is created enough. The processes of sending back signals of inhibition are auto-inhibition, short loop feedback, and long loop feedback.

All of these processes done by autonomic nervous systems silently that we do not consciously know. The activations of each process of sending backward and forward the orders to stimulate and orders of inhibition are done by the mechanism of conditioned responses. It means that the brain and organ cells remember the pattern of stimulations from the environment then create the conditioned responses inside the body that make the body safe in the environment. The people who live in Europe, Asia, and Africa have different autonomic conditioned responses with the changing of temperature. Let see how marvelous our body can create changes in the varieties of temperature in the world: average daily temperatures for the hottest major European cities is Valletta, Malta (22.3^0C) and Athens, Greece (22.0^0C); average daily temperatures for the coldest major European cities Reykjavík, Iceland (7.0^0C) and Kazan, Russia (7.9^0C).

In Africa, the hot temperature is much more different the hot temperature in Europe: hottest spot the mean temperature in Dallol, Ethiopia is 34.4°C - the highest annual average temperature on earth. In South East Asia: Singapore, The South of Vietnam, and Thailand: annual average high is 31 °C and the annual average low is 25 °C. Sometime we could not imagine how well we can live with such coldest places and hottest places on earth, but after seeing my friend travel to Europe and Africa for study and work, they adapt so well with the new environment in those places without any illness or chronic diseases. I realize how potentially our autonomic body can adapt. This is a part of our potential mind creating needed changes that we do not know anything at all.

Sometimes I wonder what happened if the potential mind works against the self. I wonder why so many people got autoimmune diseases. Why the immune systems constantly attack the normal organs of the body? Is there any relation between the autoimmune diseases, the wrong working of the potential mind, and health problems? If yes, what is the factor that the scientists are missing? After searching, I have found that all mental problems, health problems, and autoimmune diseases have some relations. In one health problem most of the time, there are so many roots or symptoms of other problems. If people with one health problem are not treated well, they will get many serious problems. Many chronic diseases cannot be treated but only reduce by modern medicines raised big questions for all scientists? Searching further, I found that these diseases have close relationships with other problems. Most problems have a strong relation with the stressed state.

Pay attention to hormone systems, the problems that scientists do not notice is the hypothalamus and other hormone organs are under the control of high brain centers. All organs relating to the creating hormones are under the high brain centers or mental state. The autonomic nervous system is controlled by the subconscious mind and mental state. From the state of mind, the high brain centers send neurohormones to hypothalamus then the hypothalamus activates the series of changes in the body. All of these processes silently work as the conditioned responses that people do not consciously know. Fortunately, if people pay attention to the body, listen to gut feelings, they can understand the changes in their body.

Let see the conditioned responses with a group of five people in one family: a couple: husband John (51 years old) and wife Marry (45 years old), the son Bob (25 years old) and Elizabeth (20 years old), and Tom (35 years old, Marry's brother, an officer of FBI). They go to a regional festival. Let's guess the feelings, emotions, and conditioned responses inside the body: muscles, face, feelings, thinking, behaviors, words of each individual in each stall in the festival they meet:

- Half price for the perfume Channel.

- Half price for Victoria bikini.

- Half price for wine: Johnny Walker, Chivas Whisky.

- A beautiful, charming girl with the note: "Free hugs, thank!"

- Discount 80% for all ancient watches, ancient coins, and ancient statues with the age from 300 years old to 500 years old.

- Ten white, cute kittens give free for anyone to love kitten because their owner has to travel abroad to work for three years.

- Half price for all comic books, fiction books of best-selling authors.
- Half price for all business books, psychology books.
- They watch the performance of an Indian man with three king cobras; these venomous snakes have the length from 2.0 meter to 3.0 meter.
- Elizabeth suddenly realizes Taylor Swift standing next to her watching the performance of a violist. Later, she hears that Justin Bieber will have a meeting with fans in the nearby club. Does she scream?

There are many assumptions and imaginative stories that help us understand the conditioned responses of other people. These also help us understand more about the reaction of other people and ourselves. The fact is there are countless changes in our body according to the emotion we have and the state of mind that we have not yet fully known. These are the example that we are happy when seeing something that we like.

With a man got severe disease, he knows that they only live for one year, two years, five years, or ten years. What is the quality of the rest of his life? After knowing about the diseases for five months, he gets news that one of his friends die in one car accident. What are the quality of his living and his friend living for the previous five months? With the same day of death, the people know that death will come and the people do not know at all have different quality thinking, emotion, feelings or behaviors that they have.

If the people at the same age of you lived in 1950 knew that the standard of living would increase substantially, and they can see the abundance that we (their children) have in 2017: car, food, house, cell phone, television, water, and swimming pool. They would think that we are ten times or one hundred times happier than people lived in 1950. The fact is no, we even feel more miserably than our ancestors did. The perception, thinking, and feelings determine all the quality of things we possess. Kids eating banquet with turkey, pork, roasted beef in 2017 do not have the feelings of gladness, happiness, and gratitude as the kids eating a bow of hot soup or noodle in 1957 or any previous difficult time. It is the same as any other possession. Without the feeling of contentment, happiness, or gratitude, any expensive products or luxury things we have will become worthless. Even worse, we may fall into the traps of greed and jealousy. Stuck in the traps of irrational thinking make us feel miserable and stressed with the thinking of possessing, giving or receiving. The actions of giving or taking do not make us stressed or died, but the negative thinking and feelings from those actions may make serious harm to us.

Back to the stress that miserable people have every day. They are maybe greedy people with a long list of wants or needs. The misery of miserable people comes from a greedy mind. The miserable signs are eat-in stress, sleep in stress, wear clothes with anger, give help with discomfort, and receive with discontentment. Miserable men live in villas with anger, sleep in a mansion with fear and uncertainty, see negative aspects of problems because of comparing with others, travel by car and airplane with fear, have a luxury life with the feeling of insecure and contempt, and play the sports game with the thinking bearing pain for victory. Moreover, they have a lot of obligations to do, help others with thinking of suffering or sacrifice, work in a good company with stress and discontent. They are the victims of the greedy mind with always wanting, never satisfying, nurturing children with the thinking of obligation, caring children with the thinking of losing, making love with the thinking of having to. They always speak about the thing they have done with the words of having to, obligation, sacrificing, hurting, suffering, burden, and responsibility. They do not have the feeling safety so that they have to try hard, stay in alerted state to protect the things that they possess. They always find the negative sides of problems. They are the weakest individuals in society. Their pain does not come from their possession but come from their thinking with the things they have. As the mind commend, the whole brain and body obey works all day, catches all unwanted things to alert them. Living with negative feelings, negative emotions, and negative thinking, the hypothalamus received the order of arousing stress state, arousing all other organs to prepare for "fight or flight." "Fight or flight" needs a lot of energy from glucose; strong muscles from pumping all blood to muscles and withdrawing blood for skin, fingers, and limbs; and all power for important organs and important functions. Countless hormones and organs are in the alerted state to support for "fight or flight." The degree of arousing the brain and alertness of the whole body depends on the degree of negative thinking or feelings they have.

These negative feelings come from negative belief systems. The belief system is the compound of countless causes and effects that they and human beings have done. Their belief system is the product of countless phenomena happened to them, created from them, and the thought they used to have in their mind. People suffering severe stress, under any unwanted situations, the brain, body, and hormones are highly activated just because of negative thinking and negative feelings: contempt, fear, panic, discontent, anger, and so on. The brain constantly sends the signals to hypothalamus then hypothalamus sends the signals for relating organs to create hormones for preparing in critical situations. The problems with the stressed people are the brain constantly sends the orders to other organs to prepare the alerted state to ready for "fight and flight", the arousing state has to fit with the degree of negative thinking and feelings they have. Unfortunately, the negative thinking and feelings come from their perception and imagination of the situation; it means and they are changing constantly, immeasurable, and unlimited. So the order of stressed mind to the body is preparing the highest alerted state with a lot of energy to "fight and flight". But the physical changes in the body are much slower and have the limit. The conflict starts to arouse between the mind with unlimited thinking and the physical body with limited abilities. When the changes inside the body reach to a threshold of the body, the organs start to send feedback via the routes of auto-inhibition, short loop feedback, and long loop feedback to the high brain centers, and other organs with the message of enough and stop stimulating. It means the body starts to against the arousing mind. The conflict may become serious if the mind becomes serious stressed; extreme stress may cause serious conflict inside the body between the brain and the organs. Attitude is crucial, negative attitude with negative feelings and thinking can stimulate the conflict between the organs inside the body. The self-destruction of the body can be activated only by the negative thought.

The brain resolves the conflict by mobilizing the immune system to destroy all cells, routes, and organs, which resist the order of preparing for "fight and flight." The immune system not only reduces action in the stressed state, but also it receives the orders from the brain to destroy some normal cells of the body which participating in regulating or preventing the order of the brain.

The stressed state needs as much as energy for the fighting as possible. The richest source of energy is glucose. Insulin secreted by the beta cells in islets of Langerhans to decrease blood glucose. So the immune systems start to attack the beta cells in islets of Langerhans. The immune systems do not kill alpha cells, delta cells and gamma cells in the islets of Langerhans.

The intestine systems reduce the activity in the stressed state but it may increase the absorption of glucose in the intestine by increasing the intestinal permeability via the border control system in the gut. Unfortunately, increasing intestinal permeability by loosening the junction between cells in the gut wall make the poison stuff can pass through. This is often described as making the gut "leaky." Increasing intestinal permeability is a big problem because strange particles go through the gut barrier can stimulate the immune systems to work to digest the poison articles, this leads to the inflammation reactions in the intestine. Increasing intestinal permeability may start the development of autoimmune diseases. People who have inflammation in the gut are the ones who have celiac disease and non-celiac gluten sensitivity. On top of inflammation leading to increased permeability, gluten accelerates this process by stimulating the release of a protein called zonulin. Zonulin independently contributes to loosening the junctions between cells in the gut. Stress increases the permeability of gut; the increased permeability starts a series of gut inflammation. Add together the orders of the nervous system, the inflammation, wheat, and the zonulin has a powerful effect on gut permeability.

Wheat has some relation with the process of the leaky gut so that many people may misinterpret that wheat may cause leaky gut.

The stressed state needs a lot of glucose for energy, so that most of the stressed people like to eat, especially sweet foods.

Some part of brains, hypothalamus, pineal gland, pituitary gland, thyroid gland, parathyroid glands, adrenal glands, pancreas, ovaries (female), and testes (male) participate in the process of creating and regulating hormones. These organs also mobilized when people fall into the chronically stressed state. So that some parts, cells in these organs may over-stimulate to create excessive hormones prepare for stress. Moreover, other parts or cells of these organs that prevent the process of preparing for fight and flight may be killed by the immune system. Because of stress, the immune system starts to attack countless normal cells in the organs of the body, gradually people infected with autoimmune diseases.

This may be the best explanation for the soaring number of people infected autoimmune diseases in the abundance living. By contemplating and observing we can know how stress, fear can deteriorate the stressed people. People can look back to your previous painful experiences, how terrible they felt after experiencing. Otherwise, you can do experiment with yourself with sleeping near the graveyard, sleeping in the emergency room of a hospital, doing something that against your religious belief, doing something that against your taboos. Do you want to try eating with fear, anger, and doubt? Can you try eating dog meat, putting a cage of the animal, which you are very afraid of in your house, inviting a strange guest to live in your house with your children? How about living with the people that you hate, sleeping with the people that you afraid, sleeping with the enemy, having sex with the enemy, living in the castle with fear and contempt, working with fear, and so on.

Stressed people do everything like eating, giving, spending, or helping with the negative feelings, stressed state, anger, and contempt. These actions and perceptions not only the products of countless phenomena they created or perceived but in return, these actions and perceptions will the causes of countless phenomena happened to them. Any actions they do and their people did also influence their quality of eating, sleeping, doing, thinking, self-healing, and self-destructing silently or obviously. The effects of countless actions and phenomena still linger in air, environment, relating people, and in themselves. Countless actions and phenomena embed in their gene, cells, atoms, energy, brain, body, belief system, habits, emotional life, spiritual life, and so on. The sage and experienced people may feel the essence of the pattern of phenomena that come in and go out from anyone.

Even with the guarantee from authorities that they will be safe in fearful situations, the negative people still have negative feelings and fall to extreme stress if they try to live in prisons if they try to sleep with the enemy. Negative people will extremely be stressed with negative thoughts in their mind with any fearful experiment. Their stressed state may activate the process of self-destroying. They are not only the victims of excessive stress chemicals but also they are the victims of their own immune systems. The hormones systems, the body, the brain, the homeostasis, the state mind, the cognitive thinking, the behaviors, the personality will be out of balanced; or even, will be extremely deteriorated. Working in the healthcare sector, physicians have seen a hundred people who suffered severe pain, severe illness, and malignant diseases that our professors do not know what caused the diseases. They cannot make any treatment except giving some medications to reduce symptoms. These cases of health problems urge physicians to find the answers.

Scientists can do experiments or record the observation of animals in a stress situation. Putting a cage of a bird next to a cage of a cat, the cat cannot catch the bird. But seeing the cat, hearing the cat, smelling of the cat can make the bird so much stress that the bird can die in several days. It is the same as all other animals. They can use sophisticated machines to detect the smallest signs of stress. I hope that one day scientists can show clearly in statistics about all problems in society with stressed life; then they can give instructions for specialists, politicians, educators, and billions of people to create a happy living environment. With enough data, scientists can conclude the effect of stress on the life of people. With their conclusion, millions of men, women, and children will be saved from countless problems and symptoms that are unknown the causes, some of these problems included mental problems, gastric problems, dermatitis.

It is not because of the food; the food now is much more nutritious and hygienic than at any previous time in human history. George Ohsawa was the founder of the macrobiotic diet and a philosopher. He understood so well about food, nutrition, and living principles, he only ate macrobiotic foods. Unbelievable, Ohsawa died of a heart attack at the age of seventy-four. In my opinion, the heart attack came from the anger, responsibility, and helplessness he had, and the overload of the work he did. He often keelhauled his students. His lifestyle and macrobiotic helped him a lot but could not save him from stress chemicals.

What are the kinds of best-selling over-the-counter drugs in Britain in 2015? People use over-the-counter to find the relief for pain, to find the comfortable from the stressful life. Unfortunately, the money spending on over-the-counter is increasing substantially annually. Is there any better way to find a healthy feeling?

Table 27: Relief uncomfortable and best-selling OTC drugs in Britain in 2015

The stress symptoms (from table 6)	Relation?	Top in Britain 2015	Cost
- Acne, dry skin, or thinning skin		Pain relief	£ 590.9 million
- Blue lips or fingernails		Cough, cold and sore throat	£ 475.5 million
- Bruising or discoloration of the skin		Skin treatments	£ 452.3 million
- Dizziness - Feeling of nervousness or		Vitamin, mineral and anti-tiredness	£ 366.6 million

anxiousness - Feeling short of breath - Headache - Hypertension - Insomnia - Mood changes, anxious, lack of focus - Nausea, vomiting, stomach pain - Numbness, weakness, or cold - Pain, burning - Pale skin or spotted skin - Slow or uneven heart rate - Sweating - Trouble breathing - Vision, speech, or balance difficulties - Weakness or tremors	Gastro-intestinal	£ 276.4 million
	Smoking cessation	£ 125.4 million
	Hay fever remedies	£ 114.4 million
	Eye care treatment	£ 69.1 million
	Sleeping aids	£ 44.0 million
	Medicated mouthwash	£ 31.5 million
	Total	**£ 2.550 million**

Table 28: The top best-selling groups of the over-the-counter and natural supplements in the United States in 2016

Kind of medications	Value
1. Cough, cold, allergy, sinus	$ 9.1 billion.
2. Vitamins and supplements	$ 6.9 billion.
3. Weight loss, nutritional meal replacements	$ 6.4 billion
4. Pain relief	$ 4.8 billion
5. Digestives	$ 4.3 billion.
6. First aid	$ 3.2 billion.
7. Eye care, ear care	$ 2 billion.
8. Incontinence	$ 1.8 billion.
9. Foot care	$ 1.2 billion.
10. Smoking cessation	$ 1 billion.
11. Intimacy health	$ 1 billion.
12. Sleeping remedies	$ 700 million.
13. Feminine care	$ 600 million.
Total	$ 35 billion

Source: https://www.statista.com/statistics/255103/value-of-the-otc-market-in-the-us-by-segment/

Below is the table of the top ten medications by sales in America. Using all of these medications, people do not recover from diseases for a short duration of time. Most patients have to use these medications for their whole life. Using medications in the entire life is the greatest burdens for the family and country.

Table 29: The top ten medications by sales in America are

Brand with active ingredient	Cost
1. Humira (adalimumab)	$8.2 billion
2. Abilify (aripiprazole)	$7.9 billion
3. Sovaldi (sofosbuvir)	$6.9 billion
4. Crestor (rosuvastatin)	$5.9 billion
5. Enbrel (etanercept)	5.9 billion
6. Harvoni (ledipasvir and sofosbuvir)	$5.3 billion
7. Nexium (esomeprazole)	$5.3 billion
8. Advair Diskus (fluticasone)	$4.7 billion
9. Lantus Solostar (insulin glargine)	$4.7 billion
10. Remicade (infliximab)	$4.6 billion

Source: http://www.webmd.com/drug-edication/news/
20150508/most-prescribed-top-selling-drugs

Unfortunately, most of these medications do not cure diseases; they only reduce the progression of chronic diseases or reduce the discomfort and pain from the diseases. Patients who have to use one of these medications tend to use it for their lifetime. What is the use when stress create the symptoms and problems, but the physicians only use these medications to reduce the symptoms and do not pay attention to the stress that patients suffer? It is useless when letting the depressive children and depressive adults take depression drugs but do not pay any attention to reduce the burden, pain, and stress they are suffering. Burden, pain, and stress come from all people they meet and all the places they go: parents, spouses, children, co-workers, bosses, employees, home, school, and workplace. Stressed people rarely trust others, so they never feel real safety, and never enjoy real happiness. They all feel of threat and no safety so that they always bring their own weapons and alert their all power to find the safety. Even during sleep, they do not dare to enjoy the deep wave sleep; they sleep with a nightmare and the state of ready fight or flight.

Total national health expenditures of America in 2015 are $ 3200 billion. What do these numbers mean?

The total GDP of twenty-two countries in 2014 in the group "Middle East, North Africa, Afghanistan, and Pakistan" are close to that number with approximately $ 3473 billion. And the GDP of forty-five countries in the Sub-Saharan Africa group in 2014 is only approximately $ 1690 billion. What an unbelievable number for America! I cannot say congratulation for their wealth or sorry for their health.

Does all their richness spend on medicines to find the feeling of joy, comfort, and happiness? If this is true, we do not want to be rich. They are rich but they do not happy. The root cause of health expenditure is stress. It comes from a lack of love, lack of connection, lack of understanding and lack of skills.

Using over-the-counter medications and prescription medications do not cure the illnesses and problems of patients. All these expensive medications only bring temporary the feeling of relaxed and comfortable for patients. They can never feel comfortable and happy. How smart do human beings be? How smart are we? On the one hand, we create stress, create tragedies, destroy nature, destroy society, destroy the family, and make countless bad phenomena to gain little feelings of gaining, rewarding.

"Sow bad thoughts, reap bad results,

Sow bad causes, reap bad effects."

To reduce the pain from bad effect, we start to use the symptomatic medication, over-the-counter medication to make us feel comfortable, to make us have the temporal joy and temporal relief. The countless bad seeds we sew still there, interacting with other phenomena. One day they will illuminate with the most power ever seen. The cause and effect are right now, when we alive, not after death.

The root cause of all other problems comes from thought. Good thoughts bring good results. Bad thoughts bring bad results. The number of people who are the victims of many problems and diseases is soaring despite huge effort have put in to prevent them. This is the indicators of the bad thought, bad feeling that these people have; it comes from the poor interaction between people. They are the victims of the modern society where there is a lack of connection, lack of love and excessive stress because of the ignorance of influencing people. Gradually, they become lack of ability; lack of ability means lack of knowledge, lack of skill and bad attitude. People with lack of ability are the most fragile people in the changing environment; they become so much stressed with the stress from the environment. All problems and phenomena happened to people do not come from the outside environment. The influence of the outside environment is so much smaller than the influence of the thought in mind to the individuals. How do you know the thought? Just observe the feeling you and surrounding people have after each time of thought or each situation. Just observe the feeling you and surrounding people have after each thought, word, and action. Most miserable people are negative people with a bad attitude, bad thought, and bad behavior.

Lack of understanding and living in fear and stress, people will even do not dare to do good things. Losing trust in the governors, people start to overreact to good things and resist governors with boycotting. Recently, people have seen some groups of people who boycott vaccination. I hope that they can gain the right knowledge of unwanted pandemic from boycotting vaccines. Seeing many cases of diseases caused by viruses in the twenty-first century like Ebola virus, HIV virus, Zika virus, all people hope that one day the scientists can create vaccines to prevent these diseases. Searching for human history, these diseases do not cause as many deaths as the diseases prevented by temporal vaccines do. One question for people who boycott vaccines: if scientists create a vaccine for HIV virus or Zika virus, do you agree to inject these vaccines?

Remove the thought that "my five-year-old child does not get a vaccination, now he is healthy." Your child does not get the vaccination is one fact. But your child is healthy is the results of countless efforts of governors, scientists, and physicians to eradicate the diseases out of your living areas. Your child get healthy is not because of not injecting vaccines, your child may die or at least paralyzed as US President Franklin D. Roosevelt if your child contacts with Poliovirus.

Will the people who boycott vaccine get the injection if scientists create vaccines for HIV, Ebola, Malaria, and dengue fever?

All the charitable works of Bill Gate are focused on the giving vaccine to the poor children in African. These small needles can create the greatest differences in children's lives. The facts about the devastating result of not using vaccines are always available. According to History of Vaccine, the Pandemic diseases have swept through human populations for millennia, causing hundreds of millions of deaths. Historians estimate that bubonic plague, also known as the Black Death, killed between 25 and 75 million people in Europe in the 1300s. Recurring waves of the illness swept through Europe until its last major appearance in England in the 1660s. Smallpox took an even higher global toll over thousands of years until it was declared eradicated in 1980. The 1918- 1919 influenza pandemic killed an estimated 40-70 million people worldwide. With some people who boycott vaccines, this huge number is useless, they are not afraid unless this pandemic falls to them. Most of the physicians worry about the life and health of their children. The life of Franklin D. Roosevelt had changed drastically if he had a chance of getting a Polio vaccine.

All results come from the thought people have. The most powerful law of human beings is the law of thought. Thoughts control the power of the mind. Thought, mind, and condition are summarized in the advice of many successful people and religious leaders.

The power of the focusing the mind, the power of thinking

"Whatever your mind can conceive and believe the mind can achieve" **Napoleon Hill**

"The outer conditions of a person's life will always be found to be harmoniously related to his inner state...Men do not attract that which they want, but that which they are." **James Allen**,

"A man's mind may be likened to a garden, which may be intelligently cultivated or allowed to run wild; but whether cultivated or neglected, it must, and will, bring forth. If no useful seeds are put into it, then an abundance of useless weed seeds will fall therein, and will continue to produce their kind." **James Allen**

"As he thinks, so he is; as he continues to think, so he remains." **James Allen**

> "Whatever we plant in our subconscious mind and nourish with repetition and emotion will one day become a reality." **Earl Nightingale**
>
> "Our environment, the world in which we live and work, is a mirror of our attitudes and expectations." **Earl Nightingale**

Many diseases in human society come from a stressed mind. If people still ignoring the warning signs, have a look at some autoimmune diseases to know the powerful destruction of the mind if we still let the mind under the negative stressed state.

Firstly, fibromyalgia is a disorder characterized by widespread musculoskeletal pain accompanied by fatigue, sleep, memory, and mood issues. Symptoms sometimes begin after physical trauma, surgery, infection, or significant psychological stress. In other cases, symptoms gradually accumulate over time with no single triggering event. Women are more likely to develop fibromyalgia than are men. Many people who have fibromyalgia also have tension headaches, temporomandibular joint (TMJ) disorders, irritable bowel syndrome, anxiety, and depression. While there is no cure for fibromyalgia, a variety of medications can help control symptoms. Exercise, relaxation, and stress-reduction measures also may help.

Secondly, fibromyalgia often goes with other health conditions. Here is the summarization of the symptoms of autoimmune diseases from www.womenshealth.gov and other medical websites:

Table 30: Summarization of some autoimmune diseases

Autoimmune diseases	Symptoms
Anti-phospholipid A disease that causes problems in the inner lining of blood vessels resulting in blood clots in arteries or veins.	- Blood clots in veins or arteries - Multiple miscarriages - Lacy, net-like red rash on the wrists and knees
Celiac disease A disease in which people can't tolerate gluten, a substance found in wheat, rye, and barley, and also some medicines. When people with celiac disease eat foods or use products that have gluten, the immune system responds by damaging the lining of the small intestines.	- Abdominal bloating and pain - Diarrhea or constipation - Weight loss or weight gain - Fatigue - Missed menstrual periods - Itchy skin rash - Infertility or miscarriages
Graves' disease (overactive thyroid) A disease that	- Insomnia - Irritability - Weight loss

causes the thyroid to make too much thyroid hormone.	- Heat sensitivity - Sweating - Fine brittle hair - Muscle weakness - Light menstrual periods - Bulging eyes - Shaky hands

    Ten Signs You May Have an Autoimmune Disease from medical websites, do you see it has any relation to the stress and symptoms of stress?

Table 31: Relation between signs of autoimmune disease and stress

10 Signs you may have an autoimmune disease	Stress symptoms	Some of the autoimmune diseases
1. Joint pain, muscle pain or weakness or a tremor	- Acne, dry skin, or thinning skin - Blue lips or fingernails - Bruising or discoloration of the skin - Dizziness - Feeling of nervousness or anxiousness - Feeling short of breath - Headache - Hypertension - Insomnia - Mood changes, anxious, lack focus - Nausea, vomiting, stomach pain - Numbness, weakness, or cold - Pain, burning - Pale	- Rheumatoid arthritis - Systemic lupus erythematosus - Celiac disease - Graves' disease - Pernicious anemia - Vitiligo - Reactive arthritis - Scleroderma - Sjögren syndrome - Type 1 diabetes - Inflammatory bowel diseases - Addison's disease - Psoriasis - Hashimoto's disease
2. Weight loss, insomnia, heat intolerance or rapid heartbeat		
3. Recurrent rashes or hives, sun-sensitivity, a butterfly-shaped rash across your nose and cheeks.		
4. Difficulty concentrating or focusing		
5. Feeling tired or fatigued, weight gain or cold intolerance		
6. Hair loss or white patches on your skin or inside your mouth		
7. Abdominal pain, blood or mucus in your stool, diarrhea or mouth ulcers		

8. Dry eyes, mouth or skin	skin - Slow or uneven heart rate - Sweating - Trouble breathing - Vision, speech, or balance difficulties - Weakness or tremors	
9. Numbness or tingling in the hands or feet		
10. Multiple miscarriages or blood clots		

"The tragedies do not happen to me; I do not care"

"The tragedies do not happen to me; I do not care." Smart people psychologically start to react seriously to any bad opinions about them. They even create many more other bad causes, bad phenomena for their grandchildren. They pretend do not see the tragedies they created. Until one day, their people start to commit suicide. With the people committing suicide, in their mind, perhaps death is better than alive. They suffer so much pain and misery from the pressures put on them and from the piercing cut from the conflict inside their bodies. The list of famous, smart and successful people who commit suicide are still expanding. They were smart; they were talented; they were powerful, but the stress human being put on them are so heavy. The stress destroyed them silently and irrationally that rare people can notice.

How do people kill millionaire men? Push them to the burden of broke or push them to bear the failure of seven-million-dollar contract or push them to bear the losses of the love ones. Take the things or people he loves the most, cut love, the cut connection from their beloved ones. Stress them with shouting and misunderstanding behaviors. How can powerful men stand? Sorry for them, the smart human beings put so much pressure on them.

How about young students, let them bear the burden of countless useless memorization, or let them the burden of isolation in school friends, teachers, school subjects, entrance tests, final tests, non-safety in the home, unsupportive parents and stressful society. Even worse, because of lacking essential skills, parents, teachers, brothers, activists, politicians want to help, they help with the greedy mind, the angry mind and the ignorant and without any understanding the students. The compound of countless unwanted events have created the worst pressure on the fragile students and make them suffer the worst stress ever even they live in "abundance" - the adults think that living in abundance.

Do you have any dogs or any pet? Let try to keep the dog in a small room for one day, five days, or fourteen days and then observe its responses and behaviors. Is there any abnormal behavior here? After keeping in the locked room, you free the dog in a park or garden then observe its wild energy, excitement, crazy acts, and silly acts. The dog is so silly and cute as a baby. The dog cannot talk, so do the small babies and infants but they have the instinct to adapt well to any environment. But all these beings have the same needs: the need for freely playing, jumping, running, chasing in the wild or natural environment. Let create more chances to make them release their wild energy. It is fine if you force to lock the pets and children in a room. According to statisticians, pets and dogs in city or urban areas have many health problems than the pets and dogs in rural areas. In the city, pets are so stressed that they got a lot of diseases as human beings do have. There are many clinics for pets in the city so many services like dental care, behavior, parasite control, nutrition, gynecology, vaccinations, and twice-a-year exams for pets, the equipment, and standard of services are the dreams of many doctors and people in rural areas. With the high standard of living, hygienic eating, and health care services, pets in the city are still get so much more problems in health than pets in rural areas and wild animals. If making a deeper investigation, we will understand what the root of the human problem is.

A. Stars and Famous people who committed suicide

- Chester Bennington was the lead singer for Linkin Park. He died in July of 2017 at the age of 41.

- Chris Benoit was a former World Wrestling Entertainment star.

- Clay Adler starred for two seasons on Music Television's Newport Harbor, committed suicide at the age of 27, in 2017.

- Dana Plato was best known for her role on Diff'rent Strokes, died in in 1999

- Dave Mirra was a legend in the world of bicycle motocross (BMX), died in2016

- David Foster Wallace age of 46, was a novelist and journalist

- Ernest Hemingway ((1899 -1961) won the Nobel Prize in Literature in 1954, killed himself in 1961.

- Junior Seau was a star NFL linebacker, committed suicide at the age of 43.

- Kurt Cobain died at age of 27.

- Lee Thompson Young was starring on Rizzoli & Isles.

- Lex McAllister was a contestant on season 14 of The Bachelor, died in 2016.

- Lucy Gordon was a British actress appeared in Spiderman 3 and Serendipity.

- L'Wren Scott was a fashion designer.

- Marilyn Monroe died at age of 36.

- Mindy McCready was a country artist, died at age of 37.

- Robin Williams (1951-2014) suffered from depression, committed suicide at age of 63.

- Simone Battle a member of American-British-Canadian girl group (G.R.L.) and an X Factor finalist, died in 2014

- Stevie Ryan The former YouTube star died on July 1, 2017.

- Vincent Van Gogh who is among the most famous and influential figures in the history of Western art. In just over a decade, he created about 2,100 artworks. On 27 July 1890, aged 37, Van Gogh shot himself in the chest.

- Wendy O. Williams was an American singer, songwriter, and actress. Williams first attempted suicide in 1993 by hammering a knife into her chest where it lodged in her sternum. However, she changed her mind and called Swenson to take her to the hospital. She attempted suicide again in 1997 with an overdose of ephedrine. Williams died of a self-inflicted gunshot wound on April 6, 1998, when she was 48.

B. Some Millionaire businessmen who committed suicide

- Christopher Foster, wealthy by virtue of his company's work creating oil rig insulation technology, committed suicide in August 2008 at the age of fifty.

- Howard Worthington a millionaire, English former businessman, who made his fortune in the steel industry, committed suicide at age of 52.

- John Lawrenson was a successful businessman who lived in a $1.8 million mansion. He was healthy and seemingly happy and had earned the right to enjoy the profits from a lucrative life in the publishing world. He committed suicide because his beloved wife was dying of cancer.

- Jonathan Wraith, a young British millionaire, was by all accounts a happy and well-adjusted young man, died at age thirty-five in 2009.

- Paul Castle, a self-styled businessman and property tycoon who had met the Queen of England and played polo with Prince Charles, killed himself in 2010.

- Peter Smedley was an enormously successful millionaire hotelier and businessman with a tinned food empire that provided him with a sizable income, also an extremely ill man, suffering from motor neuron disease. He ended his life by his own volition, at an assisted dying organization, the Dignitas clinic, in Switzerland.

- Wayne Pai was a successful Taiwanese businessman, a founder, and chairman of the securities broker the Polaris Group committed suicide in July 2008.

C. Famous people who have battled drug addiction and alcoholism

- Amy Winehouse, an Honorable British musician, died of alcohol addiction in 2011.

- Anna Nicole Smith (1967-2007) was a reality television Star.

- Chris Farley (1964-1997) was a comedian and actor.

- Dana Plato (1964-1999) was an actress.

- Michael Jackson died in 2009 of acute propofol and benzodiazepine intoxication following cardiac arrest.

- Sandra Dee (1942-2005) was an actress.

- Waylon Jennings (1937-2002) was a songwriter, guitarist, and singe.

- Whitney Houston was cited as the most awarded female act of all time by the Guinness World Records. She passed away in 2012, allegedly because of her addiction.

In a stressful environment, the best but weak ones of the group are the victims of the stressful conflict and stressful atmosphere. Good kids, good children want to help their parents or make good changes for their parents but the stressful environment not only makes them bear the pressure of cannot doing helpful things but also they may ruminate the pain of their beloved ones because of their caring heart.

> Stress from work, stress from studying, stress from living environment, stress from responsibility and stress from the family will make the good kids more and more frustrated

because of their consideration, goodness, and helplessness.

Fact: "Every sixteen minutes, someone in the U.S. dies by suicide without any visible warning signs or any talking- but rare anyone of them is gangster or prisoner"

Peace activists, nature activists, human activists, women protectors, and children protectors may have feelings of pain, hurt, crying, anger, and stress when seeing the countless destroying behaviors of bad, ignorant people. But the bad, ignorance doers do not have any concerning with their behaviors at all.

Stress belong to the characteristics and abilities of each individual. Unfortunately, they suffer pains, hurts, disappointments, crying, depression, severe stress, and committed suicides because of their consideration, goodness, and helplessness. Then all people will fall into the vicious circles of bad human causes.

References:
Adrenal gland. (n.d.). In Wikipedia. Retrieved July 17, 2017, from http://en.wikipedia. org/wiki/Adrenal_gland

American Psychological Association. (2006, February 23). Stress weakens the immune system. Retrieved July 19, 2017, from http://www.apa.org/research/action /immune.aspx

Annie B. Bond. (April 10, 2005). The Healing Power of Love – A True Story Retrieved from https://www.care2.com/greenliving/healing-power-of-love-true-story.html

ANewDayANewMe. (n.d). Oprah: Deepak Chopra. Good Thoughts Can Heal. Bad Thoughts May Kill! Retrieved from http://www.anewdayanewme.com/oprah-deepak-chopra-good-thoughts-can-heal-bad-thoughts-may-kill/

Austin Community College. (n.d.). Reproductive system. Retrieved July 19, 2017, from http://www.austincc.edu/apreview /PhysText/Reproductive.html

Axe, Josh. (n.d.). Autoimmune disease symptoms you need to know about. Retrieved July 19, 2017, from http://draxe.com /autoimmune-disease-symptoms/

beyond fight or flight. Retrieved July 19, 2017, from http://www.endocrineweb.com /endocrinology/overview -adrenal-glands

Biography. (n.d.). Famous People Who Struggled with Drug Addiction. Retrieved July 21, 2017, from https://www.biography.com/people/groups/drug-addiction

Bitette, Nicole. (2015, September 8). Ten famous people who tragically took their lives too soon. Retrieved July 21, 2017, from http://www.nydailynews.com /entertainment/10-famous-people-committed-suicide-article-1.2351758

Boundless. (2016, August 23)." How the Body Responds to Stress." Boundless Psychology. Retrieved July 19, 2017, from http://www.boundless.com/psychology /textbooks/bound less-psychology-textbook/stress-and-health-psychology-17/stress-and-the-body-87/how-the-body-responds-to-stress-328-12863/

Boundless. (2016, May 27)." The Endocrine System and Stress." *Boundless Psychology*. Retrieved July 19, 2017, from http://www.boundless.com/psychology/textbooks /boundless-psychology-textbook/biological-foundations-of-psychology-3/the-endocrine-system-36/the-endocrine-system-and-stress-483-16747/

Boundless. (2016, August 9)." Humoral, Hormonal, and Neural Stimuli." Boundless Biology. Retrieved July 19, 2017 from http://www.boundless.com /biology/textbooks/boundless -biology-textbook/the-endocrine-system-37/regulation-of-hormone-production-213/humoral-hormonal-and-neural-stimuli-803-12039/

Boundless. (2016, August 9). Hormonal Regulation of Stress - Boundless Biology Boundless. Retrieved July 19, 2017, from http://www.boundless.com/biology /textbooks/boundless -biology-textbook/the-endocrine-system-37/regulation-of-body-processes-212/hormonal-regulation-of-stress-802-12038/

Boundless.(2016, May 27)." Adrenal Glands." Boundless Biology. Retrieved July 19, 2017, from http://www.boundless.com /biology/textbooks/boundless-biology-textbook/the-endocrine-system-37/endocrine-glands-214/adrenal-glands-807-12045/

Brown, Troy. (2015, May 08). The 10 Most-Prescribed and Top-Selling Medications. Retrieved July 29, 2017, from http://www.webmd.com/drug-medication /news/20150508 /most-prescribed-top-selling-drugs

Business Pundit. (2011, November 30). Ten Millionaire Businessmen Who Committed Suicide. Retrieved July 21, 2017, from http://www.businesspundit.com/10-millionaire-businessmen-who-committed-suicide/

Category: Musicians who committed suicide. (n.d.). In Wikipedia. Retrieved July 10, 2017, from https://en.wikipedia.org /wiki/Category: Musicians_who_committed_ suicide

CDC/National Center for Health Statistics. (2017, May 3). Health Expenditures. Retrieved July 21, 2017, from https://www .cdc.gov/nchs/fastats/health-expenditures.htm

Celiac disease, non-celiac gluten sensitivity or wheat allergy: what is the difference? (n.d.). Retrieved July 19, 2017, from http://www.gluten.org/resources/getting-started/celiac-disease-non-celiac-sensitivity-or-wheat-allergy-what-is-the-difference/

Connelly Dawn. (2016, March 24). The OTC market in Britain in 2015. Retrieved July 29, 2017, from http://www.pharmaceutical-journal.com/news-and-analysis/infographics/sales-of-over-the-counter-medicines-in-2015-by-clinical-area-and-top-50-selling-brands/20200923.article

Drug Abuse. (n.d.). Thirty Famous Musicians Who Have Battled Drug Addiction and Alcoholism. Retrieved July 21, 2017, http://drugabuse.com/30-famous-musicians-who-have-battled-drug-addiction-and-alcoholism/

Durani, Yamini. (2015, May). About the Immune System. Retrieved July 19, 2017, from http://m.kidshealth.org/en/parents/immune.html?WT.ac=

Endocrine Society. (n.d.). Brainy hormones. Retrieved July 19, 2017, from http://www.hormone.org/hormones-and-health/brainy-hormones

Endocrine system. (n.d.). In Wikipedia. Retrieved July 17, 2017, from http://en.wikipedia.org/wiki/Endocrine_system

Farabee, M. J. (n.d.). The endocrine system. Retrieved July 19, 2017, from http://www2.estrellamountain.edu/faculty/farabee/biobk/BioBookENDOCR.html

Franklin D. Roosevelt's paralytic illness. (n.d.). In Wikipedia. Retrieved July 17, 2017, from http://en.wikipedia.org/wiki/Franklin_D._Roosevelt%27s_paralytic_illness

George Ohsawa. (n.d.). In Wikipedia. Retrieved July 17, 2017, from http://en.wikipedia.org/wiki/George_Ohsawa

Ghimire Nikhil. (n.d.). Top 10 great musicians who Committed suicide. Retrieved July 21, 2017, from http://www.elist10.com/top-10-great-musicians-who-committed-suicide/

Hansen, Fawne. (2015, May 29). How Does Stress Affect Your Immune System?. Retrieved July 19, 2017, from http://adrenalfatiguesolution.com/stress-immune-system/

Hater, Hilton (2016, February 17). Twenty-four Stars Who Committed Suicide. Retrieved July 21, 2017, from https://www.theHolywoodgossip.com/slideshows/19-stars-who-committed-suicide/page-4.html

Immune system. (n.d.). In Wikipedia. Retrieved July 17, 2017, from http://en.wikipedia .org/wiki/Immune_system

Limbic system. (n.d.). In Wikipedia. Retrieved July 17, 2017, from http://en.wikipedia .org/wiki/Limbic_system

List of suicides. (n.d.). In Wikipedia. Retrieved July 10, 2017, from https://en.wikipedia .org/wiki/List_of_suicides

Mayo Clinic Staff. (2017, May 02). Fibromyalgia. Retrieved July 19, 2017, from http://www.mayoclinic.org/diseases-conditions/fibromyalgia/home/ovc-20317786

Myers, Amy. (2013, April 18). Ten signs you have an autoimmune disease and how to reverse it. Retrieved July 19, 2017, from http://www.mindbodygreen.com/0-8843/10-signs-you-have-an-autoimmune-disease-how-to-reverse-it.html

Paleo Leap. (n.d.). Eleven ways gluten and wheat can damage your health. Retrieved July 19, 2017, from http://paleoleap.com/11-ways-gluten-and-wheat-can-damage-your-health/

Portella, Joy. (n,d.). Global spending on health is expected to increase to $18.28 trillion worldwide by 2040 but many countries will miss important health benchmarks. Retrieved July 21, 2017, from http://www.healthdata.org/news-release/global-spending-health-expected-increase-1828-trillion-worldwide-2040-many-countries

Ranker. (n.d.). Famous Musicians Who Committed Suicide. Retrieved July 21, 2017, from http://www.ranker.com/list/famous-musicians-who-committed-suicide /celebrity-lists

Sargis, M. Robert. (2015, April 8). An overview of the adrenal glands: Beyond Fight or Flight. Retrieved July 21, 2017, from https://www.endocrineweb.com/endocrinology/overview-adrenal-glands

Statista. (n.d.). Value of the over-the-counter and natural supplements market in the United States in 2016, by segment. Retrieved July 29, 2017, from https://www.statista.com/statistics/255103/value-of-the-otc-market-in-the-us-by-segment/

Statista. (n.d.). U.S. Sales Vitamins & Nutritional Supplements 2000-2017, Statistic. Retrieved July 29, 2017, from www.statista.com/statistics/235801/retail-sales-of-vitamins-and-nutritional-supplements-in-the-us/.

Stress (biology). (n.d.). In Wikipedia. Retrieved July 17, 2017, from http://en.wikipedia.org/wiki/Stress_(biology)#General_adaptation_syndrome

The History of Vaccines. (n.d.). Vaccines for pandemic threats. Retrieved July 19, 2017, from http://www.historyofvaccines.org/content/articles/vaccines-pandemic-threats

The World Bank. (n.d.). Health expenditure, total (% of GDP). Retrieved July 21, 2017, from http://data.worldbank.org/indicator/SH.XPD.TOTL.ZS?end=2014&start=2014&view=bar

Vaishnavi, Hema. (2015, January 19). Top 10 Famous Celebrities who Committed Suicide. Retrieved July 21, 2017, from http://listcrux.co/top-10-famous-celebrities-who-committed-suicide/?_sm_au_=iVVM1bjnTrtQ4HV5

Workman, Linda. (2016, November 2). Assessment of the endocrine system. Retrieved July 19, 2017, from http://nursekey.com/assessment-of-the-endocrine-system-2/

Awaken you wonderful we

Part VIII: Game of Mind Masters

Chapter 33: God does not bless any human beings.

As ordinary people, ordinary businessmen, ordinary organizations, ordinary citizens, all are afraid of the games like: "Game of mind masters" "Game of Thrones".

The dictators are the masters of using words, concepts, motivation, and feelings of the human mind. They create the peak emotion in the ignorant mind by the art of persuasion. Dictators code the ignorant minds with noble pictures, noble purposes, and noble ideas. When the mind at the peak, the dictators call on to take the needed actions. Watching the documentary films of World Wars II, Hitler's soldiers were so smart, proud, eager and ready for wars to protect Hitler's opinions. Millions of people had been coded so successfully that killing approximately 6 million Jews was legal action. World War II was the most widespread war in history and directly involved more than 100 million people from over 30 countries. In a state of total war, the major participants had thrown the entire economic, industrial, and scientific capabilities behind the war effort, erasing the distinction between civilian and military resources. Marked by mass deaths of people for both sides.

All people in the world were coded for war during World War II. A lot of stories about the Japanese commanders had committed suicide by their swords after failing the order of their general. They can be seen as the heroes of the army.

Table 32: The cost of human life in the human World War II

The dead	Allies	Axis
Military dead	16.000.000	8.000.000
Civilian dead	45.000.000	4.000.000
Total dead	61.000.000	12.000.000
Number of human beings dead	73.000.000 people	

The human mind is indifferent to the numbers, even the numbers of million victims suffering the pain, abusing, trafficking and stress every day. Talking to mind people need emotional stories, inspirational stories, and the novels to let the mind understand how miserable human beings had suffered. Below are the stories I collected about the miseries people create for the world. I want to give thank for the countless effort of the activists to make our societies better. I hope that we will understand who we are? Who human beings are, what they and we have created?

Chapter 34: The killing of Jews

The killing of Jews at Ivanhorod, Ukraine in 1942: A woman tries to shield a child with her body as Einsatzgruppen men aim their rifles. Perhaps this was the darkest moment in human history.

- In 1944, the Nazis from Lyon sent two vans to the French village of Izieu. Their Mission: to exterminate the children of an orphanage known as La Maison d'Izieu. On the morning of April 6, 1944, as children all settled down in the refectory to drink hot chocolate, three vehicles pulled up in front of the home. The Gestapo, led by the Butcher of Lyon, entered the home and forcibly removed the forty-four children and their seven supervisors, throwing the crying and terrified children on to the trucks like sacks of potatoes. Of the forty-four children kidnapped by the Nazis in Izieu, not a single one survived.

- One survivor of Auschwitz revealed during Klaus Barbie's trial what happened to the children: "I asked myself where were the children who arrived with us?" In the camp, there wasn't a single child to be seen. Then those who had been there for a while informed us of the reality. "You see that chimney, the one smoke never stops coming out of ... you smell... that odor of burned flesh ..."

- One of the children of La Maison d'Izieu was eleven-year-old and her brothers were sent to their deaths a few days after she wrote this letter to God:

- "God? How good You are! How kind and if one had to count the number of goodnesses and kindnesses You have done, one would never finish."

-"God? It is You who command. It is You who is justice, it is You who reward the good and punish the evil."

- "God? It is thanks to You that I had a beautiful life before, that I was spoiled, that I had lovely things that others do not have."

- "God? After that, I ask You one thing only: Make my parents come back, my poor parents protect them so that I can see them again as soon as possible."

- "Make them come back again. Ah! I had such a good mother and such a good father! I have such faith in You and I thank You in advance."

- Another child of Izieu was eight-year-old, born Oct. 30, 1935, in Vienna. After the war a letter to his parents was found - the little boy wrote:

- "Chere Maman, I send you 10000000000 kisses your son who loves you very much. There are big mountains and the village is very pretty. There are a lot of farms and we look for blackberries and raspberries and white mulberries. I hug you with all my heart."

- A baby boy was sent to be sheltered in the Children's home in Izieu. While in Izieu she wrote a letter to his mother:

- "O Maman, my dear Maman, I know how much you've suffered on my account and on this happy occasion of Mother's Day I send you from afar my best wishes from the bottom of my little heart. So far from you, darling Maman, I have done everything I could to make you happy: when you have sent packages, I have shared them with the children who have no parents. Maman, my dear Maman, I leave you with hugs and kisses. Your son who adores you!"

- "We arrived and saw smoking chimneys - we thought it was a factory."

- "Your mother and daddy ... are going to give you everything we can. We will always give you all the love we have. I love you with all my heart and soul forever and forever. Your loving daddy."

- "I love you so much my five little angles. You play, dance and sing all day make me think that our house is heaven. Until one day, they break the door when we were sleeping. Father shouted "It's the Germans, save yourself." then collapsed." I heard the cries, screams of the children that were being kidnapped, someone screaming because of raping, and... I heard the shouts of the Nazis who were carrying my children away....Then those who had been there for a while informed us of the reality." You see that chimney, the one smoke never stops coming out of ... do you smell that odor of burned flesh?"

They died peacefully with the thinking that God would test, protect and welcome them. By observing, I am grateful for the thinking there is no intelligent God, no intelligent creators, no intelligent Holy Spirits. Because if there are intelligent creatures, will they enjoy the food we worship? We may scout other for that food, kill other beings for that food, and destroy the nature of that food.

Imagine that if there are intelligent creatures, they created a kind of beings to enjoy the heaven they created: bird, flowers, forest, sun, sky, rivers, oceans, caves, animals and countless being creatures, which are gorgeous, magical, and godlike. Look at what human beings have done with the heaven of the imaginative intelligent creators: human beings destroyed all for their greed and anger; human beings burn forest, polluted air, and oceans for the note of money; they do all the evil things with other beings just for fun of mad mind, not for their basic physical needs. Unbelievably, human beings always prepared for wars and joined the World Wars with destructive weapons to bring safety and certainty to the mad mind. What will happen with the human world if there are some powerful intelligent creatures or intelligent God? Will the intelligent creatures kill these ingrate bugs?

Artists are the ones with the highest intuitive mind who can see the madness of human beings. The real artwork reflexes something real in society come from the intuitive mind. Artworks are out of words, sound, image, and normal senses, so that the real artwork is not easy to listen, watch, touch or understand. The real artwork is expressed by out of sound, out of the image, out of sensual sense, but audiences have to see, listen, and touch to feel it.

Can you describe the beauty of Picasso's painting for blind people?

Can you describe how beautiful of Mozart's music to deaf man just by showing a series of Mozart's musical notes and letting him watch the orchestra playing?

To understand the artworks, people should forget about the sensual senses, and feel by heart or intuition the perceived signals. Just half an hour of watching these songs can help readers understand how madness we are, we should know to correct.

- "What've done", "Waiting for the end", and "Final Masquerade" by Linkin Park;
- "Earth song" and "Heal the world" of Michael Jackson
- "Look what you made me do" of Taylor Swift
- "Because of you" of Kelly Clarkson

In fact, human beings have created more destruction for other beings than the songs described. Since they come to this planet as a species, they cut all down, dug all up, burnt all, and poisoned all. They have done all of these because of lacking virtues and goodness. Today, they are made by greed but they are smarter and have better technology so human beings are doing so on a greater scale than ever.

As parents, we have conditioned the safety, love, connection, significance, development, and contribution to our children. With our children, we give them life, food, unconditioned love, connection since they are the fragile infants; all these good deeds have come into their subconscious mind. Children may do not understand in words or expressions but they understand the precious feelings parents made for them. All are stored in subconscious mind that adults may not understand. Any children will say their parents are God; they need their parents the most. Thief, prisoner, politician, manager, doctor, terrorist or whoever the parents are, their kids still need the love, connection and support them. Parents are Gods and Saints; children are angels and Gods also; all are Gods. All religious leaders taught people the golden rules to treat other beings and golden rules to correct their mistakes. Some of them are the creators of the world.

Unfortunately, if mistreated they may be Satan, angels of darkness and destroyer of the heavenly world.

The way greedy human beings mistreated the heavenly world may be same as the way greedy parents mistreated their angel children. Parents with greed, lack of understanding, and under pressure will always feel angry and stressed with the unwanted behaviors of their children. Ignorance, anger, and hatred have not only made parents stay away from their children but also make their children hide their sweet words for parents and walk to the …chimney. Some of the words that children want to talk but may never dare to talk, they even painfully bury deep inside because of the ignorance of adults.

· "All these years, I have always done what I wanted to, without thinking about its impact on you. Yet, you never did anything without thinking of its impact on me. Thanks for everything mommy daddy."

· "Dad, I will never find out how you manage to love me despite all the pain I have given you. Sometimes I feel that my brutal lies and hurtful curses don't deserve the selfless love of an affectionate dad like you. I love you, dad."

· "Dad… sometimes I don't say Hi, sometimes I don't give you hugs. Sometimes I ignore you, sometimes I get annoyed at you. Regardless of my moody sometimes, I want you to know that deep down inside I love you all the time."

· "Daddy mommy, even a fleeting memory of your loving smile is enough to light up my darkest days. I love you."

· "Daddy, mommy, I want to invent the time machine so I can rewind to my childhood and hit pause, to relive all the awesome memories I share with you. I love you."

· "Every girl dreams about living the life of a princess. I have never dreamed of that because I have always been treated like a princess by you. I love you, daddy. I love you, mommy"

· "How do I describe my daddy? I just add the three letters EST after Cool, Strong and Best. I love you, dad."

· "I am going to write a letter to Facebook to put a HUG button on your profile so I can hug you anytime I want. I love you, mommy. I love you, daddy"

· "I expect a lot from all my friends because my dad has set high standards of friendship… by being my best friend since childhood. I love you."

· "I may detest your advice, abhor your suggestions and loathe your opinions. But that doesn't stop me from loving the man behind them all… dad, I love you."

· "I will never understand the kind of love you have for me… the kind that makes you want to give me a hug while I am giving you my mood swings. I love you, dad."

· "If all daddies of the world were like you, the future of all children would be easily predictable - perfect. I love you, dad."

· "If I was given a chance to start all over again, there are a lot of things I'd change about my life except one thing… my dad, my mom, who's been there for me through it all. Love you."

· "My daddy is a magnet who has pulled me away from the worst and close to the best of what life has to offer. I love you."

· "My friends binge on ice cream and chocolate when they feel down and out. I just pick up the phone and call my home with mom and dad. I love you."

· "My life is like a comic book because whenever I am in trouble, I am always saved by a hero called super dad. I love you."

· "No matter how old my daddy becomes, he will always be the first man who held me up in his arms and cuddled me as if I was the queen of the world. I love you, daddy."

· "Nothing makes me feel stronger than knowing that I have a dad who's got my back. I love you."

· "Real men are not those who kill all the bad guys and save the world in movies. Real men are those who strive to be great fathers to their children to make the world a better place - just like you. I love you, dad."

· "Superman is not a fictional character found only in comic books and movies. He is my dad who I love to bits."

· "The worst part of being your son is that following your footsteps is going to be more difficult than climbing the highest mountain. I love you."

· "When friends walk away, when life seems to come to a halt and when the world seems like the cruelest and heartless place... I think of you and everything seems perfect all over again. I love you, mom. I love you, dad."

· "You brought me every single toy that I wanted when I was young. I hope I can return the favor when I grow up by achieving every single goal that you always wanted me to. I love you."

· "You have seen me at my worst, yet you think that I am the best. I love you dad. I love you mom"

· "You have the most difficult job in the world called Best Dad. It involves dealing with the toughest customers and clients in the world called TEENAGE SON and TEENAGE DAUGHTER. We love you daddy."

· "You hug me even when I am wrong; you pat me on the back even when I fail. You smile at me even when I lie; you forgive me even when I curse. If there is anything in life that keeps me going... it's you, mom and da.!"

What has made father angry with his wife and his kids to prevent these words from them? Stephen Covey was not proud of the success he had, but he was proud to be a good father to his children. He was a father of nine and grandfather of fifty-two, he received the Fatherhood Award from National Fatherhood Initiative in 2003. I am wondering what do any one of these his nine children and fifty-two grandchildren, and great-grandchildren suffer the mental problems, health problems or social problems as most American children do?

Please awaken you, please awaken we!

Chapter 35: Some are cheated and coded

Follow the recording of historians and journalists we can easily find out the misery that cheated and coded mind have done:

Raping

An alleged rape victim was found "screaming", "hysterically crying", and alone by the side of an Ashburton road. The complainant screaming, crying and rocking backward and forwards, having allegedly been raped a short time before.

"I tried to talk to her straight after I saw that ... I couldn't even understand through her screaming and crying, but she didn't sound fine, so I started to head back when I heard her voice and how she was." Her friend told.

She continued: "She was hysterically crying, nothing behind her eyes, just looking around everywhere." And "she was terrified, she wouldn't stop crying and screaming... she was hysterical, she even uses tape to zip her vagina, tweeting her feet during sleep. Then sudden screaming, panic looking around then fainting".

The second witness broke down in tears as she described seeing the complainant sat outside the meatworks.

Her friend continued "There's crying. I don't even know how to describe it. She was curled up in a ball, rocking backward and forwards. Perhaps she got crazy. Please help her"

"It was just the most horrible thing I have ever seen in my life."

"I helped her back to the house. I remember holding her up while she screaming and panicking"

Women's hell - Please bless them!

Approximately 6,000 girls are subjected to female genital mutilation each day, and 30 percent of girls subjected to its most radical form die from the effects. Four million women are sold each year as slaves. In sub-Saharan Africa, 55 percent of HIV-infected adults are women, and teenage girls are five times more likely to be infected than boys. These numbers, gathered from a variety of sources and published by Global Women, an organization that supports the global ministry of women, are only the tip of an iceberg adrift in developing countries across the world. Perhaps they live in hell on the heaven earth. They are the sexual slaves. They can be traded for goods. Some husbands do not beat his dogs, but he can freely beat the wife crucially.

"In India, we say a woman born into poverty is twice oppressed. Her first oppression is that she is born a woman. But to be born poor as a woman adds another oppression all its own."

In Indian Society, girls are serious financial burdens to their families. When they marry, parents must pay a dowry to their daughters' husbands.

"In many cultures, she will be excluded from educational opportunities, her options for the future limited to early marriage where her life will continue as before — the 'inside person' — behind walls, inside the gates, suffering in silence."

Never there is a female dog, a female wolf, a female bird, a female pig have to care, protect or serve for its male partners like which have crucial beat her let alone stressed bearing sex with it male partners.

Rural African women work 16 to 18 hours each day, performing labor-intensive tasks such as hauling water for miles, tending crops, gathering fuel for fires, caring for their families and preparing meals from scratch. Their culture demands such work from women of all ages, including pregnant women and those who have just given birth. In addition, some tribes forbid women to eat protein-rich foods such as eggs, chicken, and milk.

In developing countries, what most husbands do?

They eating, drinking, drug addicting, demanding a lot of things, demanding sex then beating their partners. Look at the geographic of consuming alcohol, violence, gender gaps, poverty and HIV on the global we will know some part of the human world.

How have women and men been code?

Some facts and stories that women and girls are bearing the stupidity of human beings in return they are the mother of some of the next human generation: leaders, politicians, doctors, soldiers, bombers. Are we creating bad causes for ourselves?

What do religious beliefs help them?

- Often these women have been told for so long that they are worthless that they believe it too, and therefore cannot even take advantage of opportunities that come because they cannot believe they deserve better. They are ready to suffer the miseries, stress, beating, kicking on them. It's a bit like the battered women syndrome.

- With rewards and punishment, with the images of God, the threatening of society, millions of girls have been coded with the concepts, belief system. Women are coded who they are, what are their responsibilities? They have to feel right, feel good with their instincts, which God give to them.

- Wake up early in the morning prepare water, food for the whole family. Do the agriculture work, serving her husband as the boss. Women are ready to be shouted, kicked, and beaten anytime by their husband and husband's family. Depend on the husband family. Work from 5 am to 9 pm without ceasing and do not have the right of complaining.

- Maybe some misery women have to bear pregnancy, giving birth alone, caring for their infants and families alone. Some of them are rejected by the husband's family. She has to work hard as normal right after giving birth.

- Still having sex during pregnancy whether or not she wants, still having sex after giving birth whether or not she wants. 9 pm, it is time to go to sleep but that is the time of the sexual animal husbands. No complaining, no crying, no rejecting, just bearing, even stressed with sex.

- The women right in some countries are not equal to the animal right in other countries.

- "Never ever in the being world there is a dog, cat, wolf, elephant, tigers have to work and have sex as some women beings in some countries in the world. They have been coded so well to bear the misery, the stupidity of their people." Activists think.

- "In Islam or Hinduism, women have no guaranteed salvation," says Overstreet." They are not necessarily considered completely 'human' and therefore they are viewed as servants, slaves, the property of their fathers or husbands and having little value. They can be traded."

- Hindu society places a low value on women, who are worth less than a cow. It is believed that bad deeds in a former life will cause a person to be reincarnated as a woman, says Lutz. Girls are serious financial burdens to their families, as parents must pay a dowry to their daughters' husbands. "Dowry deaths" - the murder of new wives by their husbands - allow men to marry again for another, or better, dowry. In 1995, the Indian Government reported 7,300 dowry deaths. It is no wonder those steeped in Hindu culture dread giving birth to girls.

- "The killing of baby girls in India is continuing - both inside and outside of the womb - despite new legislation that bans the use of ultrasound tests in determining the sex of unborn children," says Lutz." But recent reports suggest the law is being widely violated around the country. It is estimated that up to 5 million baby girls are aborted every year in India."

- India and China hold the highest numbers of abandonment and murder of female infants and of aborting female fetuses.

- In eastern countries, women are still often valued far beneath men because of the old philosophy.

Chapter 36: Worst of the worst: concepts in the funeral rituals

Sati

Sati was a funerary practice among some Hindu communities in which recently widowed women immolated themselves on their husband's funeral pyre. The practice of Sati was considered to be religious in the history of India. The custom was seen as a voluntary act, but there were many instances in which women were forced to commit Sati sometimes even dragged against their will to the fire. However other forms of Sati exist, including being buried alive with the husband's corpse and drowning. One reason why Sati started is that it was introduced to prevent wives from killing their wealthy husbands (typically with poison) and marry their real lovers.

Although the practice is outlawed and illegal in today's India, yet it occurs up to the present day and is still regarded by some Hindus as the ultimate form of womanly devotion and sacrifice.

The term Sati is derived from the original name of the goddess Sati, also known as Dakshayani, who self-immolated because she was unable to bear her father Daksha's humiliation of her husband Shiva. Interestingly, India was not the first and only culture to adopt the tradition. Other ancient societies that practiced something similar to Sati included the Egyptians, Greeks, Goths, and Scythians.

Self-Mummification - Buddhist mummies

Practiced seemingly exclusively by Japanese Sokushinbutsu Buddhist monks, the rite of self-mummification was intended as a means of demonstrating dedication and spirituality. Priests would essentially commit suicide over an extended period of time, beginning with the ingestion over 1000 days of a nut and seed diet intended to rid their body of all its fat. They would then eat bark and drink poisonous tea over another 1000 days in order to make their body so poisonous that maggots would not infest it after the monk's death. This tea drinking did, however, have the unfortunate side-effect of causing vomiting and massive fluid loss. The final part of the process would see the monk take up their final residence within a sealed stone tomb, containing nothing but an air tube and small bell, which would be rung once each day to let those outside know that they were alive. Once the bell stopped ringing, the tomb would be sealed for a further 1000 days before the mummified priest was removed and put on display in the monastery. There are a lot of Buddhist mummies around the world. There are the two Buddhist mummies of Vu Khac Minh and Vu Khac Truong in the Dau Pagoda, Thuong Tin, Hanoi, Vietnam.

The Viking Funeral: heaven or hell?

Hindi women clearly had it tough but so did the slave girls of Viking noblemen. According to the historical account of Ahmad ibn Fadlan, a 10th-century Arab Muslim writer, the ritual following the death of a chieftain was exceptionally brutal.

Once dead, a chieftain's body was put into a temporary grave for ten days while new clothes were being prepared for him. During this time, one of his slave girls would volunteer or force to volunteer to join him in the afterlife; she was then guarded day and night and given copious amounts of intoxicating drinks. Once the cremation ceremony got started, the girl went from tent to tent to have sex with every man in the village. As the men were having sex with her or what today we would call "rape" they would say, "Tell your master that I did this because of my love for him." Following this, the girl was taken to a tent where she had sex with six Viking men. Crying, fainting or panicking did not make any meaning to the tribe. People still take the funeral ritual. After being raped, she was strangled to death with the rope and finally stabbed by a village matriarch. And the bodies of the chieftain and slave girl have placed onboard a wooden ship that was set alight. The Vikings did this to ensure that the slave girl would serve her master in the afterlife, while the sexual rites were a way to transform the chieftain's life force. No one thought of the girls. What the heaven she was living in?

What happens if one of our children, Holy Spirits is killed like this?

Chapter 37: The karma we have created for ourselves

Please forgive us. We own the mother earth too much. We own our innocent beings too much. We are too greedy, too angry and too ignorant but we think we are smart and noble. We need patience to practice, to gain wisdom and enlightenment before it is too late because we have created too much misery in life.

- In German, recently a nurse lured to park by "fake cries for help" then being beaten unconscious and sexually abused by five African men.

- The Preda Home for Abused Girls has helped hundreds of children some as young as 8 years old to overcome the hurt, pain, and anger they felt at being abused by releasing it in cry and scream therapy. In the emotional release therapy, they can freely express all their pent-up and buried pain and anguish. It pours out into the padded room where they scream and shout and cry and confront their abusers. They punch and beat and kick the cushions as they release the pent up hatred and anger at being abused.

- "Why did you do it to me, why? Why? I hate you, I hate you!" one 15-year-old screamed at her abuser. Another 14-year-old released her anger at her mother." You let him do it to me, you did not stop him," she cried out. Another 12-year old girl screamed with her lungs bursting and shouted at her mother." You did not believe me, you told me to say nothing, why did you not help me and stop him?" She screamed. And it goes on every day. Is there anyone help to stop these? They are extremely stressed; they may get crazy; they may get mental diseases. Living in stress, anger, hatred, ignorance, and indifference, they may create another Hitler, another crime, another terrorist for the modern world. Please forgive me, please help these girls.

- The 36 girls will have their therapy and scream and shout similar anger and hurt. As it pours out it makes your hair stand up and your body cringe with every new scream that cuts through the air with feelings of anger, hurt pain, and anguish.

- They cry and scream and then when finished they reveal one by one to the group and therapist what they relived in their Emotional Release Therapy. They are able to reveal for the first time those that had abused them. They are strengthened and empowered after every session. They find the courage to testify against their abusers in a court of law and sometimes win convictions.

What the church and other authorities, abusers, rapists, and parents do not want to recognize is the pain the victims continue to endure all their lives. They do not admit that the emotional wounds that they inflict on the children they abuse or allow to be abused remain with the children all their lives. It is only when we see the individual cases and hear their deepest emotional experiences can we get a glimpse of the suffering they endure during and long after the acts of sexual and physical abuse.

The lack of justice is another barrier to healing. Victims are frequently not believed and even they are blamed for allowing the abuse to happen. That is the greatest injustice of all.

Unfortunately, intelligent human beings are wrong.

From her vagina, her uterine, there is forming the world.

From her vagina, her uterine, there is forming the heaven and hell, Gods and monsters.

From her vagina, her uterine, there are forming the men, leaders, governors, singers, doctors, soldiers, policemen, scientists, and spiritual leaders.

What will happen to the world when the owners of these vaginas are suffering the severest stress, the severest misery and the severest inequalities of the human world?

What will happen to the world if the mothers of leaders, governors, soldiers, policemen, scientists, presidents, and spiritual leaders have to suffer the severest stress, the severest stupidity of human beings? Unfortunate for human beings if one day the baby of unfortunate mother will in charge of operating government, army, atomic bombs or atomic missiles.

Scratching on the trigger button of the bomb, he thinks about the misfortune he and his mother have to bear; he thinks about countless contempt moment that other humankind does it to him; he thinks about the laughing of his friends talking about raping next door girls. He feels the blood flush to his face with the thinking that no one, no governors save him and his mother before the inequality. The blood flushes again with the thinking that the money that his mother got from the selling sex had to give half to the rich and corrupt people. His girlfriend, the most beautiful and kindest girl he has ever met, treated him very kindly and differently, has died in his hand because of committing suicide to protest her parents who forced her to get married to a rich man. He thinks of countless pain and stress he has suffered to take him to this position. His blood pressure and heartbeat are soaring. He turns to the moment he met the one told that he could revenge his insults. His head is very painful with endless thinking. He can feel clearly the contempt in the saliva on his face that a powerful corrupt man spat fifteen years ago. A war of chemicals keeps on taking place in him. The voices and thoughts keep on emerging. His body is intense; his head is pain and going to explode.

Women and children are the most fragile creatures but they have to suffer the severest ignorance of the world. What will the human world be? They are formed in stress since the sperms meet eggs. They will be the receivers of countless stressful events before and after that moment, countless cortisone and other stress chemicals. They will be the fruits and illuminations of countless stress events, countless human ignorance and countless inequalities. Scientists have observed that when the mother is in stress, anger or negative emotion, the fetus brain shrink, and the fetus become less active compared with the happy moment of the mother.

And one day, these children will govern and create negative changes or misery in the world unless the sages stop these vicious circles. There will be more soldiers, more heroes, commanders, dictators and generals been born.

Chapter 38: God does not need their blood to wash the human sins.

I am sorry to tell that some activists have been killed because of other human beings with ill thoughts, ill beliefs. The human world has paid a too high price because of their ignorance. Some of them were the peace activists but after their deaths, some serious wars, violence had taken place with the countless innocent deaths.

Well-known assassination in history

1. Abraham Lincoln, U.S. President 1865. Assassin: John Wilkes Booth
2. Alexander II Tsar of Russia, 1881
3. Archduke Franz Ferdinand, probable heir to the Austro-Hungarian throne, 1914. Assassin: Gavrilo Princip.
4. Benazir Bhutto, former Prime Minister of Pakistan, 2007
5. Commodus, Roman Emperor, 192. Assassin: His wife poisoned his food and his wrestling partner strangled him in the bath.
6. Empress Myeongseong, Queen Min of Korea, 1895. Assassin: More than 50 Japanese agents under Miura Goro of the Imperial Japanese Army.
7. Indira Gandhi, Indian Prime Minister, 1984.
8. John F. Kennedy, U.S. President, 1963. Assassin: Lee Harvey Oswald
9. John Lennon, Beatles member, and activist, 1980. Assassin: Mark David Chapman.

10. Julius Caesar, Roman military leader, 44 BC. Assassin: Rome's Senate, led by Gaius Cassius Longinus, Marcus Junius Brutus.
11. King Henry IV, King of France, 1610. Assassin: Francois Ravaillac
12. Mahatma Gandhi Indian political activist and spiritual leader, 1948.
13. Malcolm X, activist, and writer, 1965.
14. Martin Luther King Jr., leader of the Civil Rights movement, 1968. Assassin: James Earl Ray.
15. Nicholas II, the last Czar of Russia, 1918. Assassin: A firing squad under command of Bolshevik officer Yakov Yurovsky.
16. Park Chung- Hee, leader of South Korea, 1979. Assassin: Kim Jaegyu, director of the Korea Central Intelligence Agency.
17. Philip II of Macedon, father of Alexander the Great, 336. Assassin: Pausanias, young Macedonian noble, one of Philip's bodyguards.
18. Reinhard Heydrich Senior Nazi Official, 1942.

Mahatma Gandhi raised the voice of non-violence in an increasingly violent world. He was gunned down on the streets of New Delhi by a university student turned activist was a tremendous blow not only to India but to the entire world. The only positive thing that can be said of his assassination is that it was fortunate his assailant was a fellow Hindu.

Chapter 39: Our gods, our Holy spirits also died because of the ignorance of his people

The death of Jesus:
Agony in the Garden, betrayal, and arrest

After the Last Supper, Jesus takes a walk to pray, and then Judas comes with an armed mob, sent by the chief priests, scribes, elders and the authorities come and arrest him. He kisses Jesus to identify him to the crowd, which then arrests Jesus. In an attempt to stop them, one of Jesus' disciples uses a sword to cut off the ear of a man in the crowd. After Jesus' arrest, his disciples go into hiding, and Peter, when questioned, thrice denies knowing Jesus. After the third denial, he hears the rooster crow and recalls the prediction as Jesus turns to look at him. Peter then weeps bitterly. In Matthew, Jesus criticizes the disciple's attack with the sword, enjoining his disciples not to resist his arrest. He says, "All who take the sword will perish by the sword"

Trials by the Sanhedrin, Herod, and Pilate

After arrested, Jesus is taken to the Sanhedrin. In Matthew 26:57, Mark 14:53 and Luke 22:54, Jesus is taken to the house of the high priest, Caiaphas, where he is mocked and beaten that night. Early the next morning, the chief priests and scribes lead Jesus away into their council.

During the trials Jesus speaks very little, mounts no defense, and gives very infrequent and indirect answers to the priests' questions, prompting an officer to slap him.

In Luke 23:7-15 Pilate realizes that Jesus is a Galilean, and thus comes under the jurisdiction of Herod Antipas, the Tetrarch of Galilee and Perea. Pilate sends Jesus to Herod to be tried but Jesus says almost nothing in response to Herod's questions. Herod and his soldiers mock Jesus, put an expensive robe on him to make him look like a king, and return him to Pilate. Who then calls together the Jewish elders and announces that he has "not found this man guilty."

Observing a Passover custom of the time, Pilate allows one prisoner chosen by the crowd to be released. He gives the people a choice between Jesus and a murderer called Barabbas. Persuaded by the elders (Matthew 27:20), the mob chooses to release Barabbas and crucify Jesus.

To be affixed to Jesus' cross (John 19:19-20 then scourges Jesus and sends him to be crucified. The soldiers place a Crown of Thorns on Jesus' head and ridicule him as the King of the Jews. They beat and taunt him before taking him to Calvary, also called Golgotha, for crucifixion.

Jesus' crucifixion is described in all four canonical gospels. In Luke 23:27-28 Jesus tells the women in the multitude of people following him not to weep for him but for themselves and their children. At Calvary, Jesus is offered a concoction usually offered as a painkiller. According to Matthew and Mark, he refuses it. The soldiers then crucify Jesus and cast lots for his clothes. Above Jesus' head on the cross is Pilate's inscription, "Jesus of Nazareth, the King of the Jews"; soldiers and passersby mock him about it. Jesus is crucified between two convicted thieves, and according to Luke one of them rebukes Jesus, while the other defends him.

The Roman soldiers break the two thieves' legs: a procedure designed to hasten death in a crucifixion, but they do not break those of Jesus, as he is already dead. In John 19:34, one soldier pierces Jesus' side with a lance, and blood and water flow out. In Matthew 27:51-54, when Jesus dies, the heavy curtain at the Temple is torn and an earthquake breaks open tombs. Terrified by the events, a Roman centurion states that Jesus was the Son of God. On the same day, Joseph of Arimathea, with Pilate's permission and with Nicodemus' help, removes Jesus' body from the cross, wraps him in a clean cloth, and buries him in his new rock-hewn tomb.

Death of Nguyen Trai (1380 - 1442)

Nguyen Trai was born in Chi Ngai commune, Chi Linh district in 1380. He followed Le Loi in the resistance war against the Ming invaders and made great contributions to the nation's glorious victories. He was also the author of a huge volume of literary works, including 110 poems and especially Binh Ngo Dai Cao (Great Proclamation upon the Pacification of the Wu), one of the country's first declarations of independence.

Nguyen Trai's death resulted from a scandal involving the young king, Lê Thai Tong, and the wife or concubine of Nguyen Trai named Nguyen Thi Lo. Early in 1442, the young king began an affair with Nguyen Thi Lo. This affair continued when the king visited the old scholar at his home. Not long after the king left, he suddenly became ill and died. The nobles at the court blamed Nguyen Trai and Nguyen Thi Lo for the young king's death; accused them of regicide and had both, along with their entire extended families, exterminated. Approximately one hundred innocent people in Nguyen's extended families executed.

Twenty years later, the King Le Thanh Tong officially pardoned Nguyen Trai, saying that he was Holy innocent in the death of King Le Thai Tong.

Most cities in Vietnam have named major streets after him and festival to pay tribute to him annually.

Being a military tactician and a poet, Nguyen Trai's works varied in many areas ranging from literature, history, geography, ceremony, and propriety; many of them were missing after his execution. Most of his poems that survive until today were collected in Uc Trai's Poems Collection. His poems, written in both ancient Chinese and Vietnamese were highly regarded by notable philosophers, poets, and politicians in Vietnamese history. Nguyen Trai's poems demonstrate wit, humility, and a conversational tone, and express his personal perception and experience.

In 1980, on the occasion of his 600th birthday, Nguyen Trai was recognized by UNESCO as a world cultural celebrity, an eminent military expert, and a talented politician.

In 2012, Festival pays tribute to national heroes. A ceremony was held on September 30 to commemorate the 570th death anniversary of national hero and world cultural celebrity Nguyen

Trai (1942-2012) at his native land in the northern province of Hai Duong. The commemoration is part of the autumn festival in Con Son-Kiep Bac, which is a complex of relics associated with the life of many Vietnamese heroes and scholars, including Tran Hung Dao, Nguyen Trai, Tran Nguyen Dan, and Chu Van An.

In 2016, according to The Hanoitimes, Con Son-Kiep Bac Autumn Festival 2016 has been taking place with a wide range of activities in the northern province of Hai Duong. A ceremony to commemorate the 574th death anniversary of Nguyen Trai, a national hero, and a world cultural celebrity, was held at Con Son-Kiep Bac relic site in Chi Linh town of northern Hai Duong province on September 16. Con Son Pagoda, also known as Tu Phuc Pagoda and Hun Pagoda, is at the foot of Con Son Mountain under the shade of dense groves of seasoned trees. Inside are statues of Buddha and national hero Nguyen Trai. A lot of traditional rituals, traditional worship has been taken place to commemorate the death anniversary of Nguyen Trai. In Vietnam, Nguyen Trai is the Holy God of Vietnamese.

The Death of Socrates

Socrates (470/469 - 399 BC) philosopher of philosophers, was a classical Greek philosopher credited as one of the founders of Western philosophy. He is an enigmatic figure known chiefly through the accounts of classical writers, especially the writings of his students Plato and Xenophon and the plays of his contemporary Aristophanes.

Plato's Socrates also made important and lasting contributions to the field of epistemology, and his ideologies and approach have proven a strong foundation for a much Western philosophy that has followed. Nothing written by Socrates remains extant. As a result, information about him and his philosophies depend upon secondary sources. Furthermore, the close comparison between the contents of these sources reveals contradictions, thus creating concerns about the possibility of knowing in-depth the real Socrates. This issue is known as the Socratic problem or the Socratic question.

To understand Socrates and his thought, one must turn primarily to the works of Plato, whose dialogues are thought the most informative source about Socrates' life and philosophy, and also Xenophon. These writings are the Socratic dialogues, which consist of reports of conversations apparently involving Socrates.

Socratic paradoxes - his legacy to help his people

Many of the beliefs traditionally attributed to the historical Socrates have been characterized as "paradoxical" because they seem to conflict with common sense. But Socratic paradoxes have a lot of similarities with the Tao Te Ching of Lao Tzu, Yin, and Yang of ancient China, and egoless and emptiness of Buddha. The following are among the so-called Socratic paradoxes:

· No one desires evil.

· No one errs or does wrong willingly or knowingly.

· Virtue is knowledge.

· Virtue is sufficient for happiness.

· Not believing in the gods of the state.

Nothing is absolute, things are equal. There is no superior or "long live the King" or "King is God" as in the eastern feudal philosophy. He had sowed the seed of democracy, the seed of continuous questioning to find the truth. He had sowed the seed for science.

Socrates paradox seems like the emptiness and egoless in Buddhism. There is no absolute. Things rely on each other to survive and perish along together: interchangeable, interdependent.

The paradox is nothing absolute to cling in. By continuous questioning, people will find the truth. You are good but not that good. You are smart but not that smart. You are intelligent but not that intelligent. You think you know but you may not know. You said you love but you do not love. You think you are kind but may not kind. So do not stop questioning. Look around you will see: many things that you think that is good are creating pain for countless people and you but you do not know.

The destination of questioning is to find out the stable things; the things that will make a meaningful life. It is a virtue. Virtue is knowledge, virtue is sufficient for happiness.

You think that you have got to your destination, fulfill your life, perhaps not because life is the continuous journey.

You think you have gained the new advancement, you have reached the highest states and you have caught something. But if look closely with questioning, I think that you have lost a lot. You have traded the forest for the wooden house. You have lost your virtues for recognition. Look at the bird you caught, it is not a bird, it is a dying creature. You have gained a degree but you have lost the attitude of lifelong learning. You may achieve a big achievement but you have lost the resources of future generations.

In gain, there is a seed of losing. In achieving, there is a seed of defeating. In sadness, there is a seed of happiness. In the pain, there is a seed of joy. Things are not static, things are not constant. Things are relative. So do not stick your mind to old thinking.

You think this is the peaceful world but there are countless girls, boys are screaming and crying but you do not know. You think you suffer the severest pain ever because of a toothache, but that pain is so tiny with the pain of young girls being raped, she is screaming, panicking and depressed that no one knows. With her, this world is not peace. You may think one girl is too small for the billions of people, so just enjoy the meal. You do not have the compassion, you do not have virtue. You think you gain but you lost the most essence of your life. She is just a young girl with an unwanted child in people's eyes. But in her eyes one year ago, Mother Teresa saw her youth, her energy, and her kind heart; mother thought she would do more than the mother can do for the human world. Now she is a schizophrenic patient, her son becomes indifferent with the human pains, like to beat others, he has some behaviors and thoughts like Hitler. They make become vital few in the world.

You think you stay till but you are traveling with extremely high speed compare with the son. You think that you are flying fast but perhaps you are still staying in in one dust of the universe.

Things are not absolute with any characters, so why you have to die or kill others for them. In the roots of wrong, there is the seed of right. In the root of, weakness there is the root of strength. You steel knife is not concrete is not solid. It can divide into atoms, electrons, neutrons, quarks, and emptiness with pure energy.

By continuous questioning, you will gain wisdom and enlightenment. The term, "Socratic paradox" can also refer to a self-referential paradox, originating in Socrates' utterance, "I know that I know nothing." So that I have to read, think and observe carefully before I make any decisions.

You will gain the enlightenment that words are cheating, words are seducing and actions can be cheating also. How can I know others? By removing all your assumptions, start to observing, and feel the attitude of the people; the virtues, and characteristics of doers. Are they greed or selfless? Do they anger, do they anger with the tiny unwanted things?" The answer will give you the clues.

Gaining wisdom and enlightenment will help you do no commit the actions that create stress for your children, your spouse, people, and your society. Changing from the self may help you create positive changes in the world.

The best way of self-help is not to sacrifice in selfish acts but is love, kindness, and consideration in helping others.

The highest of all is action with inaction, harmony with the pace of nature.

Clean food may be not clean. The dirty mind requires clean foods. Buddha with the tranquil mind, inner peace, and serving heart would eat whatever food that other people serve him when he went beg for food.

People use luxury covers, luxury cars, luxury food may not be strong ones; they may be too weak to use the luxury covers, noble words to compensate for their weakness inside. Warren Buffet does not like these covers.

Great governors do not use noble words like nationalism, heroism, sacrifice, kill for future, the smartest people, the strongest nation, kill to save the nation, kill to save the world, or to revenge for the bad reputation. Only dictators and Hitler use these.

Great parents do not use bad words for fragile children. They lie below all with the compassion heart to guide their children, to help their children from weak and fragile to the ones with strength and abilities.

Great teachers, great brother do not stay high and use skills and tricks to teach kids. They in the lowest place to use the kind heart to guide children.

The paradox in the writing is that there are too much "great" words. In fact, mother Teresa does not like to be called great. Buddha did not like to be called great. Lao Tzu did not like to be called great. And a lot of enlightened ones do not like to be called great. They do not want people to make worship of them as the act of remembering. They only want people to take the acts of kindness, use compassion heart to treat others, the old, the ill and the miserable as they have done if people want to commemorate them.

Owning for the paradox, we may understand the challenge of the leadership of Jim Rohn. We can know how to distinguish the difference between strong and rude; kind and weak; bold and bully; thoughtful and lazy; humble and timid; proud and arrogant; humor and folly. If intelligent men assume he knows everything, he will easily be cheated by the speakers. Even worse, the intelligent ones may treat cruelly the good and innocent people.

The mind has a delusive character. Any things that mind can perceive and create bearing the paradoxes. The more strong the mind think they are, the more of the number of the crowd, the easier they are deceived.

Trial and death of Socrates

Socrates lived during the time of the transition from the height of the Athenian hegemony to its decline with the defeat by Sparta and its allies in the Peloponnesian War. At a time when Athens sought to stabilize and recover from its humiliating defeat, the Athenian public may have been entertaining doubts about democracy as an efficient form of government. Socrates appears to have been a critic of democracy, and some scholars interpret his trial as an expression of political infighting. Claiming loyalty to his city, Socrates clashed with the current course of Athenian politics and society.

According to Plato's Apology, Socrates' life as the "gadfly" of Athens began when his friend Chaerephon asked the oracle at Delphi if anyone were wiser than Socrates; the Oracle responded that no-one was wiser. Socrates believed the Oracle's response was not correct because he believed he possessed no wisdom whatsoever. He proceeded to test the riddle by approaching men considered wise by the people of Athens - statesmen, poets, and artisans - in order to refute the Oracle's pronouncement. Questioning them, however, Socrates concluded: while each man assumed he knew a great deal and was wise, in fact, they knew very little and were not wise at all. Socrates realized the Oracle was correct; while so-called wise men thought themselves as wise and yet were not, he himself knew he was not wise at all, which, paradoxically, made him the wiser one since he was the only person aware of his own ignorance.

Socrates defended his role as a gadfly until the end: at his trial, when Socrates was asked to propose his own punishment, he suggested a wage paid by the government and free dinners for the rest of his life instead, to finance the time he spent as Athens' benefactor. He was nevertheless, found guilty of both corrupting the minds of the youth of Athens and of impiety: not believing in the gods of the state, and subsequently sentenced to death by drinking a mixture containing poison hemlock.

Xenophon and Plato agree that Socrates had an opportunity to escape, as his followers were able to bribe the prison guards. There have been several suggestions offered as reasons why he chose to stay.

Socrates' death is described at the end of Plato's Phaedo. Socrates turned down Crito's pleas to attempt an escape from prison. After drinking the poison, he was instructed to walk around until his legs felt numb. After he lay down, the man who administered the poison pinched his foot; Socrates could no longer feel his legs. The numbness slowly crept up his body until it reached his heart. Shortly before his death, Socrates speaks his last words to Crito: "Crito, we owe a rooster to Asclepius. Please, don't forget to pay the debt."

Death of Maudgalyayana

Maudgalyayana was one of the Buddha's closest disciples. A contemporary of disciples such as Subhuti, Sariputra, and Mahakasyapa, he is considered the second of the Buddha's two foremost male disciples together with Sariputra. Maudgalyayana and Sariputra became spiritual wanderers in their youth. Maudgalyayana attained enlightenment shortly after following Buddha. As a teacher, he was known for his psychic powers, which he used extensively in his teaching methods. He died at the age of eighty-four, killed through the efforts of a rivaling sect.

This violent death has been described in Buddhist scriptures as a result of Maudgalyayana's karma of having killed his own parents in a previous life. No one knows the purpose of the explanation of his death.

In post-canonical texts, Maudgalyayana was known for his filial piety through a popular account of him transferring his merits to his mother. This led to a tradition in many Buddhist countries known as the ghost festival, during which people dedicate their merits to their ancestors. In the nineteenth century, relics were found attributed to him, which have been widely venerated.

The Ghost Festival, also known as the Hungry Ghost Festival, Zhongyuan Festival or Yulan Festival is a traditional Buddhist and Taoist festival held in Asian countries. According to the Chinese calendar, the Ghost Festival is on the 15th night of the seventh month or 14th in southern China. Activities during the month would include preparing ritualistic food offerings, burning incense, and burning joss paper, forms of material items such as clothes, gold, money, and other fine goods for the visiting spirits of the ancestors. This month is the month of lonely spirits and believed to be haunted and particularly unlucky.

Chapter 40: How are some coded?

Reunify, reunification, Sovereignty of man, people, villages, countries, world, earth, universe, superiority, the ethnic spirit, heroism, for development, for peace, for wealth are the most sacred words to peace activists. It is the best weapon to arouse the stupid minds and motivate stupid minds.

The wars of students, families, brothers, spouses, friends, colleagues, civil, social class, religions, regions, and world are not human wars. But the wars of coded being creatures, coded minds with some needs, noble purposes, philosophy and killing behaviors, then these ignorant men will eager to take the destructive weapons to kill other beings. These wars were led by war philosophy and fighting philosophy. All participants are the followers of greatest military commanders. Billion people, young man, the intelligent, geniuses and young girls in each side eager to join in to serve their side in the wars. They are responding to the call of war.

Reading the history, seeing the documents film of millions of young men participated to serve Hitler in World Wars II with the intention to reunify the world, for the good sake. They were full of smile, eager and proud. Millions of young men in German left home to serve Hitler's opinions. I am terrified of the thinking that if I and my readers were born in German and were mature when World War II started. I am certain with 100 % that we would eager to join in Nazi army. I am terrified that if I were born in 1700, I would have had some slaves and sex slaves or I would have satisfied to become a slave.

Table 33: Their farewells of warriors

The wishes of farewell	The people who receive it	Coded purposes	What does it means	Success
May God bless you"	Nurses serve in wars	Liberation the world	Fulfill the targets	Winners will have titles, medals, big rewards, lifelong salaries and big incomes
"Have a safe trip"	Special forces	Reunification	Bomb the city successfully	
"Have a safe and sound journey"	general	The ethic spirits	Kill as many enemies as possible	Thank God!
	soldiers, sailors, marines, airmen	Sovereignty of people Sovereignty of villages or countries	Bomb atomic bomb in the right place	For God's sake
"All the best wishes to you!"			Self sacrificing is the noblest action.	Proud, joy of victory
"Best wishes to you"	Ordinary people	Sovereignty of earth		Big celebration
"Good Luck"	Companion in arms	For God's sake.	Fulfill your responsibilities	Congratulation
"God bless you"	All people involving in wars	For the goodness	Die if needed to kill enemies	The sake of goodness
"Have a sound trip"		For heaven's sake		Annual worshipping
"I trust in		Protect the world Protect the		Annual anniversary

435

Awaken you wonderful we

you" God will protect you		peace		

Hitler conditioned the mind of his people. He used a big lie. A big lie is a propaganda technique. The expression was coined by Adolf Hitler, when he dictated his 1925 book Mein Kampf, about the use of a lie so "colossal" that no one would believe that someone "could have the impudence to distort the truth so infamously." Hitler claimed the technique was used by "the Jews" to blame Germany's loss in World War I.

World War I had radically altered the political European map, with the defeat of the Central Powers, including Austria-Hungary, Germany, Bulgaria, and the Ottoman Empire, and the 1917 Bolshevik seizure of power in Russia, which eventually led to the founding of the Soviet Union. Despite strong pacifist sentiment after World War I, its aftermath still caused irredentist and revanchist nationalism in several European states.

These sentiments were especially marked in Germany because of the significant territorial, colonial, and financial losses incurred by the Treaty of Versailles. Under the treaty, Germany lost around 13per cent of its home territory and all of its overseas possessions, while German annexation of other states was prohibited, reparations were imposed, and limits were placed on the size and capability of the country's armed forces.

The ethic spirits, irredentist and revanchist nationalism, heroism, the greedy mind with the feelings of inequality, the stress between European nations, the art of seducing the mind by Hitler, and the intention of dominating the world by other countries have triggered the World War II.

Chapter 41: How did Hitler seduce the mind of millions of people and soldiers?

The answer can find in his quotes:

1. "All great movements are popular movements. They are the volcanic eruptions of human passions and emotions, stirred into activity by the ruthless Goddess of Distress or by the torch of the spoken word cast into the midst of the people."

2. "All propaganda has to be popular and has to accommodate itself to the comprehension of the least intelligent of those whom it seeks to reach."

3. "Anyone can deal with victory. Only the mighty can bear defeat."

4. "As a Christian I have no duty to allow myself to be cheated, but I have the duty to be a fighter for truth and justice."

5. "As soon as by one's own propaganda even a glimpse of right on the other side is admitted, the cause for doubting one's own right is laid."

6. "By the skillful and sustained use of propaganda, one can make a people see even heaven as hell or an extremely wretched life as paradise."

7. "Demoralize the enemy from within by surprise, terror, sabotage, assassination. This is the war of the future."

8. "For there is one thing we must never forget… the majority can never replace the man. And no more than a hundred empty heads make one wise man will an heroic decision arise from a hundred cowards."

9. "Germany will either be a world power or will not be at all."

10. "God is not moved or impressed with our worship until our hearts are moved and impressed by Him."

11. "Great liars are also great magicians."

12. "He alone, who owns the youth, gains the future."

13. "Humanitarianism is the expression of stupidity and cowardice."

14. "I do not see why man should not be as cruel as nature."

15. "I go the way that Providence dictates with the assurance of a sleepwalker."

16. "I use emotion for the many and reserve reason for the few."

17. "If freedom is short of weapons, we must compensate with willpower."

18. "If you want to shine like sun first you have to burn like it".

19. "It is always more difficult to fight against faith than against knowledge."

20. "It is not the truth that matters, but victory."

21. "Keep a very firm grasp on reality, so you can strangle it at any time."

22. "Life is like a mirror, if you frown at it, it frowns back; if you smile, it returns the greeting."

23. "Make the lie big, make it simple, keep saying it, and eventually they will believe it"

24. "Mankind has grown strong in eternal struggles and it will only perish through eternal peace."

25. "Money glitters, beauty sparkles and intelligence shines."

26. "Never trust a person who isn't having at least one crisis."

27. "People may not always believe what you say, but they will believe what you do."

28. "Strength lies not in defense but in attack."

29. "Struggle is the father of all things. It is not by the principles of humanity that man lives or is able to preserve himself above the animal world, but solely by means of the most brutal struggle."

30. "Success is the sole earthly judge of right and wrong."

31. "The broad masses of a population are more amenable to the appeal of rhetoric than to any other force."

32. "The doom of a nation can be averted only by a storm of flowing passion, but only those who are passionate themselves can arouse passion in others."

33. "The great masses of the people will more easily fall victims to a big lie than to a small one."

34. "The great strength of the totalitarian state is that it forces those who fear it to imitate it."

35. "The greater the lie, the greater the chance that it will be believed."

36. "The leader of geniuses must have the ability to make different opponents appear as if they belonged to one category."

37. "The only preventative measure one can take is to live irregularly."

38. "The very first essential for success is a perpetually constant and regular employment of violence."

39. "The victor will never be asked if he told the truth."

40. "There must be no majority decisions, but only responsible persons and the word 'council' must be restored to its original meaning. Surely every man will have advisers by his side, but the decision will be made by one man."

41. "Those who want to live, let them fight, and those who do not want to fight in this world of eternal struggle do not deserve to live."

42. "Through the clever and constant application of propaganda, people can be made to see paradise as hell, and also the other way round, to consider the most wretched sort of life as paradise."

43. "To conquer a nation, first disarm its citizens."

44. "What good fortune for governments that the people do not think."

45. "What luck for rulers that men do not think!"

46. "When diplomacy ends, a war begins".

47. "Who says I am not under the special protection of God?"

48. "Whoever lights the torch of war in Europe can wish for nothing but chaos"

49. "Words build bridges into unexplored regions."

50. If you tell a big enough lie and tell it frequently enough, it will be believed.

References:

Admin. (2015, January 7). 50 Famous Quotes by Adolf Hitler. Quote Sigma. Retrieved September 22, 2017, from http://www.quotesigma.com/50-famous-quotes-adolf-hitler/

Adolf Hitler. (n.d.). BrainyQuote.com. Retrieved August 19, 2017, from BrainyQuote.com Website: https://www.brainyquote.com/quotes/authors/a/adolf_hitler.html

Big lie. (n.d.). In Wikipedia Retrieved September 22, 2017, from https://en.wikipedia.org/wiki/Big_lie

Buddhist mummies. (n.d.). In Wikipedia Retrieved September 22, 2017, from https://en.wikipedia.org/wiki/Buddhist_mummies

Children of Izieu. (n.d.). Retrieved September 22, 2017, from http://www.auschwitz.dk/Star/Izieu.htm

Cloud Mind. (2015, October 28). 25 Unusual Death Rituals from Around the World. Retrieved September 22, 2017, from http://cloudmind.info/25-unusual-death-rituals-from-around-the-world/

Cullen, Shay. (2017, February 10). Hear the Cries of Victims of Sexual Abuse. Retrieved September 22, 2017, from http://www.preda.org/fr-shays-articles/hear-the-cries-of-victims-of-sexual-abuse/

Danelek, Jeff. (2012, May 31). Top 10 Most Important Assassinations In History. Retrieved September 22, 2017, from http://www.toptenz.net/top-10-most-important-assassinations-in-history.php

Dang, Son, et al. (2012, October 2). Festival Pays Tribute to National Heroes. Vietnam Travel Guide. Retrieved September 22, 2017, from https://www.vietnam-travel.org/news/festival-pays-tribute-to-national-heroes.html

Ghost Festival. (n.d.). In Wikipedia Retrieved September 22, 2017, from https://en.wikipedia.org/wiki/Ghost_Festival

Hanoi Times. (n.d.). Con Son - Kiep Bac Autumn Festival Opens in Hai Duong. Retrieved September 22, 2017, from http://hanoitimes.com.vn/travel/festivals/2016/09/81e0a8ec/con-son-kiep-bac-autumn-festival-opens-in-hai-duong/

James, Patrick. (2010, March 18). The 15 Most Infamous Assassinations in History. Retrieved September 22, 2017, from https://www.good.is /articles/the-15-most-infamous-assassinations-in-history

Jesus. (n.d.). In Wikipedia Retrieved September 22, 2017, from https://en. wikipedia.org/wiki/Jesus

Maudgalyayana. (n.d.). In Wikipedia Retrieved September 22, 2017, from https://en. wikipedia.org/wiki/Maudgalyayana

Nguyễn Trãi. (n.d.). In Wikipedia Retrieved September 22, 2017, from https://en. wikipedia.org/wiki/Nguyễn_Trãi

Socrates. (n.d.). In Wikipedia Retrieved September 22, 2017, from https://en. wikipedia.org/wiki/Socrates

Talkvietnam. (2016, September 17). World cultural celebrity Nguyen Trai remembered. Retrieved September 22, 2017, from https://www.talkvietnam .com/tag/nguyen-trai-temple/

Part IX: A Stressed World with Rainbow of Stress

Chapter 42: Stress syndrome and the rainbow of stress

"As within so without
As above so below"

****

We get information by all senses, then the information processed in the brain in the way called thinking. We have conditioned responses from the perceived information. The responses start with a conclusion in the mind, self-talk, the changes in the body: muscle, urine, eye, heartbeat, the pattern of d the decision also have in emotion, feelings, talk, decision, and action. All of these are the temporal illumination of the countless events before that. From the moment of illumination, the future and destiny are formed. The talk, emotion, feeling, and action called causes are temporary. But the effect of causes remains for thousands of years. In history, the causes only were remembered by the memory, talking and recording of people. But in modern society, with the digital recording devices and high awareness of ordinary people, countless events and phenomena are recorded and replayed help people think better about the causes and effect, real and myth; fact and rumor. It speeds human being to the realization of the universal truth.

The human brain develops over time through the process of thinking from the baseline of the animal brain. The animal's brain also has the function of thinking, but, maybe the process of recording and responding takes place silently and are not recorded and verbalized transmit to the next generations. But the development of neo-cortex helps the brain understand what is happening inside the brain. The human brain knows what is happening inside the brain, the process of translating and sending back and forth of information. The brain decoded information into other qualitative and quantitative characters. The perceived information can be described in assumption of varieties like space, sound, smell, picture, color, height, wide, rhythm, kinetic, logical and illogical way. The ability in recognizing and mastering each of these varieties can be called the intelligence. All of the varieties we use to describe the world are just the assumption. We think the world with the varieties. It created the term "mind". The neo-cortex develop different regions to take charge of remembering the kind of varieties of information.

The human world is the product of the interaction between mind and environment. The human world is the relative truth, which is the product of reflection of the ultimate truth on the mind of human beings. The human world depends on the perception and assumption of individuals. All the products of mind are relative. Ideas of birth and death, being and nonbeing, above and below, coming and going, sameness and difference, defilement and purity, increasing and decreasing, can all be called relative truths. They are concepts that we use in daily life which are very important to understand the relativity of the things and events in the world. Perception, concepts and relative truths are just the reflection of the ultimate truth in the human mind and human understanding. Thich Nhat Hanh teaches that at the level of relative truth, these pairs of opposites are everywhere you-me, mother-son, husband-wife, people-animals, and animals-tree. At the level of relative truth, there is discrimination and separation. And if stick to the discrimination and separation, people may think they have separate self and ego, then they start thinking that they have the right to greed and anger. Time is also a relative truth to describe the relativity of moment taken place at the events. The perceived world or relative world of a girl, a twin brother, a king, a husband, and a wife is never the same.

Thich Nhat Hanh adds that when we observe more closely, we see something different, we see the ultimate truth that things are really inside of each other, everything is in everything else, and everything interpenetrates. Because of interdependence, to live harmoniously and happily, people should follow the teachings of the old about the principles, virtues, and values.

Human beings have to use some premises to create some branches of sciences. It is just the worldwide universal assumptions of specific subjects of human beings. An object, a phenomenon in the world can be decoded with the assumption of quantitative and qualitative varieties, and then it will be taught for other people.

In elementary school, students are taught basic calculation: one plus one is two; one tree plus one tree is two tree; one man plus one man is two men; and the shape of the absolute circle, triangle, and square. Physic and chemistry in high school also based on the absolute assumptions, pure chemical: pure iron, pure sodium, and pure aluminum to have the chemical equation and physical equation. These are the basic steps to prepare for people to understand higher in universities. Simple equation, simple world taught in elementary school becomes a quantum equation and the quantum world in higher education and specific sciences. This is the natural process of learning. To adopt higher education, students have to take the essence of previous education then remove all the old assumptions taught in elementary school and high school to adopt the quantum theory of the real world. On the way of pursuing knowledge, the old assumptions and religious beliefs may prevent students from understanding and apply new knowledge. Medical students, biology students, and all students will hardly to understand the basic theory: theory of evolution to examine all phenomena, applications of theory and the finding of paleontologists if students still believe the Seven Days of the creation of the world.

The best way to describe or taught other people about a new phenomenon is related to the known information. It is easy to teach an American about the characters of snow but it is very difficult to teach African man about the characters of snow if he has not known any things relate to snow before. It is easy to explain the lemon and its flavor for the young children if they have eaten a lemon.

Human world and human knowledge are just the assumptions to help people think better and have a better life. The feelings of happiness, of joy, of safety, are the best conditions to help the brainy mind function better. So the most effective way of studying and remembering is the good condition for the mind function and combination of all senses and intelligence in studying. The best condition for studying is feelings of happiness, joy, and safety, use all intelligence to decode the phenomena in humorous and imaginative ways of space, sound, smell, picture, color, height, wide, rhythm, kinetic, logic and emotion. When all parts of the brain participate in the learning process, students will get the most from learning and remember better. Children can learn so many things that adults cannot imagine if adults nurture curiosity in children and create a good condition for the mind function.

The more we study, the more we will reach the conclusion that the world is relative, things are relative. There is nothing in the world similar to other things. They only have the same quantitative and qualitative characters but not the same. Because there are millions or countless varieties in an event or object that human beings do not realize, do not understand. These are the different varieties of different objects.

Never human being can create the same egg from one egg. Watching the two Sony televisions manufactured from one batch of one brand in the showroom, we do not realize the difference between the two televisions but they have a lot of different that we do not know. From one inch of the television screens, we may think they are the same inch. But the fact is not, the inch is not one solid dot, but it created from the countless different atoms of carbon, hydro, oxy, and metal atoms. These atoms may be formed from the death of different stars billion years ago. Each second of watching the televisions, we may the television generate the same qualities of the image, but in quantum physic, the image from one second watching two televisions are not the same. In one second, there are billions Planck Times. Each Planck Time, there are countless changes and interactions between the atoms and electrons that generate the different photons that we do not recognize. The human mind will assume that are the same televisions to make it better in the process of thinking, but it is not true in reality.

The human mind is relative. The state of somebody's mind is the meetings of countless phenomena before. These phenomena may have direct or indirect relation with those people that they do not know. It is true with the state of the world and the event of the world. They are the meetings of countless phenomena that human beings do not know at all.

But the ignorance, ego, selfish, negative mind, greed, and anger have prevented people from the ultimate truth; and made people make countless errors and destructions in the world. The whole world is in stressed. Next session is discussing the problems and its causes in the world.

Chapter 43: The geographical of diseases in the world

Cardiovascular diseases in Europe:

It is not fat food, trans-unsaturated fatty acids, and smoking, which majorly cause heart diseases. To some extents, food only contributes to the small part of physical health. It is time to search for the mental state, happiness, and state of mind of these people

According to the British Heart Foundation, the United Kingdom has more heart diseases than Germany, Belgium, and France. Even British consumption of saturating and trans fats less than these three countries.

Even more confusing are the people of France. Although the French smoke more, eats more fat, and consume only slightly more fruit and vegetables than the British do, the French have the lowest heart death rate in the European Union - only about one-quarter of the British rate. This is the notorious "French Paradox".

Although French hearts appear to be the healthiest and best preserved in Europe, they are certainly among the worst on the risk factors of diet and smoking.

The Spaniards, Finns, Italians, and Portuguese all eat less harmful fat and consume more fruit and vegetables than the French - yet die in greater numbers from heart disease.

According to the United Nations, in their report called the UN Chronicle, The Atlas of Heart Disease & Stroke, Japan has one of the lowest rates of coronary heart disease in the world, but the Japanese were found to have a gradually increasing risk after moving to North America, eventually approaching that of those people born there.

The highest rate of heart disease on the planet fluctuates a bit from year to year, but the annual winners seem to rotate around Eastern European populations in Ukraine, Bulgaria, Russia, and Latvia. Those Ukrainians, with a whopping 891 heart attacks per 100,000 populations, are hard to beat on dietary risk factors alone

Cardiovascular diseases in Canada:

In Canada, when it comes to our likelihood of suffering a heart attack, the geography of our country also plays a role - along with income. New data from the Canadian Institute for Health Information show that the rate of heart attacks in Canada's lowest-income neighborhoods was 255 per 100,000 populations, compared to 186 per 100,000 in the most affluent ones. That is a significant 37% difference. One explanation is, when people do not compare, and do not compete, and do not stressfully chasing the money, they will feel much happier and less much get a heart attack. Important gaps in heart health still exist between socio-economic groups, as well as between geographic regions in Canada. If we make a deeper investigation, we will see that the vital of the irrational mind with the thinking of happiness and contentment. The strong proof is the most surprising evidence from The Canadian Institute for Health Information suggests that where people live has the most significant impact on heart attack rates, followed by neighborhood income; these factors were more impactful than cardiac risk factors cited traditionally - like diet and exercise.

The good news for treatment is the state of mind is more important than person's income, according to the report, is that regardless of a person's income or place of residence, both the care they received and their treatment outcomes were similar no matter where in Canada they lived.

Cardiovascular diseases in China:

The situation in China: No one can escape from cardiovascular disease prediction in China. They are more stressed even the standard of living increase substantially.

It seems to help with the pandemic of heart diseases. According to official data, in China, about 230 million people have cardiovascular disease.

One in 5 adults in China has a cardiovascular disease.

In 2010, 154.8 per 100,000 deaths per year are estimated to be associated with cardiovascular diseases in urban areas and 163.1 per 100,000 in rural areas.

This number accounts for 20.9% /17.9% (urban/rural) of China's total number of deaths per year. People have enormous differences in standard of living and living environment but they still have nearly the same level of heart diseases.

Projected annual cardiovascular events are predicted to increase by 50% between 2010 and 2030 based on population aging and growth alone in China. Projected trends in blood pressure, total cholesterol, diabetes (increases), and active smoking (decline) would increase annual cardiovascular disease events by an additional 23%, an increase of approximately 21.3 million cardiovascular events and 7.7 million cardiovascular deaths.

Cardiovascular disease in China appears to have been spurred largely by increases in high blood pressure, according to a new study from Harvard T.H. Chan School of Public Health. The factor relating to stress and stress relieving factors: increasing body mass index (BMI), decreasing physical activity, a high prevalence of smoking, and the unhealthy diet has also contributed to the growing burden of cardiovascular disease — the leading cause of death in China.

Other results of stress living have been accompanied by marked increases in high cholesterol, obesity, and type 2 diabetes among the Chinese population.

"China is facing a rising epidemic of cardiovascular disease and it shows no sign of abating," said senior author Frank Hu, professor of nutrition and epidemiology at Harvard Chan School." It's imperative to continue to monitor the problem, which has serious social and economic consequences. The author also advised: "Prevention of chronic diseases through promoting healthy diet and lifestyle should be elevated to a national public policy priority."

It is time to look back the teaching of the ancient Chinese philosophers, and the profound of Chinese ancient pearls of wisdom to find out the real answer.

Cardiovascular diseases in the United States and its characters:

Because of different instincts and roles in society, men with pressure stress and women with ruminating stress develop a different kind of heart diseases.

Men are more stress than women are because of their instinct and responsibility.

Coronary artery disease, the type that causes heart attacks and is generally known as heart disease, is the leading killer in the United States., and men have much higher rates of it than women do.

One factor is that a heart attack often happened during night sleep. This is also the time of incubi and nightmare. How and why does it happen? My assumption is that during sleep, the cognitive mind is not activated; only the brain areas in the limbic system that control the anatomic nervous system activate. If people do anything wrong or illegal, or stressfully, which they consciously know or do not know, the limbic system or subconscious mind maybe over-activated because of the feeling of non-safety or danger. Stress chemicals arisen all day and significantly high during sleep because of fear, they may overact during sleep, and they may have experience of incubi (pressure on the heart because of the stress chemicals' effect on the heart) or they may have nightmare, stressed sleep, tired sleep, and worst of all is stroke.

Why Japanese men have far less heart disease than American men do?

Japanese men have far less heart disease than the American doe. In Japan, the percentage of men who smoke is 35.4%, more than double the rate of 17.2% in the United States.

Their average systolic blood pressure of Japanese men is 130.5, compared to 123.3 in the United States.

The cholesterol level averages of Japanese men: 201 mg/dl compared to 197 mg/dl in the United States.

The rate of diabetes in Japan is 7.2%, compared to 12.6% in the United States.

Surprisingly, the rate of coronary heart disease among Japanese men is less than one third that of the United States at 45.8 (per 100,000 per year), while American men have a rate of 150.7. Scientists will fail to figure out the cause of these diseases if they still attach with their old assumption about the diseases and do not investigate others factor like culture and characters of Japanese men and culture and character of American men. Suffering all the assumption risk factors for heart diseases and stress, but the differences in culture, characters, family, peaceful living understanding, relationship, and government have helped Japanese men more content, calm and happier than American men; that is why the environment living has helped Japanese men reduce the burden of risk factors. Japanese men have less stress in their family and in society. They are the ones who interact with others quite well, harmoniously, calmly and peacefully. Calm mind, good mental state and others advantage from abundant living have made Japanese people are the outliers in the battle of heart diseases.

Japanese men smoke cigarettes at twice the rate of American men, have higher cholesterol and higher blood pressure, yet they have about 30% the rate of heart diseases as in the United States. Note that their rate of diabetes is about 60% that of the United States.

The United States obesity rate is 33%; in Japan, it is 5%. As obesity is not the direct link to heart disease, obesity is other factors to measure the stress of populations.

Men in Japan, despite smoking much more than American men, and despite higher cholesterol and blood pressure, have a rate of heart disease 70% lower than American men do.

The problem of Japan

Any people in the world also surprise when seeing, reading, or hearing the stories told about the discipline of Japanese: children, adults, officers, and citizens. The order, disciplines of society still available in natural disasters and tsunami. Unfortunately, Japan has typical problems, most suicides are men, 71% of suicide victims in 2007 were male. They suicide perhaps mainly because of their disciplined, pressure from responsibility, and boring cultures. Japan may be a small disciplined military organization. So that the remedy for them is the humor, fun, irrational smile, cheerful, and supporting and caring for all people for each other, the best way to learn is by observing the angel babies.

In 2009, the number of suicides among men rose from 641 to 23,472 with that aged 40-69 accounting for 40.8% of the total

Suicide was the leading cause of death among men aged 20-44. Males are two times more likely to cause their own deaths after a divorce than females are. Nevertheless, suicide is still the leading cause of death for women age 15-34 in Japan.

Stress and diseases in Animals:

Research the habits and diseases of the animals we will understand the role of a calm mind and aggressive mind in the body.

Elephants are the big animals but the kind, calm ones, not the angry and aggressive ones. So that they can live longer, they do not suffer from stress. Look at how peaceful, calm and slowly they walk. The muscles do not much tension as the muscle of the aggressive and angry ones.

Large dogs are more aggressive and anger to fight than small dogs. It is true with the cat. That is why large dog and cat do not live as long as the expectation of the researchers.

Only about 5% of elephants die from cancer. This is staggeringly low when you consider that one in five humans will die from the disease. It against as human used to think, in theory, this ought to be a simple numbers game. The more cells an organism has and the longer it lives, the more likely it is that one of its cells will succumb to a random cancer-causing mutation. Elephants have trillions of more cells than us and live a long time, yet they have lower cancer rates. This is called "Peto's paradox", after the scientist Richard Peto, who noticed that cancer prevalence is not correlated with body size. The same is true of large dogs. Larger dogs are more prone to cancer. Cats can get many forms of cancer.

If elephants rarely get cancer, bowhead whales seem to get even less. That is surprising because, in theory, they should have a high risk of cancer. As well as being one of the largest animals alive, they are also among the longest-lived, sometimes surviving for over 200 years. That means their cells have plenty of opportunities to mutate and become cancerous, but they hardly ever do. The peaceful style of living, the calm and good brain state make the whale and elephants are getting a lower risk of cancer that the expectation of scientists. Giant bowhead whales have leisure life, has the pace of nature.

The naked mole rat, live under the ground make them absolutely feel safe. They live slowly and peacefully. The style of living helps them live much longer. Naked mole rats look pretty weird: they are wrinkly and hairless, with enormous front teeth. But they also live for up to 30 years, which is ancient for such a small animal. What's more, they have a natural defense mechanism against cancer. After several decades of observation, no naked mole rat has been observed developing a tumor.

Why is the rate of cancer increasing in beluga whales and sea lions? Perhaps they are still in the fear of killing. They live under stress more than before. Environmental pollutants are the coincident factor in countless stress human have created for wildlife animals. Thirty years ago, a Canadian marine biologist noticed something mysterious was happening to beluga whales in the St. Lawrence Estuary. Decades of over-hunting had decimated the population, but several years after the government put a stop to the practice, the belugas still hadn't recovered." They were dying of cancer," said Daniel Martineau, now a professor of pathology at the University of Montreal. The white whales were victims of intestinal cancers caused by industrial pollutants released into the St. Lawrence River by nearby aluminum smelters.

In the St. Lawrence region of Quebec, people who worked in smelters near the cancer-stricken belugas have reported many cases of lung and bladder cancers linked to coal tar exposure at the factories. Other residents of the region have higher rates of the digestive tract and breast cancers than people who live elsewhere in Quebec and Canada.

Chapter 44: The stressed world

How factors: love, connection, ability, and stressful environment affect longevity?

Researching the life of people with highest life expectancy, we will hardly find the proof for economy affect directly on longevity.

Jeanne Calment died at age of 122 years. Calment suggested that her longevity was to have credited her calmness, saying, "That's why they call me Calment." After her admission to the nursing home *"Maison du Lac"* in January 1985 at the age of 109, she initially had a highly ritualized daily routine whereby. Seated in her armchair she did gymnastics wearing her stereo headset. Her exercises included flexing and extending the hands, then the legs, and her caregivers noted that she moved faster than the other residents, who were 30 years younger, despite her blindness.

In nursing home:

Lack of love, lack of connection, lack of compassion make the old are more stress and do not have much enthusiasm in life. They do not die because of hungry, cold, pressure but because of the boring lifestyle.

According to the statistic of the length of stay in nursing homes at the end of life of the old, if the old come to the nursing home, the chance of the old living in the nursing home is nearly zero percent. It means that if your healthy 60-year-old enter the nursing home, the chance for them to live to 70 years old are very rare let alone they can live to 78 years old as the USA life expectancy.

Length of stay in nursing homes at the end of life of the old is less than 120 months. Most of them died during the first six months and the first thirty months.

The statistic shows that the health of the old in the nursing home has some relation to the love, caring and visit of their children, grandchildren.

There are stories that before the important day like national holiday, birthday and New Year, the death rate of the old reduces substantially. Perhaps, the hope, the wait, and expectation the important event with the reunion with their family members make them healthy enough to live.

Alarming the distribution of stress results all over the world:

It is lack of love, lack of connection, lack of ability, lack of understanding, and lack of compassion that cause people to live with lack of guiding by virtues, lack of gender equality, misunderstanding phenomena and causes countless bad causes. Worst of all, everyday life is covered by greed, hatred, anger and ignorance, and lots of violence, contempt for interaction, lots of violence in the act of helping others.

Let look at the geographical global distribution of some factors by the search on Google. Readers can easily search the articles and images on Google.

1. Age-standardized suicide rates per 100000 populations, both sexes, 2012 around the world.

2. Alcohol consumption by per capita consumption (liters) around the world

3. The attitude of population toward foreign visitors: most and least welcoming to foreigners

4. Average daily suicide rate per month around the world

5. Child poverty in the developed world

6. Corrupt across the world visualized: countries and territories ranked on perceived public sector corruption in 2014.

7. The discrepancy in education around the world

8. The discrepancy in secondary education around the world in 2015

9. Distribution of the diseases by countries around the world

10. Economic inequality around the world

11. Global gun deaths

12. Infant mortality rate per 1000 birth around the world

13. The probability of dying from the four main non-communicable diseases between the ages of 30 and 70 years, comparable estimates around the world in 2012

14. The rate of chronic hepatitis B virus infection around the world

15. The best and worst countries to be a mother

16. The best and worst places to be born

17. The distribution of heart diseases, diabetes around the world

18. The global overview 2014: people internally displaced by conflict and violence around the world

19. The health and chronic diseases of newborn babies depend on the month they are born.

20. The prevalence of heavy episodic drinking or binge drinking among male drinker around the world in 2004

21. The rate of equal education between male and female around the world

22. The rate of mental illnesses of adult and children around the world

23. The rate of suicide and homicide around the world

24. Geographic distribution of death sentences in the United States and around the world.

25. Women in politics around the world

26. World map of annual cannabis use

The health and chronic diseases of newborn babies depend on the month they are born. The chronic diseases babies will get in the future will not the same as the diseases that adults get the most that month. This is the indicator that the stress puts on the pregnant women will have an influence on the fetus and the chronic diseases children will get in the future. Chronic diseases children might get depend on the development of the fetus, the stress, the stage of fetus suffering stress, the abilities of parents, the stress after being born the fetus have. It has countless varieties so I hope that science will.

27. Age-standardized death rates due to cardiovascular diseases in 2013 around the world.

28. Age-standardized suicide rates per 100000 populations, both sexes around the world in 2012.

29. Consanguinity (%) around the world

30. Distribution of child and adult mortality around the world.

31. Education index around the world 2009.

32. Gini index or inequality in the distribution of and economic wealth among a population around the world.

33. Global gun deaths per 100000 populations around the world.

34. Gross enrolment ratio, primary, gender parity index (GPI) around the world in 2016.

35. Mental disorders span the globe: "Prevalence of mental disorders: anxiety, mood disorders, impulse-control, and substance abuse around the World.

36. Prevalence rates of intimate partner violence by WHO region in 2010.

37. The equality of receiving education between men and women around the world.

38. Worst of all is the "stroke mortality per 100000 populations around the world in 2010

"Intimate partner violence" The strange people first meet treating well, nicely, kindly and respectfully each other as the independent beings. After a hard time of courting, they become lovers with the serving heart. Getting married they have an assumption of becoming husband and wife. After getting married, what is the hell here! The social assumptions, social paradigms put on them that make the husband has the total right to demand many things from the wife. Even the wife, from the independent being, becomes the possession of the husband. The strange man after getting married, coded by social paradigms become the dictatorial man, he has a total right to treat whatever ways he like with his wife - a strange woman previously.

Watching the "Distribution of unsafe abortion per 1000 women aged 15 to 44 years around the world" and "Prevalence rates of intimate partner violence by WHO region in 2010" to understand better how ignorant human beings have rightly made with other human beings.

39. Distribution of unsafe abortion per 1000 women aged 15 to 44 years around the world

40. Prevalence rates of intimate partner violence by WHO region in 2010

Global burden of disease study & the Lancet, 2014 with the leading causes of death are Heart diseases, Lower respiratory infection, HIV/AIDS, Violence, Malaria, Diarrhea, Preterm birth, Birth defects, Stroke, Road injuries, and War. Looking at "The distribution of leading causes of lost years of life around the world in 2013" will give us a deeper understanding of the causes.

41. Differences in national homicide rates exist within regions and between regions.

42. Distribution of trafficking of females around the world.

43. Prevalence of female genital cutting around the world scaled 2011

44. The distribution of leading causes of lost years of life around the world in 2013

Going everywhere in the world, you will experience physical and/or sexual violence by a partner or sexual violence by a nonpartner." What is happening, what is the curse for human beings when the prevalence of women suffered intimate partner violence by WHO rouse around lowest is 23.2% in high income countries and highest are 36.6% in the African region, 37.0% in the Eastern Mediterranean Region and 37.7% in South-East Asia Region; it means one in three women. This is the tipping of the iceberg; we will have to suffer more if we do not eradicate the root.

People in the stressed world find drugs like "cocaine, cannabis, amphetamine stimulants, opioids, solvents and inhalants, sedatives" to relieve pain and find temporary good state. Let look at "What drugs countries seek treatment for." And "World Wealth level around the world in every year"

45. What drugs countries seek treatment for

46. World Wealth level around the world every year

The pattern thinking of human beings can be found in the allocation of their asset on investment, spending, education or buying the protective weapon. We will understand the real world we are living because "all in one and one in all". The spending of the United States on military in 2015 was $596.5 Billion that account for 54% of all spending of the United State in the year of 2015. All the major areas for stability and development like education, Medicare & health, veteran's benefits, housing & community, international affairs, energy & environment, science, social security, unemployment & labor, transportation, and food and agriculture was less than the spending on the military.

> "Do not ask me about the stability and development when people spend major resources on a minor military, and spend minor resources on all other major sectors"

Death rate, suicide rate, homicide rate, the percent of gender committed suicide rate, the kind diseases, health problems, teenager's problems, mental problems, social problems and quality of life are the reflection of the big hidden problem in society.

It is the lack of virtue, goodness, kindness, and integrity in society. The stress in society.

Seasonal stress in the developed world

The months of less stress in all developed countries is the summer holiday.

During the summer holiday, children may not suffer much stress and boring at school from the study and test. They have time to go out and play. During this time, the rate of injuries is increased and teenage death is higher than in other months.

Also, do adults arrange free time same as school summer holiday for the whole family to go somewhere for holiday? The words relating to stress like "pain, anxiety, stress, depression, and fatigue" searched on the internet from the United States drop substantially during national holiday and summer holiday.

During the summer month, people suffer the least stress to the rate of deaths per 100000 people reduced substantially in every country compared with other months.

Look at the mortality % of yearly average in the countries: United States, Japan, Italy, France, Spain, Canada, Australia, Sweden, Greece, New Zealand, and Cyprus. Low in the summer holiday, the rise during autumn and get the peak in the winter then go down in spring.

The pattern of the monthly death of the group one: United States, Japan, Italy, France, Spain, Canada, Sweden, Greece, and Cyprus have nearly the same pattern of fluctuation of monthly deaths because they have the same summer vacation time around June to September. The death rate around these months: June to September is the lowest in the years.

Luckily, the low stress in the summer vacation can affect the death rate by comparing the monthly death rate of group one with group two. In group two: Australian and New Zealand, they have the same pattern of death rate, but both countries have the opposite pattern of monthly death rate compared with group one. It is because the time of summer vacation of Australian and New Zealand is from the end of December to March. So that the death rate from December to March is lowest in the year, and the death rate from May to September is the highest in the year.

The pattern of the monthly death rate of these developed countries and the death rate and injury rate during the summer vacation tell us a lot about the pattern of stress in human society. It is the seasonal stress.

Furthermore, the peaks of death, the suicide rate in America and all other developed countries are in the spring and autumn. These times are the times of important examination of students in schools and universities around the developed world.

The important fact is all the previous researchers have failed to indicate the correlations of temperature, wealthy, longevity, the standard of living, geographic factors with the fluctuation of death rate around the year.

Does formal education is putting stress on children and stress on society is still an open question needed to answer in the future.

Young people committed suicide account for a big portion of the suicidal number. Do these young people stress with the old education, money and reward culture?

Recording of the death rate in the last ten centuries in Europe shows that from 1000 to 1600, the death rate of summer, spring, and fall was always higher than the death rate of winter. Until the seventeenth centuries - the era of the first industrial revolution - the death rate of winter started to over the death rate of summer, spring, and winter. Do formal education and lifestyle living of industrialization have any contribution to the monthly death rate?

There is a high number of people fail in the attempt of committing suicide. However, with the popularity of using guns in some countries, the percentage failing in committing suicide by using a gun to commit suicide is very rare. According to the article "Gun control could save veterans' lives" of Perry Stein in Newrepublic.com, in 2006, the Israeli Defense Forces made a relatively simple policy change that required soldiers to leave their weapons at their bases when they headed home for the weekend. The result: a staggering 40 percent drop in the suicide rate among soldiers aged 18-21, according to a November 2010 study.

"All in one, one in all" normally, if the young kid stressed from problems arisen from family, school, society, and friend, parents and other will invisibly fall to stress too. Stress will degrade the health of all people day after day.

Cancer and seasonal stress because of stressed mind in the United States.

Look at the geographic distribution of wealth, health, hygiene, social problems, health problems, mental problems in America, we will understand the illogical pattern of stress caused by the mind and condition living that effect to human beings.

The distribution of "food environment index" and "severe house problems" do not match with the mental problems, health problems, social problems, and teenage problems mean that mean stress and mental state do not have a direct correlation to the quality of food, eating, and physical living as most people assumed.

47. Geographical food environment index in the United States

48. Geographical severe house problems in the United States

Stress problems, stress diseases belong to the mind so it has illogical patterns. Irrational stress or stress paradox is the best explanation for the American paradox of distributions of wealth, health, diseases, social problems, teen problems, mental illnesses, and death rate.

They have suffered the outcomes of stress.

Stress comes from: lack of love, lack of connection to all other beings, and lack of ability to deal with problems and stressful situations; these lacking lead lack of understanding, lack of compassion, and lack of virtues, characters, and integrity. Over time, people distrust all things, events, and news. They live all day in fear, doubt, suspension, frustration. Their mind is full of discontentment, stress, confliction, and irritation. Where there is little trust, people start to be the slave of greed, anger and self-centered. Countless problems arise because the mind does not find peace and safe in society. The result is people are exhausted because of useless work like preparing, alerting, suspecting, and accumulating for self-protecting. These people are very weak and hurt inside. Even when the people at home, they do not feel safe let alone higher feelings of happiness. The mind starts to activate destructive stress state to prepare for the fight and flight and destroy all others feedback signals or balancing correction. Instead of healing, the minds of stressed people blindly destroy themselves.

49. The rate of cancer per 100000 people by the state is high in the southeast of America.

50. Report of urbanization by state: high in South of America

51. Cancer mortality rates by county in the United States

52. Geographic of incidence rates for all cancer in America 2006-2010

53. Crime rates by state, 2008

54. Map of the United States showing the mean number of mentally unhealthy

55. Prevalence of serious psychological distress among adults aged ≥18 years, by state, United States, 2007

56. Mean number of mentally unhealthy days during past 30 days among adults aged ≥18 years, by state, United States, 2009

57. Map of diabetes prevalence by county from 2004 to 2012.

58. Map of United States. Divorce per 1000 people.

59. Homicides per 100000 populations by state.

60. Percent of obese adults (body mass index of above 30)

61. Heart attack death rates, 2011-2013 adult, age 35+, by county.

62. Age-adjusted average annual deaths per 100000 populations.

63. County-level prevalence of frequent mental distress among U. S adults: 2003 -2009 from Centers for Disease Control and Prevention.

64. The inequality make discontent mind can see in the percent state population living in poverty by state

65. Childhood poverty rates, by the state also high in urban areas.

66. The ratio of population to mental health providers is high in the southeast areas.

67. Hazard distribution and frequency in the world

Food environment index is poorest in less developed areas in American. Astonishingly, the distribution of food environment index seems to contrast with the health index of the population. This is the clue that food is not a key factor that influences the health of people.

The other factor is "severe housing problems" are higher in less developed areas. This is proof that physical condition living does not influence much of the mental problems, social problems, and health problems as people usually assumed.

Discontentment comes from the fact that children in poverty are severer in urban areas.

The percent of preventable deaths per 100000 is American is highest with black American, and lowest in Asian American and Hispanic American. This fact may suggest to us that Black American are suffered the worst consequences of stress in society, and the Asian and Hispanic are suffered minor consequences of stress in society. Consequences are the combination of the love, connection, stress and ability of the individuals.

January is the month of death, and the trend is increasing year after year. There are seasonal fluctuations in United States deaths. I think it matches the seasonal stress in the United States. Let look at top 10 American children's health concerns from C.S Mott children's hospital national poll on children's health, 2011

Table 34: Top 10 American children's health concerns, 2011

Top U.S. children's health concerns Child health concern % rated as "Big problem" in 2011	Top 10 U.S. Children's health concerns rated by Hispanics Health concern, % rated by Hispanics as "Big problem" in 2011
1. Childhood obesity, 33%	1. Drug abuse, 49%
2. Drug abuse, 33%	2. Teen pregnancy, 44%
3. Smoking and tobacco use 25%	3. Childhood obesity, 44%
4. Teen pregnancy, 24%	4. Child abuse & neglect, 38%
5. Bullying, 24%	5. Stress, 38%
6. Internet safety, 23%	6. Driving accident, 37%
7. Stress, 22%	7. Bullying, 37%
8. Alcohol abuse, 20%	8. Smoking and tobacco use 35%
9. Driving accident, 20%	9. Internet safety, 34%
10. Sexting, 20%	10. Sexually transmitted infections, 33%

Source: C.S. Mott Children's Hospital National Poll on Children's Health, 2011

The county with the highest level prevalence of frequent mental distress among United States Adults: 2003 - 2009 is the Southeast United States or urban areas.

Heart disease death rates, 2008 -2010, adults, by county, highest in the Southeast United States or urban areas.

Percentage of people in poverty for the past 12 months, by state in 2011; the 2011 United States poverty average is 15.9 %. The Southeast states have a high percentage of people live in poverty. The gap between standard living makes the poor become more discontent and more stressed when they compare with rich people. Arizona has 19% of people in poverty, Mississippi with 22.6% of people in poverty.

According to Huffington Post, people live in urban areas of southeast America have the healthy life expectancy at age 65 is 13 years or less, whereas, people live other less developed areas have the life expectancy at age 65 is higher; some areas with 15 years or more.

Seasonal stress in America

Stress month of America is the January and February because it is the time to pay the debt by credit card. The financial burden is so heavy for them because they have overspent on the shopping season and Black Friday before Christmas and New Year.

Americans are so much stressed after overeating, overspending, and discontent with stressful work after the long holiday so that the flu season in America in January and February. There are a lot of incidences of deaths, flu, and strokes at the beginning of the year more than another month of the year. Even the weather of spring is better than the weather of winter.

The incidences of death rates and heart diseases in The United States during the beginning of the year are significantly higher than another month of the year and similar to with other developed countries.

Americans are so much stress with the burden put on them so that the month of heart diseases is February.

American misery index of 2014 searched on the Google

Look at the daily misery index, 2014 by the keywords searched on Google are depression, anxiety, pain, stress, and fatigue. The fluctuation of the searches is also the fluctuation of stress in the United States in 2014, retrieved from "The Google misery index: The times of year we're most depressed, anxious and stressed" by Christopher Ingraham on The Washington Post:

The searches rise in the spring and fall, ebb during the summer months, and drop sharply during holidays. Christmas is the least miserable days of the year, with Christmas Eve and New Year's Day.

The rhythm of stress during the week:

Peaks and valleys in the raw reflect the rhythm of the workweek. People are more stressed on weekdays, less so on weekends. Weekends are the best day of the week:

Pain and anxiety peak on Mondays, these numbers suggest that people literally hurt more on Mondays or afraid of boring stressful work.

Stress and depression are high on Tuesdays. Fatigue is high on Wednesday.

Searches for all terms drop sharply going into the weekend and then edge back upward on Sunday.

The gap between weekends and weekdays shrinks in the summer months (summer holiday): those peaks and valleys are a lot closer to each other in July than they are in March and April.

The annual trend in searches for "seasonal affective disorder," we will find that these peak in December and January. But the broader terms like "depression," "anxiety," and "stress," all show a pronounced dip in December. It means that shopping, preparing, planning, waiting and expecting, and enjoying the important and exciting days of the year make people happier than other days.

At the daily level, Thanksgiving, Christmas Eve, Christmas day, and New Year are all among the year's least-miserable or least stressed days.

After long and expensive holiday has made people more frustrated with work, but they have to bear the financial burden of the overspending credit card for the shopping season, Black Friday, and the spending during the holiday has made the people suffer the worst stress. These may be the trigger of the stress that they have suffered for a long time.

Randomly, on Wednesday, April 23rd, 2014 the large upper-level of stress words searched were accompanying cold front draped across the Central United States on April 18. Formed

April 15, 2016, and dissipated April 23rd, 2016. With snowfall, ice accretion, and rainfall near 51 cm around the Houston, Texas areas. Damage $ 2.7 billion. On 23rd April 2016 was the highest search with the stress words.

4/7/2016 is the National Day of America. People enjoy and celebrate so the stress words search on Google is the lowest.

Perhaps, people glad and treat well with each other on Valentine day, so the Saturday after valentine day of 2016, the stress words search on Google is the lowest.

Days of New Year, Thanksgiving, and Christmas was the happiest day of American. So the stress words search on Google is the lowest.

Reading this article, the facts show the reader enormously how fragile modern people are! People in the wealthy countries and all over the world are fall to the rhythm of stress on society. There are no direct root causes, stress is the accumulation of countless bad behaviors. Rare anyone can escape from the effect of stress. All people are affected by stress directly or indirectly. Worse of all, the infants, babies, the young, the old, the weak are the most fragile creatures affected first, then all people in society and the whole world will suffer later directly and indirectly. The sages will show the way to get out the spiral of stress.

The South African Stress and Health (SASH) study

By observing, you will see people living in the city with a lot of facilities do not make them happy if they have a discontent mind. Even worse, by comparing with other, discontent mind can fall to extreme stress.

People of South African are more stress than Nigerians are. Perhaps they do not accept or deal well with the problems as Nigerians do. They do not deal well with poverty and inequality as the Nigerians do. Lack of skills, abilities and discontent mind make them suffer more stress than Nigerian.

Especially, people in cities are lack of connection with people and nature so that they fall to more stressful and mental illness compared with the people in rural areas.

People and children in cities are better facilitated and fed than the people and children in the rural areas so that they lack some vital skills to deal with stress, people in cities are more stressed and get more mental illness than people live in the city. It is the skill, ability, and environment that directly and indirectly cause people stressed.

The Western Cape, which has the highest prevalence of common mental disorders, was the first region of South Africa to be colonized and has a high level of urbanization. In contrast, rural provinces generally have lower rates of common mental disorders, with the lowest rates in the Eastern Cape.

South Africa has a relatively high 12-month prevalence of anxiety and mood disorders when compared with the other countries in the World Mental Health Survey. Only Belgium, France, Germany, New Zealand, The Netherlands, Colombia, Lebanon, and the USA have higher rates of anxiety disorders than South Africa. And Belgium, Lebanon, Colombia, The Netherlands, France, Ukraine, Israel, New Zealand, and the USA have higher rates of mood disorders than South Africa. Hopeful that in the near future, scientists will find out detail the varieties in the cause and effect of stress on people.

Only 1 in 10 Nigerians had a lifetime DSM disorder, compared with 1 in 3 South Africans. Compared with Nigerians, twice as many South Africans had lifetime anxiety disorders, 4 times as many had lifetime mood disorders, and almost 6 times as many had substance use disorders. Reasons for differences in the prevalence of mental disorders in high- and low-income countries belong to the varieties stress states in the mind of people.

A recent study conducted by international research company Bloomberg, ranked South Africa as the second "most stressed out" nation in the world, following Nigeria. El Salvador was ranked third." The high-stress levels have been linked to mental illnesses such as depression and anxiety, and can also lead to substance abuse. In severe cases, these problems can lead to a person becoming suicidal," says Viljoen, but if make the deeper investigation, people will be astonished by the results of stress and the causes of stress that they are making and bearing.

The problem of the rich: substance abuse

Psychiatric illness on the rise: South Africa already has high rates of substance abuse with, for example, alcohol alone being the third-highest contributor to death and disability among citizens, according to a 2014 study published in the *South African Medical Journal*.

Dominique Stott from the Professional Provident Society, an insurance company for graduate professionals, said: "Rates of major mental illnesses such as schizophrenia seem to be stable but cases of depression and anxiety are certainly escalating." Perhaps, stability in major mental illness is own for the raising high standard of living, healthcare, and insurance so that they can treat the mental illness sooner and better. But the case of depression and anxiety are escalating because these above factors do not have any influence on the poor habitual living, poor cultural living, the stressful lifestyle and the poor abilities of the individuals.

Season of stress, not the season of heat and cold kills people

Summer break in the United States - Around 10-11 weeks, either from the end of May to early August, early June to Mid-August, or the end of June to the day after Labor Day in early September, or late June to the day after Labor Day - depending on region and state.

The death rate in Canada by month from 2007 to 2011 is the same. Whereas the incidents of injury are increased substantially during these months, and the teenage deaths during these months do not reduce as the total death.

During these summer days, just the small fluctuation of the hot temperature below 35 C° degrees can make changes in the number of deaths in developed countries. Temperature with 35 C° degrees is the normal temperature during the summer of people in developing countries in South East Asia, India. And it can be seen as the cool temperature in India and Africa. People in these developing countries usually live with a shortage of electricity and water during the hot summer.

Lack of vital things leads them to lack the adaptability with the small changes in temperature. The temperature is not the cause of deaths; perhaps, it is the trigger to worsen the stress of stressed people in western countries.

People died more because of diseases caused by stress despite the fact that the standard of living and healthcare have increased substantially.

Worldwide Facts

Over 80 percent of the world's deaths from heart disease occur in low- and middle-income countries. Stress is the product of poor interaction with too many problems and inequality. These lead to the discontent mind.

Stress is illogical. The mind is irrational.

These can explain the paradox that the French diet is high in dairy, fats, and red meat, these factors known to increase heart disease risk.

According to Oishimaya Sen Nag from Worldatlas.com,

The top five countries with the highest rates of heart disease deaths are:

1. Russia

2. Bulgaria

3. Romania

4. Hungary

5. Argentina

The top five countries with the lowest rates of heart disease deaths are:

1. France

2. Australia

3. Switzerland

4. Japan

5. Israel

Rainbow of stress

Because of the difference in the social status, social recognition, social gender advantages, religions, instincts, abilities, talents, and skills of different gender so that men and women suffer different stress outcomes spread on the rainbow of stress.

In America, suicide rates with age from 15-24 years old people, the number of males committed suicide substantially higher than the number of females.

- Nation sport in America caused different fatalities per 100000 students in high school after-school club activities from 1998 to 2007. It depends on the kind of fierce competitive sport or cooperative sport:
- "Fatalities per 100000 students are highest in Judo and Rugby", and lowest in tennis and table tennis.
- The sports like basketball, soccer, baseball have an average number of fatalities per 100000 students.

Cancer alarm at the firehouse, does it relate to stress at work? The answer is yes. Let see some clues. Stress in fighting fire is the factors that may multiply the effect of air quality of burning building. No one can imagine how stressful, how horrible, how hard in the battle with the fire of firefighters. Firefighters, their friends, the lives of people may die if they make mistake and fail.

During the firefighting, their bodies surge with the highest level of stress chemicals than the workers of other jobs that rarely anyone can imagine.

The study of Harvard researchers also showed that younger firefighters had more cases of certain types of cancer, such as bladder and prostate, than expected, that chances of lung cancer increased with time spent at fires, and the chances of dying from leukemia increased with the number of fire runs. These may be the indicators of skills, abilities, and state of mind of the young firefighters.

Harvard researchers led by postdoctoral fellow Emily Sparer, researchers including students from Harvard and MIT have teamed up with local fire departments to tackle a healthcare mystery: How does the firehouse itself increase cancer risk among firefighters?

The research showed an elevated rate of cancer diagnoses and deaths for firefighters, mainly for the digestive, oral, respiratory, and urinary disease. In addition, firefighters were about twice as likely to develop malignant mesothelioma, rare cancer related to asbestos exposure.

Heal thyself

There are facts that breast cancer survivors cite in preventing a recurrence. The major contribution to the long-term breast cancer survivors relates to the mind like positive attitude, diet, healthy lifestyle, exercise, stress reduction, and prayer. All of these factors help to make the people happier, less misery, less stress than normal. These factors make the mind in the good state and happy state so that the potential mind will correct the immune system and activate the healing function of the bodies. The human mind and human bodies have the most sophisticated and most effective function of protecting and healing the body that people not yet know.

Table 35: Attributions of cause and recurrence in long-term breast cancer survivors, 2001

Factors	Percent
1. Positive attitude	60%
2. Diet	50%
3. Healthy lifestyle	40 %
4. Exercise	39%
5. Stress reduction	28%
6. Prayer	20%
7. Complementary therapies	11%
8. Don't know	5%
9. Luck	4%
10. Tamoxifen	4%

The source: D. E Stewart et al., "Attributions of cause and recurrence in long-term breast cancer survivors," 2001

Chapter 45: Nature does not answer or revenge human beings

Luckily, nature does not care about human mistakes, human cruelties. Nature is just changing faster owning for the contribution of human beings. The slow pace of nature and evolution has created a heaven on earth through billion years. Slow but steady. How the miracle in nature that human beings do not know entirely. But one thing I know about the miracle of nature: all sophisticated creatures spices, bugs, flowers, animals, viruses, bacteria, and all the things people see, hear, and touch are the outcomes of revolution of raw materials in nature. Coal, gas, oil and countless residuals, fossils are the remaining of the previous creatures accumulated for billions of years. Human beings and the human world also are the products of nature evolved for billions of years. Look at your body and your children's body: how miraculous are the eyes, ears, intestine systems, heart, kidney, and brain! I am astonished seeing the creatures of nature. I am surprised seeing the wonder of nature. The moment of "Ah", "Wow", "Incredible", "Awesome," the bright wide opened eyes, and smiling faces cannot enough to describe how miraculous nature and what exactly hidden inside nature?

Unfortunately, nature takes billions of years to create a suitable environment for the development of human beings and temporal creatures. Each time of changing from the one ecosystem to the other ecosystem lead to the massive destruction of all beings. Dinosaurs started and dominated the earth for nearly 200 million years. Human evolution has only started for 65 million years, and the history of human beings is only 12000 years. Unfortunately, the changes caused by the human being are so enormous that nature starts to have some changes: hurricane, earthquake, landslide, storm, eruption volcano, the ozone layer, atmosphere, etc...

In 2017, the Hurricane Irma in the United States is twice as powerful as every World War II bomb dropped. Hurricane Harvey equal to one million Hiroshima Bombs per Day. We are too fragile and too weak with any changing of nature or ecosystems. If human beings still greedy like before, no one can have an exact answer for how long human beings will survive.

Look at the "natural disasters reported from 1900 to 2007" on Planetindistress.com we can easily draw out some facts: the natural disasters was stable low during 1900- 1940 fluctuated around 10 to 20 disasters a year, but since 1950, the number of disasters has astonishingly soared and reached to 500 natural disasters in 2000. If the natural disaster keeps soaring at this rate in the 21st century, billions of people will be the victim of natural changes and no one can warrant the safety of any other people.

Writing this book, a lot of events and crisis happened to the world with unknown causes. Most astonishing one is the two powerful earthquakes struck Mexico in just one month. From CNN, for the second time in two weeks, a powerful earthquake struck Mexico, toppling buildings, cracking highways and killing hundreds of people. The magnitude-8.1 quake struck off Mexico's southern coast on Thursday night; it's been described as the strongest earthquake to hit Mexico since 1932.

Chapter 46: The hidden correlation

There is always the correlation between all events happened to people, society, countries, and the world. The name of events, the description of the events, and the characters of events may not the same, but they all bear the same pattern. The pattern comes from the quality of the interaction of all creatures, beings, and elements in it. There are no single separate people, self and, ego, and beings. The world is interdependent. We are inter-beings. The quality of our life depends on the quality of life and the quality of all people despite that we cognitively know about their existence or not. The world is mysteriously interdependent, the virtues, pace of nature, Tao, and principles are the hidden laws control the interdependent world; these are the core in the teachers of all great philosophers, great religious leaders, and great educators.

Each time, people commit cheating, violating virtues, or doing against principles, they may do not cognitively care about the behaviors. But their potential mind can sense the smell, sound, and images of danger or non-safety. Each time they commit mistakes, their unconscious mind will sense the threatening which destroys the satisfaction of their basic needs, they make their mind fall to the more and more state of stress. All the luxury covers, wealthy cannot compensate for the weakness inside, cannot be satisfied with the hunger inside of beings. The more they neglect, the bigger the stressed mind. The mind may be stressed because it understands the effects of the bad actions but it cannot send the message to the cognitive mind, cannot create gut feelings strong enough to catch the notice of cognitive mind, and it cannot stop the countless bad actions... Until no one can help them.

Do you want to try the feelings of danger and un-safety?

- Try to cheat someone for money.

- Try to pickpocket someone's money

- Try to cheat on the exams

- Try to treat anyone

> And best of all is from the experiences: remember the feelings, pain, embarrassment, and uncertainty when you accidentally or purposefully making harm other, breaking the expensive pot or any behaviors that you know that it is against the common senses.

References:
Amerian psychological Association. (2011, January). Stressed in America. Retrieved September 19, 2017, from http://www.apa.org/monitor /2011/01/stressed-America.aspx

Amerian psychological Association. (n.d.). Report Highlights: Stress in America: Paying for our health. Retrieved September 19, 2017, from http://www.apa.org/news/press/releases/stress /2014/highlights.aspx

Ashtari, Shadee. (2014, June 24). Higher Gun Death Rates In States With Weak Gun Laws And High Ownership: Report. Retrieved September 19, 2017, from http://www.huffingtonpost.com /2014/06/24/states-gun-death-rates_n_ 5523570.html

Batts, Shelley. (2007, January 18). The Geography of Wealth and Pollution. Retrieved September 19, 2017, from http://scienceblogs.com/retrospectacle/2007/01/18/the-geography-of-wealth-and-po/

Burgreen, R. John. (2016, November 29). What have we been doing to end poverty? Retrieved September 20, 2017, from https://www.quora.com/ What-have-we-been-doing-to-end-poverty

Centers for Disease Control and Prevention. (2013, October 4). Mental health: Surveillance Data Sources: Health-Related Quality of Life—Behavioral Risk Factor Surveillance System. Retrieved September 20, 2017, from https://www.cdc.gov /mentalhealth/data_stats/nspd.htm

Cohena, S., Janicki-Devertsa, D., Doyleb, W. J., Millerc, G. E., Frankd, E., Rabine, B. S., and Turner, R. B. (2012, February, 27). Chronic stress, glucocorticoid receptor resistance, inflammation, and disease risk. Retrieved September 19, 2017, from http://www.pnas.org/content/109/16/5995.full

Coutsoukis, Photius. (2005, August 18). map of deaths from Urban Air Pollution. Retrieved September 19, 2017, from http://www.allcountries.org/ maps/urban_air_pollution_maps.html

Fisher, Max. (21013, August 12). 40 maps that explain the world. Retrieved September 20, 2017, from https://www.washingtonpost.com/news/worldviews/wp/2013/

08/12/40-maps-that-explain-the-world/?utm_term= fc9563d753e6

Galimberti, Katy. (2016, September 22). 5 easily-spread illnesses that peak in fall, winter. Retrieved September 20, 2017, from https:// www.accuweather.com/en/weather-news/fall-winter-illnesses-flu-noro/34682492

Gammon, Crystal. (2009, August 27). Cancer in wildlife, normally rare, can signal toxic dangers. Retrieved September 19, 2017, from http://www.environmentalhealthnews.org/ehs/news /wildlife-cancer

Global Burden of Disease Health Financing Collaborator Network, Campbell M., Chapin A., Eldrenkamp E., Fan V.Y., Haakenstad A., Kates J., ..., Murray C.J.L.(2017, April 19). Future and potential spending on health 2015-40: development assistance for health, and government, prepaid private, and out-of-pocket health spending in 184 countries. Retrieved September 19, 2017, from http://www.thelancet.com /journals/lancet/article/PIIS0140-6736(17)30873-5/abstract

Harvard T. H. Chan. (2016, August 15). China facing an epidemic of heart disease, stroke. Retrieved September 20, 2017, from https://www.hsph. harvard.edu/news/press-releases/china-heart-disease-stroke-epidemic-hu-li/

Harvard T. H. Chan. Department of Social and Behavioral Sciences (n.d.). Cancer Prevention with the Boston Fire Department. Retrieved September 20, 2017, from https://www.hsph .harvard.edu/social-and-behavioral-sciences/cancer-prevention-with-the-Boston-fire-department/

Harvard University. (2017, June 6). Anxiety and physical illness. Retrieved August 26, 2017, from https://www.health .harvard.edu/staying-healthy/ anxiety_and_physical_illness

Herman, A. A., Stein, J. D., Seedat, S., Heeringa, G. S. Moomal, H., And Williams, R. D. (2011, October 12). The South African Stress and Health (SASH) study: 12-month and lifetime prevalence of common mental disorders.Retrieved September 20, 2017, from https://www.ncbi.nlm. nih.gov/pmc /articles/PMC3191537/

Hogenboom, Melissa. (2015, October 31). The animal that does not get cancer. Retrieved September 19, 2017, from http://www.bbc.com/ earth/story/20151031-the-animal-that-doesn't-get-cancer

Jeanne, Calment. (n.d.). In Wikipedia. Retrieved September 19, 2017, from https://en.wikipedia.org/wiki/Jeanne_Calment

Kersley, Richard. (2016, November 22). The Global Wealth Report 2016. Retrieved September 19, 2017, from https://www.credit-suisse.com/corporate/en/articles/news-and-expertise/the-global-wealth-report-2016-201611.html

Key, Jane. (2016, July 6). These Sick Animals Could Be Key to Understanding Cancer. Retrieved September 19, 2017, from http://news. nationalgeographic.com/2016/07/these-sick-animals-could-be-key-to-understanding-cancer/

Kivimäki, M., and Kawachi, I., (2015, August 04). Work Stress as a Risk Factor for Cardiovascular Disease. Retrieved September 20, 2017, from https://link.springer.com/article/10.1007/s11886-015-0630-8

Kosatky, Tom. (2005, July 1). THE 2003 EUROPEAN HEAT WAVES. Retrieved September 20, 2017, from http://www.eurosurveillance.org /ViewArticle.aspx?ArticleId=552

Lee, L., Roser, M., and Ortiz-Ospina, E. (2017). 'Suicide'. Published online at OurWorldInData.org. Retrieved September 20, 2017, from https://ourworldindata.org/suicide/

Macmillan, Susan. (2015, July 23). UK chief scientific adviser visits Kenya: Part 3: The dual rise of the global livestock sector and antimicrobial resistance. Retrieved September 20, 2017, from https://news.ilri.org/2015/07/23/uk-chief-scientific-adviser-visits-kenya-part-3-the-dual-rise-of-the-global-livestock-sector-and-antimicrobial-resistance/

Maier, Rachael. (2014, February 28). Heart Disease Statistics. Retrieved September 19, 2017, from http://www.healthline.com /health/heart-disease/statistics

Mangan, P. D. (2016, October 10). Why Japanese Men Have Far Less Heart Disease. Retrieved September 20, 2017, from https://medium.com/the-mission/why-japanese-men-have-far-less-heart-disease-badbc3841322

Martin, Sean. (2017, September 19). WARNING: Italian SUPERVOLCANO is becoming 'more dangerous' as magma builds beneath surface. Retrieved September 19, 2017, from http://www.express.co.uk/news/science /856092/volcano-Campi-flegrei-eruption-Naples-Vesuvius-Pompeii

Martin, Sean. (2017, September 7). Hurricane Irma twice as powerful as EVERY World War Two bomb dropped. Retrieved September 20, 2017, from http://www.express.co.uk/news /science/851240/hurricane-Irma-path-NOAA-track-models-update-Florida-US-World-war-two-bomb

Military budget of the United States. (n.d.). In Wikipedia. Retrieved July 17, 2017, from https://en.wikipedia.org/wiki/Military_budget_of_the_United_States

Mortimer, Caroline. (2015, June 10). How your birth month affects what diseases you will get. Retrieved September 19, 2017, from http://www.independent.co.uk/life-style/health-and-families/how-your-birth-month-affects-what-disease-youll-get-10310792.html

Nag, S. Oishimaya. (2017, April 25). Countries With Highest Rates Of Cardiovascular Disease Deaths. Retrieved September 19, 2017, from http://www.worldatlas.com/articles/countries-with-highest-rates-of-cardiovascular-disease-deaths.html

National Poll on Children's Health. (2011, August 15). Drug Abuse Now Equals Childhood Obesity as Top Health Concern for Kids. Retrieved September 19, 2017, from http:// www.mottnpch.org/reports-surveys/drug-abuse-now-equals-childhood-obesity-top-health-concern-kids.

National Poll on Children's Health. (2013, August 19). Top Child Health Concerns: Obesity, Drug Abuse, and Smoking. Retrieved September 19, 2017, from http://www.mottnpch.org/reports-surveys/top-child-health-concerns-obesity-drug-abuse-and-smoking.

National Priorities Project. (2015, May 28). Cost of National Security Retrieved July 29, 2017, from https://www.nationalpriorities.org/cost-of/

National Priorities Project. (n.d.). Military Spending in the United States. Retrieved July 29, 2017, from https://www

.nationalpriorities.org/campaigns/military-spending-united-states/

Nield, David. (2015, October 15). These Animals Don't Get Cancer, And Scientists Think They Could Hold a Cure. Retrieved September 20, 2017, from https://www.sciencealert.com/these-animals-can-t-get-cancer-and-scientists-think-they-could-hold-a-cure

NOAA Fisheries West Coast Region. (n.d.). 2016 Elevated Califorena Sea Lions Strandings in California: FAQs. Retrieved September 19, 2017, from http://www.westcoast.fisheries.noaa.gov/protected_species/marine_mammals/sea_lion_UME.html

Orenstein, Peggy. (2008, June 29). Stress Test. Retrieved September 19, 2017, from http://www.nytimes.com/2008/06/29/magazine/29wwlnlede-t.html? mcubz=3

Park, Alice. (2015, June 08). See What Diseases You're at Risk For Based on Your Birth Month. Retrieved September 19, 2017, from http://time.com/ 3913118/birth-month-disease-risk/

Planet In Distress. (2012, May 18). Increasingly frequent disasters and the fulfillment of prophecy. Retrieved September 10, 2017, from https://planetindistress.com/2012/05/18/increasingly-frequent-disasters-and-the-fulfillment-of-prophecy/

Powell, Alvin. (2017, August 14). Cancer alarm at the firehouse. Retrieved September 19, 2017, from http://news.harvard.edu/gazette/story/2017/08/harvard-researchers-examine-firehouse-cancer-threat/

Reeves, C. W., Strine, W. T., Pratt, A. L., Ahluwalia, I., Dhingra, S. S., McKnight-Eily, R. L.,..., and Safran, A. M. (2011, September 2). Mental Illness Surveillance Among Adults in the United States. Retrieved September 20, 2017, from https://www.cdc.gov/mmwr/preview/mmwrhtml/su6003a1.htm

Rogers, L. Heather. (2016, Dec 12). Heart disease and the stress hypothesis in the mid-twentieth century: a historical review. Retrieved August 26, 2017, from http://www.scielo.br

/scielo.php?script=sci_arttext&pid=S0102-79722016000104301

Schneiderman, N., Ironson, G., and Siegel D. S. (2008, October 16). STRESS AND HEALTH: Psychological, Behavioral, and Biological Determinants. Retrieved September 20, 2017, from https://www.ncbi. nlm.nih.gov/pmc/articles/PMC2568977/

School holidays in the United States. (n.d.). In Wikipedia. Retrieved August 26, 2017, from https://en.wikipedia.org/wiki/School_holidays_in_the _United_States

Shah, Ajit, and Chandra, Mahmood. (2010, Jun). The relationship between suicide and Islam: a cross-national study. Retrieved September 20, 2017, from https://www.ncbi.nlm.nih.gov/pmc/articles/PMC3134910/

Sheldrick, Giles. (2017, June 21). Is your health written in the stars? How your birth month affects diseases you could get. Retrieved September 19, 2017, from http://www.express.co.uk/life-style/health/819685/health-horoscopes-birth-month-affect-diseases-you-could-get

Spencer, W. Roy. (2017, August 25). Hurricane Harvey: 1 Million Hiroshima Bombs per Day. Retrieved September 19, 2017, from http://www.drroyspencer.com/2017/08/hurricane-harvey-1-million-hiroshima-bombs-per-day/

Stewart DE1, Cheung AM, Duff S, Wong F, McQuestion M, Cheng T, Purdy L, Bunston T. (2001, April)." Attributions of cause and recurrence in long-term breast cancer survivors." Retrieved September 19, 2017, from https://www.ncbi.nlm.nih.gov /pubmed/11268144

The Death Penalty Information Cente. (n.d.). Arbitrariness. Retrieved September 19, 2017, from https://deathpenaltyinfo.org/arbitrariness

The effect of the summer 2003 heat wave on mortality in the Netherlands. Retrieved September 19, 2017, from http://www.eurosurveillance.org/ViewArticle.aspx?ArticleId=557

The relationship between suicide and Islam: a cross-national study Ajit Shah, Mahmood Chandia J Inj Violence Res. 2010 Jun; 2(2): 93-97. doi: 10.5249/jivr.v2i2.60 PMCID: PMC3134910

Thomas, Carolyn. (n.d.). Heart disease: which countries have the highest and lowest rates? Retrieved September 20, 2017, from https://myheartsisters. org/2010/07/17/heart-disease-countries/

United Nations News Centre. (2017, September 19). At UN, Central American leaders urge 'rethink' of a system used to classify development status. Retrieved September 20, 2017, from http://www.un.org/apps/news/story.asp?NewsID=57585 #. WcIbuJAX7IU.

United Nations News Centre. (2017, September 19). Bolivia's Morales, at UN, says natural resources, basic necessities must be viewed as human rights. Retrieved September 20, 2017, from http://www.un.org/apps/news /story.asp?NewsID =57583#.WcIcj5AX7IU

United Nations News Centre. (2017, September 19). Citing Rise in Weather-Related Disasters, Secretary-General Calls for Faster, Bolder Action to Build Green Economy, at Leaders Dialogue on Climate Change. Retrieved September 20, 2017, from http://www.un.org/press /en/2017/sgsm 18697.doc.htm

United Nations News Centre. (2017, September 19). No alternative to international cooperation, stresses Austrian minister at UN Assembly. Retrieved September 20, 2017, from http://www.un.org/apps /news/story.asp?NewsID=57584# .WcIciJAX7IU

United Nations News Centre. (2017, September 19). Repair 'world in pieces' and create 'world at peace,' UN chief Guterres urges global leaders. Retrieved September 20, 2017, from http://www.un.org/apps/news/story.asp?NewsID=57549 #.WcIbrZAX7IU

United Nations News Centre. (2017, September 19). Secretary-General Stresses Political Solutions in Addressing Nuclear, Terrorism, Migration Issues, as United States President Warns Pyongyang. Retrieved September 20, 2017, from http://www.un.org/press/en/2017/ga11947.doc.htm

United Nations News Centre. (2017, September 19). Secretary-General Urges Support for Proposed Global Environment Compact to Ensure Well-Being, Dignity, Prosperity of All. Retrieved September 20, 2017, from http://www.un.org /press/en/2017/sgsm18696.doc.htm

United Nations News Centre. (2017, September 19). Transfer of power essential to strengthen democracy, Sri Lankan President tells UN Assembly. Retrieved September 20, 2017, from http://www.un.org/apps/news/story.asp?NewsID=57582#.WcI clpAX7IU

United Nations News Centre. (2017, September 19). Women's Economic Empowerment 'a Human Rights Issue', Secretary-General Tells High-Level Panel, Saying Labour Force Excludes Half Those of Working Age. Retrieved September 20, 2017, from http://www.un.org /press/en/2017/sgsm18695.doc.htm

Walsh, Bryan. (2004, May 10). Asia's War with Heart Disease. Retrieved September 19, 2017, from http://content.time.com /time/world/article/0,8599,2047659,00.html

World Economy. (n.d.). In Wikipedia. Retrieved July 10, 2017, from https://en.wikipedia.org/wiki/World_economy

World Health Organization. (2012, April). Spending on health: A global overview. Retrieved September 19, 2017, from http://www.who.int/ mediacentre/factsheets/fs319/en/

World Health Organization. (n.d.). Cardiovascular diseases: The situation in China. Retrieved September 19, 2017, from http://www.wpro.who.int /china/mediacentre/factsheets/cvd/en/

Xu, jiaquan. (2016, January). Mortality Among Centenarians in the United States, 2000—2014. Retrieved September 20, 2017, from https://www.cdc.gov/ nchs/data/databriefs/db233.htm

Part X: Paradoxes of Mind and the Science of Achievement

I understand that I am not myself. I am just the meetings and illuminations of countless events happen to and in me. Knowing that the mass of the earth has not been increased or decreased much for billions of years, the only changing thing in the earth is the constant interacting of the materials in earth has created sophisticated substance and then life. I know that my physical body, feeling, thinking, brain, consciousness, and mind are changing constantly, never cease of changing. Owning for changing, I grow from a fetus to a baby; owning for changing, I grow from a baby to a teenager, and I am now. In the process of constantly changing, I take countless substances, ideas, philosophy to embed in my brain, genes, and body. I also know that I have expelled countless things and phenomena in life in each previous Planck time. The live and development are the results of countless interactions, of giving and receiving, of bearing and forgiving, of stubbornness and letting go, of the moment taking the breath away, of loving and sharing, of understanding and enlightenment. There is nothing exist solely. Things and beings are emptiness and egoless. It means that things are interdependent. Things rely on others to exist. The illumination of meeting phenomena can create countless other phenomena. To understand the phenomena we called cause and effect. The fact is there is no single cause or single effect; definition and separation only help the mind understand but the real life is not separate like that. Life operates follow Yin and Yang. Causes are effects; effects are causes. Otherwise, inside causes, there are the seed effects, and inside effects, there are the seeds of causes. Wrong understanding of the mind is a stubborn attachment to the absolute things or attach to the separation of things. Worst of all is the attachment to the ego or nothingness, from the wrong understanding created countless bad cause for society. The result that bad causes create in life is not simple small as we logically think. Life is illogical logic. We do not know much about the logic of life. A small bad cause can create catastrophic destruction. Human beings still bear the beating of parents and adults to children or the raping of children and slaves ten years ago, hundred years ago, and thousand years ago. The inhumane acts in the history may have created dictators, corrupt politicians, thieves, killers, murders, Hitler, atomic bombers, terrorists, corrupt philosophers and corrupt leaders. Present are the product of countless events, phenomena in the past. The future will be the results of countless events in the present also. Looking at all data about human beings, the sages can predict what the future will be.

Chapter 47: Real learning

Forget the role of formal education. Forget about the degree. The result of a good education is measured by action and contribution. No matter how smart you are, no matter what degree you have, no matter how big you shout. Show what you have done, what you have done for others, what you have done for your people. And what is the attitude, drive, and emotion you have when you do. Do you greed, do you anger, do you understand others?

Measure by attitude, characters, and contribution, we will realize that real learning does not totally depend on formal education. It will depend on the characters of educators, of parents and every people they contact; and the ability of love, kindness, compassion, and purpose of learners. Most of the educators, religious leaders, contributors, self-made billionaires, and millionaires like Bill Gate, Warren Buffer, Stephen Covey, mother Teresa and top people who contribute for the development of the world do not come from the knowledge of formal education. They are the product of self-education with kind, compassion and serving heart and principles. The world needs doers, trainers, and educators who have kind, compassion, and serving heart, the world does not need empty talkers. The destination of learning is the enlightenment that Socrates, Buddha, Lao Tzu, and Benjamin Franklin pointed out: understanding the paradoxes of life to have wealth, health, abundance, happiness, and inner peace. Learn from the process of learning from fragile, weak children, with them learning is the natural and joyous process. How hard to teach the normal function, behaviors, language, and activities for autistic children? All these processes have been taking place so automatically and silently in the healthy children that we do not know.

Table 36: The process of learning

The process of learning	Gain what	Conditional personality
Information, facts	Know what	Patience
Data		Compassion
Knowledge and theory		Love Simplicity Kind and serving heart
Skills and massive action	Know-how	Good attitude
Wisdom	Understand why others and nature. The science of achievement, goals, visions, purposes and massive actions	Curiosity Imagination Initiate Empathy Enthusiasm Creativity
Enlightenment	Master the art of life and happiness. Master the paradoxes of life and the self: act without conditions, act without purposes, act without expectations, unconditioned love, and selfless actions.	Discipline Dedication Taking responsibility Selfless purposes

Chapter 48: What do create human beings?

All things in the universe create human beings; but there is no separate thing or a single thing, which created human beings. Darwin was right with the opinion that human beings are in the evolution scales as all other species. Under nature, we are equal to all other species. Human beings were luckier than other spices because of the weakness so our ancestors united to live, to protect and to fight. Then they had more time for thinking and contemplating. The neo-cortex started to develop. In the neocortex, each region taking charge of each human activity and skill, the mastery of specific skills will determine the specific intelligence of the individuals. Neo-cortex mainly crystallizes the information deeply embed in the limbic systems and all brain; to describe information in the brain, people use the limited sensual signals to describe and communicate information with other individuals: tongue with taste, the eye with sight, the ear with sound, nose with the smell, and skin with touch. Words and language is only one small part of all vehicles human use to communicate information inside the brain with others. Only a small part of the world is caught by all sense as a signal of information, only smaller part of information is embedded in brain call subconscious mind, the much smaller part of information is reflected in the neocortex and understood by neocortex, then only smaller part of information can be described in words, rhythm, images, flavors, and smell; and most of all there are countless factors can affect this process of thinking. This is the reason that people say people have relative views before each event.

In the experiment on mice, scientists ring the bell before creating a shock to the deaf mice. After several times of creating the responses, scientists just ring the without creating shock, astonishingly, the deaf mice have conditioned responses as if they are being shocked. All the process of realizing recording, recalling and taking out information inside the brain formed the concept of consciousness, awareness, and thinking. The quality of awareness depends on the connection of all parts of the brain and body. The better of the connection, the better the mind, brain, and consciousness are. The quality of the connection inside the brain and body depends on the frequencies of using the mind, the state of mind, body, and brain. The brain is a part of the natural world so to create a good state of mind people should study and follow the principles in nature to create a good environment for brain and body. These principles taught well in all teachings of the sages, who had close contact with nature. It is time to correct human errors by following the teaching of the old.

All techniques in Neuro-Linguistic-Programming (NLP), setting goals, visualization, and affirmation help to set up a new paradigm of thinking and the vivid visions as the order of to the powerful brain to make the mind, brain, and body function better. It is setting the goals, embed visions and outcome that focus the mind and brain so that the frequencies of individuals meet, see, encounter increase astonishingly, even more, the individuals will achieve that visions so much faster. Embedded goals, visions, and values seem like the giant filtering cover all individuals' senses and silently direct the mind to focus on achieving. Most of the time, the results people get fit with their goals, desires, visions, and wishes, so that people may illusively think that God will give them all the thing they ask, there is invisible creators ready to support whatever people ask, or even some people may think they are the centers which attract all the thing they want or demand described in the law of attraction. It is not true, it is the law of mind and the law of thinking that determines the human world.

The whole world, including human beings and all spices, are interdependent. If Aliens pick any one of us, move to the stars or planets years of light far away to examine, they will get nothing exact as we are today. Countless data about me could not create persons like me. Human beings are interdependent.

Billions of atoms, substances inside our body come from billions of sources. Some come from the sperm of rapists, the saliva of corrupt men, the blood of animal hundred years ago, and from the skin cells, blood cells of religious leaders. And the thinking we have also the products of people before us, and the thoughts of the following people. No one, no computers can predict exactly what will happen in the next human economic crisis, or tomorrow lottery result let alone predict the events in the next ten or hundred years. Scientists only can make the prediction of the probability of the events in the future based on the current events and dominating philosophy.

Next sections are the teachings of the sages, successful men, religious leaders that embed in me, creates my changes and create my thinking and my philosophy to write these books for needed people.

Chapter 49: Paradoxes of the mind

Psychology focus on paradoxes of the mind to overcome it

The teaching of successful men:

1. You do not believe what you see, you only see what you believe

2. When anger, people do not hear the evidence, they only hear things for themselves.

3. Smart people do not need a piece of advice, stupid ones will not take it.

4. Harper Lee taught: Many receive advice, only the wise profit from it.

5. John C. Maxwell taught: Pride deafens us to the advice or warnings of those around us.

6. Benjamin Franklin taught: Believe none of what you hear, and only half of what you see. And to succeed, jump as quickly at opportunities as you do at conclusions.

7. Aesop taught: The smaller the mind the greater the conceit.

8. Saint Augustine taught: faith is to believe what you do not see; the reward of this faith is to see what you believe.

These are some characters of our mind, to save energy, the lazy mind tends to jump to a conclusion very quickly. The mind falls to irrational and emotional thinking. When jumping to a conclusion, this conclusion will become an expectation. This expectation will be the guidance for the mind in the situation. The mind unconsciously accepts things and information support the expectation and rejects things in contrast to the expectation. With the information the mind gets and the expectation, the mind will stimulate the emotion; this emotion depends on the matching between information and expectations. If they match well, people will happy; if they do not match or have a big gap, people will angry.

With anger and conclusion in the mind, the subconscious mind does very well to scan the environment to find the supporting or threatening signals to the anger and conclusion. The huge potential power of brain misleads by anger and stubborn conclusion. Individuals close all gates for understanding. Individuals who are lazy in thinking tend to cling to this emotion and conclusion, the mind closes with other contrasting ideas. It is very difficult to advise them; especially people in anger and in stress.

Most people jump to the conclusion very quickly with shallow thinking and any evidence people catch at that moment, it is like forming their own belief about the situation. From that on, people do not believe what people see, they only see what they believe. It is like a process of programming our mind, programming the perception of the environment. If we come to conclusion, we will get the facts and information which tends to fit with that conclusion. Peter Drucker – father of modern management - advised that we should remove assumptions before coming to the situation. Just start by observing and asking questions. Warren Buffet does not use the charts, the diagrams of statistics because he knows that the results may be distorted by the understanding and assumptions of the analyzers.

When a hasty man comes to a new situation, he may jump to a conclusion quickly, and may easily fall to angry state if the conclusion does not match with his assumption. The state of mind will change just according to the matching with the assumption. Then the mind will obey the negative emotion, it scans for the wrong things, the negative faces of the situation. Most of the time the mind will get the information to feed the angry emotion, but he may think that this information comes from rational thinking. He lets the ego win, it starts latching on, demanding. An extremely negative source of energy runs through his bodies and people around. It may run throughout the home, every corner, present in every interaction. Family members, especially small kids always fall into a state of insecurity, tension or fear if they have hasty parents. This can create stress state unless the conscious mind awakes to have a good understanding of what is happening, to make him withdraw from the situation then start with the process of thinking with the imaginative questions. Time and withdrawal make him calm it down, change from emotional thinking to logical thinking naturally.

Stressed state, with the arousing of stress chemicals, creates a lot of side effects described in table three. Stress is the source of family problems, social problems, and health problems. Stress creates countless negative phenomena will still leave bad tracks an individual's actions; negative phenomena will appear when they are working, studying and thinking. People who live in a stressful environment have to work to have a feeling of safety. However, this safety is always in the hands of others who have a big ego and the irrational emotion, which are constantly fluctuating. This safe is hard to achieve, no matter how hard the individuals try. The basic human needs are not satisfied. The mind uses the giant potential of the brain to scan the environment to find the safety of the owners. Unfortunately, for individuals living in a stressful environment, they can never find safety, never find peace of mind; at home, they have to watchful and alerted as if they are in dangerous places. All-time, energy, and money are wasted on useless work, useless argument, and worthless wars. Stress makes people exhausted with countless activities, and hopeless in finding peace and happiness. Stress creates a vicious circle of problems. Family members are tired, exhausted and stressed. There are not enough words to explain the effects of chemicals of stress, which run through the body and brain every day and night. Stress consumes a lot of energy and resources to find safety. Excessive stress chemicals make a lot of unwanted effects. Stress releases oxidants, wasted products that may harm the organs and cells: the brain, the nerves, cardiovascular system, and immune system. Worst of all, the brain of people suffered chronic stress may make the order for the immune system to attack any organs participating in regulating stressed state. When these negative chemicals circulate in the body more often, the organs in the body create more receptors to receive or resist them and change some normal functions to adapt to the stressed state. The trails formed, and the adaptation causes the body and the organ to deviate from the natural rhythm, which causes changes and pathological processes that deplete the body. Some of the diseases diagnosed by physicians are the results of stress in the body lasted for many years. Doctors will prescribe symptomatic medications that work instantly, but do not cure the root of illness. Some patients prefer to reduce the chronic discomfort symptoms instantly with symptomatic medications, this lead to abuse of symptomatic medications and many of its side effects. They fall into the vicissitudes of drug side effects and drug abuse. From the point of view of a pharmacist, it will more effective for patients with chronic disease, besides taking symptomatic medication, they also need practice sports, meditation, yoga, volunteering; love and caring actions; which help to create peace of mind and stillness of mind. In a good mental state of mind, the potential brain will focus to correct any damages better than symptomatic medication.

It will be useless if people use medicine and symptomatic medication for their diseases but still have to live under stress. The negative perceptions about the environment make negative patterns appear in every thought, word, action, and behavior. They are the victims of the mind, the victims of the self. So that there is no medicine or remedy can cure their problems.

If we do not understand the mind, do not understand people, environment, the obvious differences between people, the obvious difference between genders, we will meet countless conflicts in life, suffer endless stress no matter who we are.

How do we rule the mind?

1. Abraham Lincoln taught: When I am getting ready to reason with a man, I spend one-third of my time thinking about myself and what I am going to say and two-thirds about him and what he is going to say.

2. Aristotle taught: It is the mark of an educated mind to be able to entertain a thought without accepting it.

3. Will Smith taught: Money and success do not change people; they merely amplify what is already there.

4. Mother Teresa taught: Be faithful in small things because it is in them that your strength lies. We think sometimes that poverty is only being hungry, naked and homeless. The poverty of being unwanted, unloved and uncared for is the greatest poverty. We must start in our own homes to remedy this kind of poverty.

5. Lao Tzu taught: Being deeply loved by someone gives you strength while loving someone deeply gives you courage.

For effective of using the mind, we need to entertain with thought but should not accept it immediately, remove all doubts and expectation, do not cling to our own expectation, check our beliefs, open to new ideas and theory, and get the real understanding of mind. When in the situation of making a decision, we need to awaken to know the thought and feelings, emotion comes and goes within our mind; we need to contemplate, question all the passing by phenomena. Practicing meditation can help us realize the constant changing of mind, feeling, body, objects of the thinking so that we can gain real understanding. Owning for understanding we can know how to deal with problems effectively.

Preparing, compassion, unconditional love, understanding, and removing all assumption will help us find out the win-win solutions in all conflicts.

The fact is our knowledge is a drop in the ocean knowledge if we know that, we will have an open mind, welcome new possibilities. Do not cling much to our own conclusion, our own expectation. If we cling to this, it will make us close the mind, experience extreme pain for our self and others.

Life has cause and effect, obeys the law of cause and effect. With the guiding of Lao Tzu, I think the relationship of cause and effect not direct but indirect, not visible but invisible; not obvious but subtle; not measurable but immeasurable; cannot be seen but must be felt; not be caught by chasing and grasping. It caught by sitting, contemplating in stillness, and a clear mind. This is the way of effortless but most effective - the way of nature. Perhaps, these are the answer for the failure of dealing with the problem in family and society. Even we spend a lot of resources with high technology, a lot of effort to figure out the cause of problems. We jump in with an expectation to try to find visible and direct causes. Come in with expectation, we easily jump to any conclusion go around, which seem obvious, understandable and meet our expectations. We catch them, list in the book called the Causes. Then spend much more effort to find the quick fix for the problem with the Causes. We have carried out in large scale with a lot of human resources, technology, and billion dollars. Unfortunately, year after year, the problems become much worse. The number of people suffering problems in health, diseases, troubles in the community is soaring, and with the trend out of control. The big paradox for scientists is mental diseases and suicidal death, which is high in rich countries, despite, the living standard is the dream of people in developing countries.

Money and success do not change people. Money only makes you go faster to your destiny. The answers are simple; the solutions are simple. The answers are in the teaching of Great men, Great women, Great philosophers, Buddha, Christ, Socrates, and so on. We can easily find out their belief, their thinking by the recording of their actions: the way they solved conflicts, the way they overcame themselves, the way they got out failures. They left teachings for us to study, practice to have a good life. Their actions have same basic patterns. If we act in these patterns, someday some of us will be someone else like them.

People make others feel safe, energized and happy by satisfying the need of wanted, loved and cared. According to John Maxwell, they are up-lifters or multipliers, these multipliers are capable of meeting the above needs of others, they forge good actions into habits; serving people make them feel happy, tranquil and joyful. They have the habits of highly successful people. These habits summarized in Stephen Covey's book: Seven habits of highly effective people. I highly recommend you read this book.

The story of old philosophers to teach the young: there is a good wolf and bad wolf are fighting in every people, and the wolf that people feed the most will win in that battle. In dealing with a person, the way of your approaching will feed the good wolf or bad wolf in that person. The wolf will appear in action and becomes bigger in both persons. You and that person will have the habit of calling out the good wolf or bad wolf according to your pattern of behaving. Mastering the seven habits of highly effective people and the art of winning with people, you will feed the good wolf in others and ours simultaneously.

In fact, ineffective families and effective communities, the actions of people are always driven by big visions, by principles, and by noble, selfless purposes. Highly successful people always act with empathy, compassion, sharing, caring, love and forgiveness. These actions make a huge difference in people's lives and their spiritual life. People rarely feel stressed by selfless actions. They will have feelings of warmth and happiness, and sense of the good seeds growing bigger inside. There are much fewer health problems, mental problems, and social problems in families, communities. The difference in the quality of thinking and interacting is the answer for all social phenomena, social laws, and Pareto principles. They are the outliers.

The uncontrolled mind is lazy in thinking, it stores thoughts, and automatic call out when situation come by subconscious mind in a blink. The untrained mind likes familiar things, familiar route, and familiar work. When individuals in their familiarity, their minds do not have to do much, the mind lazy in thinking; all things done by the subconscious mind with high accuracy; this is our comfort zone. We do not have to think much so we do not grow much in our comfort zone, all actions are automatic and controlled by the subconscious mind.

When out of comfort zone like come in a new environment, study new skill, get a driver license and go to new school and in a new job, our minds have to do a lot to test the information. Conscious mind analyzes the pattern of information, it analyzes by relating the unknown thing with the known ideas in mind; can be known by connecting the dots in mind. Then it sends to the subconscious mind to memorize. In new areas, there are many new things that the mind does not understand much. the mind has to work hard to process information by all senses. People need connection, love, support, and understanding to make the mind has feelings of safety, motivation, and enthusiasm. With the feeling of safety, motivation, and enthusiasm, our children can learn any skills they want. Can you drive? This skill was not popular in 1910. Can we flight airplane? This skill was out of the imagination of people in 1910. Can you use a computer, code the computer? This skill was out of the imagination of the best students in 1960. Many terms, concepts of management, leadership and many others that our high school students study and practice every day were not known by the smartest people in the first of 20th century. Even with the readers of this book, anything you possess is the dream or out of the imagination of the richest people lived in 1950. Most of our ancestors lived all their lives with the hope of having enough to satisfy the basic physical need of family members. At these moments, we cannot fly with a private engine the like iron man; we cannot fly with a flying board, flying cars, flying motorbike. I think all of the difficulties we can imagine about the flying machines our children will master in the near future. We are living in the fastest changing society ever in human history. In near future, there will have countless skills, careers, machines that we cannot imagine. Our children will master all of these new skills in the future. The more we support, the more we believe, the faster our children can master. Please, do not retrain ourselves, our children, and surrounding people with the limit of our temporary opinions, beliefs, and taboos.

The characters of untrained mind are described in many psychology experiments with are described in books like Blink - The power of thinking without thinking of Malcolm Gladwell; Thinking, Fast and Slow of Daniel Kahneman and Predictably Irrational - The hidden forces that shape our decisions of DanAriely, and many other psychology books. The mind tends to grasp the familiar things in the hook effect. In a question or negotiation in an unfamiliar area, if individuals recommended with a number directly or indirectly, these individuals will tend to choose a number around the recommended number. If you buy a red car, you will see a lot more red cars on the road compared with previous time, the red car now becomes your familiar's things; the conscious mind and unconscious mind will pay attention to it.

The mind is lazy in thinking when we give people three kinds of jam to buy in a stall on the pavement, and other time we give people twelve kinds of jam to buy; the numbers of people who buy jam with three samples higher than the numbers of people with twelve samples. The mind can process information, find out the familiarities or differences then make the decision easier and better with several samples than with many more samples. With several samples the mind easier to match them to familiar things to decide and the certain of decision is much stronger; it means that it is safer and easier for the mind when chosen with a small number of samples. With many samples, people may take a lot of thinking to choose, even worse, after choosing, people may think they make the wrong decision because of buying this jam, not buying that jam - the paradox of choices.

When individuals have specific emotion, feelings or specific decisions before a situation, all information and decision after that tend to match with the previous emotion. Researchers let one group of people hold a cup of warm water and another group of people holds a cup of cold water for five minutes then they let them read a paragraph about a man and answer a questionnaire about the man. The people hold warm cup have to answer that he is a kind and good man; on the contrary, the people hold cold cup have the answer that he is a bad and rude man. Only holding the cup for five minutes, people have the pattern of thinking that match with the pattern of things they hold. The mind is easily delusive. They tend to catch the information that fit the nearest state of mind or feelings. The mind of these people unconsciously clings to nearest feeling. People do not believe what they see; they only see what they believe. Therefore, answer about the character of the man in paragraph influenced by the state created just five minutes before reading. The ability of logical and rational thinking is affected. Only awaken people who know what appear and disappear in mind will not be affected by previous feelings. They know the process of detachment. Experts described in Blink know how to detach the previous assumption by the process of collecting information to make a good judgment.

In another experiment, a group of young men called to chat with young girls. Name of girls was mixed and give accidentally to the men. With a man called a girl with an interesting name like Elizabeth and Victoria the conversation was much more interesting than the conversation the man called a girl with the normal name like Susan or Nancy. The first impression of the name makes men thought that she was interesting, then he sent interesting signals, kind words, and a nice voice to the girl; the girl catch the hidden message then has the corresponding response consciously and unconsciously. The interesting name makes the conversation much more interesting than the conversation with the normal name.

When we hate someone, our subconscious mind only scans for anything wrong from these individuals to confirm our hatred. We do not know this process of the mind. People with prejudices and assumption only live with the previous experience they do not pay attention to the present moment, to the beautiful reality. Most of the time, we will find out information to confirm the hatred. To some extent, the invisible signals send out from us also bring the pattern of our assumption, the unconscious mind of opposite people caught it and then send back the corresponding responses. Most of the time, we will find out the evidence to support our assumption. Even we may promise that we will not find faults, we will meet to find a solution for the conflict, but our subconscious mind knows its job and does it unconsciously, it catches the irritating signals and silently sends signals forward and backward between relating people that we do not realize consciously.

Motion and gesture of body can create the state of mind and feelings. For example, the position of sitting with head put down on the table for fifteen minutes and the position of the shaking head up and down or jumping can change the state of mind, feelings, and hormones in the body. Researchers found that with people sitting in tired position for fifteen minutes, they test the saliva of these individuals and find out there is more cortisone in this saliva. With the person with active position, jumping, singing they find there is testosterone in the saliva. In nature, the powerful animals stand with large shoulder, raising the chest; the gesture gives to show the power. On the other with weak and frighten animals, they tend to shrink the body, sit quite in preserve position, watch out with all things; they are in a mild stressed state. Many motivators and speakers use the technique of affirmation with shaking body, jumping and shouting to change the audiences' emotion and their state of mind in the direction that the speaker wants. With the positive feeling and positive state of mind, people are happier, taking more action and learn more effectively. On the other hands, negative people have negative gesture; with this position, the body sends the pattern of signals to the mind as if it is in the real negative state. The mind sees the negative gesture as if the individual falls in danger. Pretend and assumption now becomes reality, negative chemicals start to increase in the body.

If people use the imagination, focus the mind on the positive experience, focus on the abundance they have, the pride moments, achievements, as long as it is vivid as real with sound, smell, size, color, and emotion. The mind can relive these moments and activate a happy state with happy chemicals. Focusing the mind is the effective technique people use to change immediately the state of mind. When they feel that they are in low energy, they are not enthusiastic in actions. They change their focus to positive things, they relive the positive moments. Thinking, visualizing, self-affirmation and acting may change the state of mind, then from the mind, the whole body change. Focusing the mind can make them live in a happy state and positive attitude. It is as if they are feeding the good wolf inside, they tend to open to things, look to bright sides, take more action with enthusiasm. They create results and these results help a lot to build their self - esteem.

With negative people, they usually focus on the negative thing, they focus on things they do not have; they are envy to other people. They are discontent individuals; always find faults even best. With envy, discontentment and lot of demand, they are rarely satisfied with life, have no peace inside or quite a moment. They lose the present moment by letting the mind chasing to unwanted things, unwanted moments and unwanted ideas or the things in the past, in the future. Rarely, they live in present. They have a habit of focus the mind on the lacking things that harmful to their needs. They fall in stress state by themselves. The unwanted things create irritating, nourishing with the negative of self-talk, lacking advice, support, and love of people around. Just by thinking, they can fall into extreme stress. The mind cannot figure out this is imagination or real life. They unconsciously wear the glasses of stress to see life; it creates a downward trend for the state of mind. Focusing on lacking, unwanted experience and negative side make individuals fall into extreme stress state, they even make evil behaviors and get mental diseases on the wealthy and abundant life. Surprisingly, some of them are smart and rich. These people are the examples that the condition of living and possession do not create real happiness. They fall into countless circles of stress just by thinking. Just pay attention, examine the state of mind and body, the feelings of pleasure or discomfort to know the time of stop and time of changing the thinking. Positive thinking same as positive attitude, negative thinking the same as a negative attitude, attitude is the difference maker in creating a successful or unsuccessful life.

Most of our minds are elusive with the hook effect and previous emotion. The mind tends to misinterpret emotion from one thing to another thing, from one person to another person, form one situation to another situation. These are the not the awaken minds. Un-awakened people tend to bring anger from home to work or bring anger from work to home. Their mind pulled up and down with emotion and assumptions unconsciously. If they live mindfully, look deep into each separate things, they may understand the difference between these things and cut out wrong thoughts, wrong behaviors on time. By mindfulness, they know how to stop the untrained mind, how to overcome the illusive thinking and the traps of irrational thinking.

Our life affected by our thinking. What we think about the most, the mind focuses the most. Our state of mind change according to our thoughts, it creates emotion and leads to action. Motivators use the technique to change the state of participants by the story, by the exercise of imagination, by changing the focus of the mind to some point of views or by vigorous actions: jumping, shouting, singing, shaking hand. These techniques can change the whole state of mind and body of participants, create the peak of emotion; from the peak of emotion create peak performance. Emotion is the energy of action; to get a good result, people need high emotion. The bad result comes from poor emotion or low energy. When people pay attention to emotion, awake to control the mind, realize the state they are in, they can know how to control the mind. The science of achievement is the science of mastering the mind. The mind has much impressed with the event with high emotion, with nearest personal experiences, and to the nearest impression. These impressions called out first as the material to judge the information they receive. Recall impressions can save the brain from overwork, save energy; it is lazy of thinking. The lazy of the mind, found in a lot of researches about people's behavior, called irrational thinking.

The illusion of the mind found in the experiment called: "a love suspension bridge". Across the deep valley, there is a suspension bridge, there was one girl on the one side of the bridge, when young men went across the bridge, if right after they came to another side of the bridge, the girl came to introduce, gave them her card and asked the man call her latter. Another time, if young men came across the street, the men rested for about 30 minutes then the girl came to introduce and give him her card. Researchers found there were more calls in the first situation than the second situation. This is the illusion of the mind. When men passed the suspension bridge, changing the state of mind from extreme fear to safety, they may have a happy state because of safety, when this state was high, a young girl appeared, they tend to match this girl with happiness and safety. With the later experiment, the happy state calmed down, and the mind could figure out clearly they were safe on earth on the side of the bridge, the girl appears, the mind does not have illusion the girl with happiness or safety or arousing a state of mind. I think if the girl stood on the side of the bridge with the man before he passed the bridge, or on the middle of the bridge and gave a card to man, she would not get any call because the man was too afraid with passing over the bridge.

Most of the people have these characters of the mind. We tend to do in an irrational way. If people do not understand the separation, we will be led by irrational thinking. We tend to mix the feelings and assumption from this to that. Illusion mind will make us easily misinterpret things with the influence of crowds and the environment. We will easily have the habits, beliefs, and taboos from the environment that we do not notice at all. We will misinterpret our own problems caused by date of birth, the star on the sky or other event and people irrationally. In Vietnam, most young boys and young girls like to see the foretellers to see if they match each other, whether or not they will happy in the future before getting married. There are many couples separated because of the bad saying of foretellers. Even worse, there is some couple like to intervene in giving birth to deliver their child at the lucky hour.

- The old teaching: People will success if they come to act quickly as they come to a conclusion.
- Napoleon Hill taught: Whatever your mind can conceive and believe the mind can achieve.
- The trap of thinking will make people easily jump to the wrong conclusion. Then they cling to these beliefs. Their unconscious mind and conscious mind will obey the orders to pick up the proofs.

The fact is human mind easily fall into the illusion of the environment. If we do not mindful, we may quickly get the assumption, belief from the environment. We will put these assumption, belief, and emotion in other things that we do not consciously know. With the wrong assumptions, we move on the wrong road, unfortunately, because of attachment, strong emotion, irrational thinking, the illusion of the mind, and big ego, we do not know that we are wrong. We do not know the time to stop and time to return. Shallow people tend to think their problems, stress caused by outside conditions so that they usually blame others for the problems they are rarely taking responsibility. It means that we are wrong and immature but we do not know. Especially the women, they do think more emotionally and illogically than men do, it is the reason why women are more difficult to understand by the men. That is why most philosopher, great men said they do not understand much about women. Because women have their own logic, irrational thinking, so they are the creatures that men should love but should not understand.

The human mind is difficult to understand. Wrong thinking, wrong assumption and lack of understanding are the sources of all problems

Stephen Hawking taught: While physics and mathematics may tell us how the universe began, they are not of much use in predicting human behavior because there are far too many equations to solve. I am no better than anyone else at understanding what makes people tick, particularly women. Oscar Wilde taught: "Women are made to be loved, not understood."

Because of attachment to assumptions, emotional acting, irrational thinking and the illusion of the mind, we misunderstand a lot of things and situation. We unconsciously cause a lot of problems for other people at work and in the family. The mother or father act according to emotion usually carry the anger, upset from work to home; they are easier upset with their children if they are upset at work. They are easier anger with whomever they contact as if they stressed. Stress, anger and negative feelings spread unconsciously over their activities. The illusion makes them blindly believe that if severe injury and loses happened are the inevitable things to gain real happiness. The illusion makes them blindly creating hurt under the mask of love and noble purposes. People need to know themselves to get enlightened. Getting a lot of problems mean they should stop to think, meditate, to upgrade their thinking, reach awaken state to stop their endless vicious behaviors.

We know that the mind is delusive, so instead of loading the mind with the wrong concept and condition children's mind with the rewards and punishments with the ideas.

> You cannot succeed; you are too weak to do any things; society is a dangerous place; money is the root of evil; that job is only for smart people, not me; how dumb I am; you see how stupid you are; we are born poor so live well with the poor is our fate; you do not have that talent; you are a girls so you have to do the job of most girls do; I love you I want to become this or do that; you have same religion as us

> since you are born, you cannot change that; I love you I want to study medicine; you do not have talent in doing business; no one can teach me anything anymore.

Let's try to make the mind the children can get this information with the reward and punishment.

> He can do this, so can you; everybody is a good teacher; he has no leg, he can succeed so can you; if you have clear goals, you can make it; what your mind can conceive and believe, you can achieve; you see how talented you are when you get good grade in primary school, the talent is still in you, you can develop that talent to have a good life; do not let other bad opinions become yours; when you think you can or cannot, you are right; you can choose your own belief; do all with your whole heart, you will success; you have so much potential; God trust in you; you have so much potential, let discover it.

With love, connection, unconditional support, compassion, positive attitudes, understanding, strong characters, and self-discipline, miracles will happen to the children and people that the parents do not have to try hard.

All experiments, researchers have failed in proving the relationship between success and happiness with measurable factors like intelligence or IQ, wealthy, richness or luxury possession. The outliers do not think that a man can succeed because of his knowledge and degree. The outliers have a high instinct in the pattern of action and attitude in the action to know that the doer will succeed or not. Blink: the power of thinking without thinking of Malcolm Gladwell, the author recommended the "Love Lab" at the University of Washington, where psychologist John Gottman has been thin slicing the way couples interact since the early 1980s. In no more than 15 minutes of observation, Gottman can predict with 90 percent accuracy whether a couple will be together in 15 years. Astonishingly, the outliers can predict more precisely by intuition with just thin slicing than sophisticated machines with the wrong assumption. Thin slicing is a neat cognitive trick that involves taking a narrow slice of data, just what you can capture in the blink of an eye, and letting your intuition do the work. The things outlier focus is the attitude of the couple to each other: do they show contempt signal to the partner? Outliers do not focus on the wealthy, abundance living of the couple at all.

The bigger, the better, the more expensive the partners require rings, presents, and bags, and perfume the more conditional love they will demand or other words, the more greedy they are after married, they will more and more disappointed, angry and stressed because of the unsatisfied greedy demands. Love becomes hate, service becomes demand; no one can save them if they are not awake. Greedy people will be stressed and miserable no matter how rich they are. It is so funny to see a greedy man complains about food that he does not like on the table of ten delicious foods. It is so funny to see a guest complains about food he does not like in a buffet party of hundred foods. He may eat with cortisone and epinephrine. The reader can find supportive facts from:

- "What the cost of your engagement ring may say about your marriage" by Taryn Hillin from Huffingtonpost.com,

- "The pricier the ring, the likelier the divorce" By Marketwatch from Nypost.com;

- "Expensive engagement rings linked to higher divorce rates" by Robert Montenegro from Bigthink.com.

When people enlightened they will have the sense of artist. They may see miracles in every normal natural thing. They may see the boring and sheer waste in the luxury shiny things. The artist can see the imageless, since the senseless, hear the soundless and feel the hidden feeling. They see things by their intuitive mind then contemplate to understand it or let it freely express. What is the price of the photo of a beautiful girl? What is the price of the picture that a painter painted a beautiful girl? Perhaps, it is only $5, or $10, or $50. That is the cheap price of the seeable message. But I do know that several paintings by Picasso rank among the most expensive paintings in the world. *Garçon à la pipe* sold for $ 104 million at Sotheby's on 4 May 2004, establishing a new price record. *Dora Maar au Chat* sold for $ 95.2 million at Sotheby's on 3 May 2006. On 4 May 2010, *Nude, Green Leaves, and Bust* were sold at Christie's for $106.5 million.

The miracle of nature:

People will awaken that to enjoy the supreme art, highest art, they have to see, sense, hear, and feel the invisible, senseless, soundless messages. They have to understand the paradox of life, the threshold of sensual senses.

There was a story that a businessman was eager to show a Zen master of his beautiful garden. The garden was very tidy, clean and beautiful with trees and flowers. Walking in the clean, beautiful garden on the brick road, the Zen master said: "it is beautiful but not really beautiful." The businessman curiously questioned. The Zen master said "the garden lacks natural traits" then he walked to the stack of leaves near the brick road and cast all the yellow, red and green leaves. Large areas of garden become more astonishingly beautiful naturally. Zen master said: "When you take small children to this garden, the things attract their attention is not the tidiness and cleanliness of the garden as you think. Children will be attracted to the green leaves, red leaves, and yellow leaves on the road then ask why endlessly. Children will be attracted to the bugs run on the garden, the worm moving under the red leaves, the noise of the frog under the water; the shape, smell and color of the rocks and dust. Children will want to ask you a hundred question about why is nature like that, what is under the earth, will the trees eat earth. But the cleanliness and tidiness of the garden and the cleanliness of the clothes will prevent children from real playing, studying, and fastening children in the boring walk as if you fastening your dog with a chain when walking on garden and jungle. Just suitable clean and tidy is good, but too much is bad. Most of Zen master, monks live healthily is because of temperate living, live in mindfulness, and live close to nature. We do not care much about the cleanliness of food, air, and water as modern people care, did Buddha not care also. Zen masters and monks only care much about major things lead to happiness, liberation and help others. With other minor things, we do not care much about, only good enough, eatable and drinkable is fine. The man with a mind full of old assumptions will never understand the miracle, mysteriousness, and sophistication of the earth, rocks, and bricks under his feet; he will never have the surprising moments take his breath away because he does not interested in the surrounding miracles."

Life is paradoxical, in tidiness there may have the mess and boring; in cleanliness, there may be has hidden negativity, hidden failure, and hidden unproductivity. Things that quick satisfy the sensual senses will easily get bored. The product of intuitive mind has so much hidden information that hardly people understand it all even they have watched it ten or twenty times. But the products of an intelligent mind can easily catch a glimpse. In mess and irrational, there may have real peace, real order; and best of all, children can imagine, play, learn by dirty trying and dirty failing and grow well in mess. The buds start to grow well and stand firmly on a messy firming ground. Albert Einstein was a messy man.

Robots with artificial intelligence can only replace a worker in the position of logical automatic work. Never the robot with artificial intelligence can write the emotional song, a symphony, and paint a cubist picture; it means that artificial intelligence can never replace the artist in creation. The demand for people with high IQ, logical mind, logical intelligence, managerial skills, technical skills, formal education, a good degree, and good certificate for the logical work will be very low in the future because most of these jobs will be replaced by robots with artificial intelligence. But the demand for people with high intuitive intelligence, creative mind, emotional intelligence, leadership skills, artistic mind, positive attitude, and creative skills will be very high in the future because robots with artificial intelligence cannot replace people in the creative works. In the connection world abundant of information and knowledge, employers will value people who have a good attitude, listening skills, integrity, lifelong learning, and self-learning more than people who have the master degree and doctoral degree with the bad attitude, lack of integrity and cannot acquire a new skill and new knowledge.

Having the enlightened mind, you may see your body is not your body, your hand is not your hand, it is the continuous illumination of the body, cells, atoms, genes, thinking, acting, attitude and behaviors of your ancestors, Buddha, your Holy Spirit, and God. Your body, people's body and the body of God, Holy Spirit, all living beings, and all living creatures do not have any separation; all are the continuations of countless phenomena, people, and events before. All is in one and one is in all. So the best way for us to commemorate and make worship to human ancestors, Holy Spirits, God, and Buddha is by treating our bodies and people's bodies and living creatures as the Holy bodies with kindness philosophy. Treat our body as the temple, and treat other's body as a temple also. Treat other living creatures with the natural way of kindness are the best ways of honoring our God, ancestors and Holy Spirits. If we see and sense our hands without an image, we will easy to realize the hidden inside our hands is the hands of mother, father, and ancestors. Observe deeply, we will see we are the continuations of the previous lives and of Holy Spirits.

When we see our hands in imageless, hear our voice in soundless, we can see we have a lot of similarity with our ancestors, our Holy Spirits. We will realize we are the continuations of our Holy Spirits, our Gods. Buddha and God are the hidden part of our body, they are the only the visible sensible of our invisible parts. It is scientifically true to say "God is in me, God is in our heart." "Buddha in me, Buddha is in my heart." "I am the continuation of my ancestors, Holy spirits." "There is always invisible God, invisible parents in me; joy and happiness are already in me."

"Born and died is only to talk about the physical and visible body. We still can understand the thinking, acting, talking, caring, influence, and love of God and Buddha. Watching the growth of a corn seed into a corn tree, I can sense there is invisible seed corn in the corn tree. The seed corn did not die; it is just changing from the seed into the tree. There will be no corn tree if the corn seed consciously resists the changing. In corn seed, there is an invisible corn tree also." Thich Nhat Hanh taught, start to bring back the mind to the body, start to observe all phenomena in imageless, soundless, and senseless, we can see miracles in life, right here at this moment, at present.

So that to show respect to our ancestors, we need to honor our body, keep it clean and make our body as a vehicle to continue doing God's goodness. Right understanding makes us see the body as the temple and natural religion is kindness religious.

If we violate the natural way of treating or integrity, kindness and common sense, even no one know, but our potential knows it, and its danger may bring; the mind sense the smell of non-safety, the danger, and threatening, the potential mind may be irritated and out of balanced. The imbalance of the brainy mind may silently intervene all the of people's activities and creating misery that they do not know. Until one day they cannot cope with the unknown pain, misery, and problems put on them and they may illusively think that they have fates or destiny. Sadly, any wrong assumption or any excuse for the problems will make the powerful mind accept it as the fact of life; moreover, the excuse will prevent the individuals from thinking, imagining and acting.

Close your eyes, close all your sensual senses, quiet the mind, you may sense the miracle, indescribable feelings, and unimaginable information. Forget your old knowledge, forget your assumption, calm down the mind, live mindfully to taste the real indescribable joy, happiness.

Studying placebo effect reveals the unknown character of the mind:

> "Be care the feeding of your mind" is the teaching of all the sages, great men, successful men, trainer, and speakers.
>
> "Sugar pills with placebo effects and the real pills with nocebo effect make me question the benefit of many drugs, supplement foods, taboo, rituals, and spiritual living."

Mechanisms of the placebo effect

Studies of the "placebo effect" often fail to adequately identify confounding factors, caused by many factors, some interesting factors relate to the mind:
- The natural course of the diseases including spontaneous improvement, fluctuation of symptoms;
- Conditional switching of placebo treatment
- Biases, including scaling bias, answers of politeness, experimental subordination, conditioned answers;
- Experimenter and observer biases including misjudgment or irrelevant response variables;
- Psychological effects including psychosomatic phenomena, expectation effects.
- Placebos May Trigger Hormone Responses: taking the placebo triggered a release of endorphins. Endorphins have a structure similar to morphine and other opiate painkillers and act as the brain's own natural painkillers. Researchers have been able to demonstrate the placebo effect in action using

brain scans, showing that areas that contain many opiate receptors were activated in both the placebo and treatment groups. Naloxone is an opioid antagonist that blocks both natural endorphins and opioid drugs. Using naloxone, placebo pain relief is reduced.

One day, a person has about 60000 thoughts, each thought is the series of chemical, hormones, electric signals in brain and body. We can detect what happens in mind by reading physical signs of body, face, organs. These thoughts will determine the acts of hormones systems in brain, body. What if all these thoughts are negative or positive and compound for days, weeks, months, years or decades.

Expectations Can Influence Placebo Responses

Other possible explanations include conditioning, motivation, and expectation. In some cases, a placebo can be paired with an actual treatment until it comes to evoke the desired effect, an example of classical conditioning. People who are highly motivated to believe that a treatment will work, or who had a treatment work previously, may be more likely to experience a placebo effect.

A prescribing physician's enthusiasm for treatment can even impact how a patient response. If a doctor seems very positive that treatment will have a desirable effect, a patient may be more likely to see benefits from taking the drug. This demonstrates that the placebo effect can even take place when a patient is taking real medications to treat an illness.

Negative Effects of placebo: nocebo

A phenomenon opposite to the placebo effect has also been observed. When an inactive substance or treatment is administered to a recipient who has an expectation of it having a negative impact, this intervention is known as a nocebo. A nocebo effect occurs when the recipient of an inert substance reports a negative effect and/or a worsening of symptoms, with the outcome resulting not from the substance itself, but from negative expectations about the treatment. A patient might report having headaches, nausea or dizziness in response to a placebo.

Chronic fatigue syndrome

It was previously assumed that placebo response rates in patients with chronic fatigue syndrome (CFS) are unusually high, "at least 30% to 50%", because of the subjective reporting of symptoms and the fluctuating nature of the condition.

Power of branding: Studies revealed If a person is given a placebo under one name, and they respond, they will respond in the same way on a later occasion to that placebo under that name but not if under another.

Placebo in the treatment of pain and illness:

One way in which the magnitude of placebo analgesia can be measured is by conducting "open/hidden" studies, in which some patients receive an analgesic and are informed that they will be receiving it (open), while others are administered the same drug without their knowledge (hidden). Such studies have found that analgesics are considerably more effective when the patient knows they are receiving them.

It was found that placebo-induced analgesia depends on the release of endogenous opiates in the brain and that the placebo effect can be undone using the opiates antagonist naloxone.

The placebo effect can be achieved in several ways: by using pharmacological preparations or simulation of operating or other procedures. This phenomenon is associated with the perception and expectation of the patient. To achieve the effect of placebo it is an essential degree of the suggestions of the person who prescribe a placebo, and the degree of belief of the person receiving the placebo.

The expected effect of a placebo is to achieve the same effect as the right remedy. Achieved placebo effect depends on the way of presentation. If a substance is presented as harmful, it may cause harmful effects, called 'nocebo" effect.

The placebo effect is not equal in all patients, the same as the real effect of the drug is not always equal in all patients.

How do placebos work? In 1978, Dr. Jon Levine and colleagues at the University of California, San Francisco, gave 40 patients who had had their wisdom teeth extracted placebos for their pain. Most, but not all, experienced a reduction in pain. An hour later, the scientists gave some of the patients another placebo and the rest naloxone, a drug that blocks the brain's natural morphine-like compounds, called endorphins. Patients given naloxone felt much more pain than those given saline. That was strong evidence that the basis for the placebo effect on pain lies in the brain's production of endorphins and other opiates. "This study was the first to show that placebos relieve pain by activating the brain's natural painkillers," says Beauregard.

Explained by Deepak Chopra:

Deepak Chopra M.D., who has taught at medical schools such as Harvard and Boston University, served on panels with the National Institutes of Health, explained that whenever we have a thought, our bodies make a chemical that goes along with that thought. And with every feeling that we have, our bodies are producing chemicals that reflect those feelings. That is because the cells in our brains, our immune system and *every* cell in our body, contain chemical receptors that are listening to our internal dialogue. This is important because when you are having a good day and feeling happy, your body is producing happy chemicals which protect us against cancer, like imipramine, which is an antidepressant, and immunomodulators, like interleukins and interferons. On the other hand, if you are feeling angry, or worried, sad and depressed, your body will receive those toxic signals and release "sad" chemicals throughout your body. Anger, more than anything else, causes inflammatory disorders and guilt and depression is correlated with cancer.

Mismatching conditioned responses: conditioned the mind.

The research was done at the University of Alabama medical school in Birmingham by Brent Solvason, Dr. Vithal Ghanta, and Dr. Raymond Hirahito. Mice were exposed for three hours at a time to the odor of camphor. The scientists showed that exposure to this odor, by itself, had no detectable effect on the immune system. But in the experiments, some of the mice were also given injections of a synthetic chemical called poly I:C (for polyinosinic-polycytidylic acid), which is known to enhance the activity of natural killer cells. The exposures were repeated nine times in a strategy similar to that of the Pavlovian conditioning in which dogs were given food every time a bell rang. In each session of the immunity experiments, the mice were exposed to the odor and given injections of the chemical.

Then, in the 10th session, the mice were exposed only to the odor of camphor. They received no injections at all. Nevertheless, every mouse showed a large increase in natural killer cell activity. The effect, Dr. Spector recommend it is the same mechanism as Pavlov's experiments in which animals could be made to salivate simply at the ringing of a bell. In the new case, the animals' brains evidently activated the immune defense without waiting for the poly I:C, just as the dogs had begun to salivate in the Pavlovian experiments without waiting for the food to appear.

Chapter 50: Science of achievement: mastering the mind by goals, visions, virtues, and principles

"With the delusive mind, it is better to make the mind have illusion with worthwhile achievements, noble purposes, big thinking and powerful characters"

****

Understanding the characters of the mind and the potential of the brains, we know how to focus the mind to achieve success in life. One of the best ways to become a success is by setting goals. Goals and visions are the product of cognitive thinking and contemplating in the neocortex. The first start of doing, setting goals and revising goals will remind the emotional mind of limbic systems what is the most important. Knowing the goals and visions, the whole brain: neocortex and limbic system, the whole mind: cognitive mind and emotional mind, conscious mind and unconscious mind will work harmoniously all day to help people achieve their goals. Obsessed goals and visions will focus the direction of thinking, control the direction of subconscious mind and control the power potential of the brain and all other resources. Observe the love of the mother to her infant, we will understand how obsessed goals control our thinking. Miracles of human potential happened during the wartime, obsessed with the visions of liberation were so strong that many soldiers as normal men and women could focus all their energy, thinking and power of the brain to carry the largest amount of goods, carry the heaviest amount of goods, and move under the toughest conditions that normal people can imagine. During peacetime, the directors want to make movies to record these miracles with these people, but these soldiers cannot redo the previous action.

Everything still is the same, but the obsessed desires, obsessed goals are not the same so they cannot redo the activity they have done.

By focusing, light in laze beam can cut steel; soft water can cut steel also. One ordinary individual has clear goals can achieve far more than genius without goals. The goals are the guiding stars for people use the potential mind to make a plan, take action, do the checking and make adjusting to reach the goals. Genius can know the way, but success cannot reach by knowing, it only can reach by taking massive actions toward goals. Goals, visions, and principles are the most effective tools to control the powerful mind, to overcome the sensual temptations and desire of satisfying the Self. People on the first stage of personal development and ordinary people can feel difficult and annoyed with setting goals. On the other hand, most successful people I know, they consider goals, visions, principles, and code of conducts as vital tools for their life. These are the tools help to direct the mind, the potential brain, the five senses, and emotion to achieve worthwhile achievement.

From reward and punishment to achievement:

> People like gain and pleasure as the reward; they avoid pain, uncomfortable as the punishment. This is the instinct of human beings and all other animals. With human beings who can use cognitive thinking, with imagination and visualization, pain and gain, reward and punishment are just the illusions of mind, the subjective perceptions. There is no same formula for all people.
>
> Without goals, without visions, without principles, without codes of conduct, and narrow thinking, people like the immediate gain, satisfy the short-term gain. They do not care or have any gut feelings about the consequences of long-term pain that they and their society have to suffer in

the future: they like short-term gain and do not care about the long-term pain. Most of the time, they will suffer severe stress in the future because of selfish actions. Billions of selfish people have appeared and disappeared that you and I do not know at all.

With goals, visions, principles, codes of conduct and broad thinking, people enjoy short-term pain, temporary failures, and the pain from acting to gain long-term gain in the future. With these tools, these people have different points of view of pain and gain compare with normal people. They may like the short-term discomfort, love short-term pain because they know these discomforts are inevitable to reach the noble vision. Their brain makes them may feel joyful and happy with the temporary pain; they may have discomfort and gut feelings with any easy temporary gain. They have the stillness of mind in the midst of chaos. They gain a good state of mind: tranquil, peaceful, still and happy because they have gained the right understanding. Reading the biography of President Abraham Lincoln, we will understand the difference in the perception of failure. With him, there was no definition of failure as we usually think. When not reaching the goals, fail, fail and fail, do not blame, think, stand up, adjust, and take massive action.

With these tools goals, visions, principles, codes of conduct, and broad thinking, people can go further, go faster than normal people can imagine. They are the movers, the creators, the innovators in the human chapter in the book of living creatures.

We have read a lot about how to succeed, how to gain the achievement. I want to use the advice of successful people to recite the things that lead to success. Understanding the work of the brain, the work of the mind, we can easier understand these teaching.

1. Brian Tracy taught: All successful people men and women are big dreamers. They imagine what their future could be, ideal in every respect, and then they work every day toward their distant vision, that goal or purpose. If you raise your children to feel that they can accomplish any goal or task they decide upon, you will have succeeded as a parent and you will have given your children the greatest of all blessings. People with clear, written goals, accomplish far more in a shorter time than people without them could ever imagine. And Goals allow you to control the direction of change in your favor.

2. Denis Waitley taught: Learn from the past, set vivid, detailed goals for the future, and live in the only moment of time over which you have any control: now. When you are in the valley, keep your goal firmly in view and you will get the renewed energy to continue the climb. Goals provide the energy source that powers our lives. One of the best ways we can get the most from the energy we have is to focus it. That is what goals can do for us; concentrate our energy.

3. Elbert Hubbard taught: Know what you want to do, hold the thought firmly, and do every day what should be done, and every sunset will see you that much nearer to your goal.

4. Henry Ford taught: Obstacles are those frightful things you see when you take your eyes off your goal. If you think you can do a thing or think you can't do a thing, you're right.

5. Jim Rohn taught: Whoever renders service to many puts himself in line for greatness - great wealth, great return, great satisfaction, great reputation, and great joy.

6. Les Brown taught said: Review your goals twice every day in order to be focused on achieving them.

7. Mahatma Gandhi taught The best way to find yourself is to lose yourself in the service of others. Service which is rendered without joy helps neither the servant nor the served. But all other pleasures and possessions pale into nothingness before service which is rendered in a spirit of joy.

8. Napoleon Hill taught: The starting point of all achievement is desire. Cherish your visions and your dreams as they are the children of your soul, the blueprints of your ultimate achievements. Desire is the starting point of all achievement, not a hope, not a wish, but a keen pulsating desire which transcends everything.

9. Peter Drucker taught: Management by objective works - if you know the objectives. Ninety percent of the time you do not.

10. Tony Robbins taught: Setting goals is the first step in turning invisible into the visible. People are not lazy. They simply have impotent goals - that is, goals that do not inspire them.

11. W. Clement Stone taught: All personal achievement starts in the mind of the individual. Your personal achievement starts in your mind. The first step is to know exactly what your problem, goal or desire is. And definiteness of purpose is the starting point of all achievement.

12. Zig Ziglar taught: If you want to reach a goal, you must see the reaching in your own mind before you actually arrive at your goal.

In a constantly changing society, sometimes we receive advice that we should remove previous knowledge and assumptions. So what should we follow, what is the guidance for us to follow? In the teaching of successful people, things that we should follow are the big visions, big goals, guiding principles, and codes of conduct or virtue. These are the guidelines for the unconscious mind work effectively.

Our own subconscious mind will scan all day to detect the threats or opportunities to help us getting goals. It will send us the gut feelings if we know our goals, desire clearly enough. People without goals see difficulties in opportunities; people with a clear goal in mind will see opportunities in difficulties. People having goals, they see many opportunities to help us to achieve goals; with them, failure is temporary, not permanently. Visions and goals are our long-term views, they help us to concentrate time and resources; on the other hand, they prevent from wasting our energy on temporary and small things. Clear visions and goals are formed by the neocortex. Reviewing visions and goals regularly, we send information about important things to the limbic system. When the limbic system understands and becomes obsessed with these visions, the whole brain's power will work to help people achieve their goals. With clear, definite goals, emotional mind and cognitive mind will become the servants of people. Goals become guiding stars to direct the powerful energy of our mind.

With clear and worthwhile goals, just by imagining regularly the visions of achieving goals can put people in the happy state with lots of energy to decide and take action; they may are unstoppable with worthwhile goals. That is the reason why successful people advise others to spend time contemplating to figure out their important goals, to figure out what are the most important results for them. This is like the second habits of end thinking. Once we find out important things to us, we should review them regularly to make the conscious mind and unconscious mind focus on acting and adjusting to achieve the goals. Setting goals and reviewing goals regularly is the conscious activities to condition the unconscious mind with the responses toward the goals.

People are ignorant when they think they know everything, they reject any different thing. Worst of all, they do not know about their ignorance. They tend to stubborn and rigid with the shallow conclusion, wrong assumptions. They are easily stubborn with whatever conclusion and emotion pop up in their mind. This is the track to failure and misery.

What are your goals for life? If all areas of your life will be perfect in the next 10, 20 years, what will they look like? When spending the time to think about these kinds of question about clear visions, important things in the future. With a clear vision, we will have guidance for the giant inside our brain.

Success is the number game. Success is the accumulation of choices, decisions and massive actions following the principles. Success leaves tracks; most outliers know the tracks of success. Having an open mind, opening to new theories, removing old assumption, sharpening the ability, guiding with principles, paying attention to compassion, love, connection in every action, gaining peace of mind and understanding, humble, funny and childish as Einstein, these characters will inspire every bodies to play, work, and innovate to achieve worthwhile achievement. Do not harm others; do not distort our perceptions by our emotion, do not distort our perceptions by previous conclusions and our selfish expectation, always remind yourself of the law of cause and effect.

Human beings are in the process of continuous improvement with gaining higher ability by mastering knowledge, mastering skills and having a positive attitude. We gain wisdom through knowledge about life, environment, and nature. Each time of reaching higher knowledge, we have to remove all our old knowledge. The more we study, the more we know that we do not know much. It is not because we become more stupid by studying, it is because we have broadened the eye, upgrade our thinking, and reach a higher state of mind. We now understand more the quote of Aesop: The smaller the mind the greater the conceit. However, the highest state of mind gained by learning is enlightenment. Enlightenment makes us understand the essence of life, from the understanding we will take selfless actions. It is true, selfless actions, not selfish actions.

Once more about the paradox of intelligence, Peter Drucker taught: "My greatest strength as a consultant is to be ignorant and ask a few questions."

References:

A.H. Maslow, Critique of self-actualization theory, in: E. Hoffman (Ed.), Future visions: The unpublished papers of Abraham Maslow (Thousand Oaks, CA: Sage, 1996), pp. 26–32

Alter, Charlotte (November 26, 2014). Deepak Chopra on Why Gratitude is Good For You. Time. Retrieved December 16, 2014.

ANewDayANewMe. (n.d). Oprah: Deepak Chopra. Good Thoughts Can Heal. Bad Thoughts May Kill! Retrieved from http://www.anewdayanewme.com/oprah-deepak-chopra-good-thoughts-can-heal-bad-thoughts-may-kill/

Annie B. Bond. (April 10, 2005). The Healing Power of Love – A True Story Retrieved from https://www.care2.com/greenliving/healing-power-of-love-true-story.html

Bar-On, Reuven, & Parker, James D.A. (2000). The handbook of emotional intelligence. New York: Jossey-Bass.

Blatner, A. (1995). The place of drama in education–A child psychiatrist's viewpoint. Youth Theatre Journal. (Also on this website.)

Books:

Boye Lafayette De Mente (January 1, 1976). Cultural Failures That Are Destroying the American Dream! – The Destructive Influence of Male Dominance & Religious Dogma!. Cultural-Insight Books. p. 42. ISBN 978-0-914778-17-2.

Brualdi, A, C. (1996) 'Multiple Intelligences: Gardner's Theory. ERIC Digest', Eric Digests, [http://www.ericdigests.org/1998-1/multiple.htm. Accessed June 15, 2008]

Bruner, J (1960) The Process of Education, Cambridge, Mass.: Harvard University Press.

Chopra 1991, pp. 54–57; Joanne Kaufman, Deepak Chopra – An 'Inner Stillness,' Even on the Subway, The New York Times, October 17, 2013.

Cohen, J. (2001). Social emotional education: core concepts and practices. In J. Cohen (Ed.). New York: Teachers College Press.

Cohen, Jonathan. (Ed.) (1999). Educating minds and hearts: Social Emotional Learning and the passage into adolescence. New York: Teachers College Press. www.teacherscollegepress.com

Cooper, Robert; & Sawaf, Ayman. (1996). Executive EQ: Emotional intelligence in leadership and organizations. New York: Grosset/Putnam.

Deepak Chopra. The Huffington Post. Retrieved April 25, 2016.

Deepak Chopra; Sanjiv Chopra (2013). Brotherhood: Dharma, Destiny, and the American Dream. Houghton Mifflin Harcourt. pp. 5–. ISBN 0-544-03210-1. Retrieved April 25, 2016.

Deepak Chopra; Sanjiv Chopra (2013). Brotherhood: Dharma, Destiny, and the American Dream. Houghton Mifflin Harcourt. p. 194. ISBN 0-544-03210-1. Retrieved April 25, 2016.

Dr. Elaine (February 23, 2016). Mind Body Spirit Mind Body. Retrieved from http://drelaine.com/are-you-giving-your-heart-the-most-critical-nutrient-it-needs/

Elias, M.; Zins, J. E., Weissberg, R. P., Frey, K.S., Greenberg, M.T., Haynes, N. M., Kessler, R., Schwab-Stone, M. E., & Shriver, T. P. (Eds.). (1997). Promoting Social and Emotional Learning: A guide for educators. Alexandria, VA: Association for Supervision and Curriculum Development (ASCD). around $22.00. The first chapter is available on the web. http://www.ascd.org. E-Mail Member@ascd.org

Ellin, Abby (2010-08-06). With Tony Robbins, Self-Help Author. The New York Times. ISSN 0362-4331. Retrieved 2017-07-18.

Gamel JW (2008). Hokum on the Rise: The 70-Percent Solution. The Antioch Review. 66 (1): 130. It seems appropriate that Chopra and legions of his ilk should now populate the halls of academic medicine, since they carry on the placebo-dominated traditions long ago established in those very halls by their progenitors

Gardner, H. (1991) The Unschooled Mind: How children think and how schools should teach, New York: Basic Books.

Gardner, Howard (1999) Intelligence Reframed. Multiple intelligences for the 21st century, New York: Basic Books. 292 + x pages. Useful review of Gardner's theory and discussion of issues and additions.

Gardner, Howard (1999) The Disciplined Mind: Beyond Facts And Standardized Tests, The K-12 Education That Every Child Deserves, New York: Simon and Schuster (and New York: Penguin Putnam).

Geoffrey Brewer (November 1993). Is this guy for real?. Sales & Marketing Management. p. 92.

Goble, F. (1970). The third force: The psychology of Abraham Maslow. Richmond, CA: Maurice Bassett Publishing. pp. 62.

Goleman, Daniel. (1995). Emotional intelligence. New York: Bantam.

Goleman, Daniel. (1998). Working with emotional intelligence. New York: Bantam/ Doubleday/Dell

Heller, Karen (1 December 2014). Tony Robbins, Self-Help Guru, is Larger Than Life. Washington Post. Retrieved 18 July 2017.

http://www.ascd.org/readingroom/books/2002novick_toc.html

Jeanne Garbarino on November 15, 2011. Cholesterol and Controversy: Past, present, and Future. Retrieved from https://blogs.scientificamerican.com/guest-blog/cholesterol-confusion-and-why-we-should-rethink-our-approach-to-statin-therapy/

Jeffrey Brown (May 13, 2013). Chopra Brothers Tell Story of How They Became Americans and Doctors in Memoir. PBS News Hour. Retrieved January 7, 2015.

Kahneman, D. (2011). Thinking, fast and slow. New York: Farrar, Straus and Giroux.

Kremer, William Kremer; Hammond, Claudia (31 August 2013). Abraham Maslow and the pyramid that beguiled business. BBC news magazine. Retrieved 1 September 2013.

M.,, Wills, Evelyn. Theoretical basis for nursing. ISBN 9781451190311. OCLC 857664345.

Maslow, A (1954). Motivation and personality. New York, NY: Harper. ISBN 0-06-041987-3.

Maslow, A.H. (1943). A theory of human motivation. Psychological Review. 50 (4): 370–96. doi:10.1037/h0054346 – via psychclassics.yorku.ca.

Maslow, A.H. (1964). Religions, Values and Peak-experiences. Columbus, OH: Ohio State University Press.

Maslow, A.H. (1980). The Farther Reaches of Human Nature (An Esalen Book). New York, NY: Penguin.

Maslow, A.H. (1987). Motivation and Personality. (3rd ed.). New York, NY: Harper & Row.

Maslow, A.H. (1987). Motivation and Personality. (3rd ed.). New York, NY: Harper & Row.

Maslow, A.H. (1999). Towards a Psychology of Being. (3rd ed.). New York, NY: John Wiley & Sons.

Neal Hall (30 June 2005). Robbins posed as waiter to meet future in-laws, court told: Father-in-law says his daughter, millionaire were 'really good friends' in August 2000. Vancouver Sun.

Neuro Associative Conditioning. www.sportshealth4u.com. Archived from the original on January 30, 2009. Retrieved July 18, 2017.

Novick, Bernard; Kress, Jeff; & Elias, Maurice. (2002). Building Learning Communities with Character: How to Integrate Academic, Social, and Emotional Learning. On the ASCD web page

Prescott, K. (Ed.). (1995). Teaching pro-social behavior to adolescents: A directory of processes and programs used in Australian schools. Torrens Park: Australian Guidance and Counseling Association.

Recommended reading:

Robbins, Anthony J. (2002). Business Leader Profiles for Students. pp. 390–394.

Salovey, P., Bedell, B. T., Detweiler, J.B., & Mayer, J.D. (1999). Coping intelligently. In C.R. Snyder (Ed.), Coping: The psychology of what works (pp. 141-164). New York: Oxford University Press.

Salovey, Peter, & Sluyter, D. (Eds.) (1997). Emotional development and emotional intelligence: Implications for educators. New York: Basic Books.

Schnall, Marianne (2012-04-29). An In-depth Interview With Life Coach Tony Robbins. Huffington Post. Retrieved 2017-07-18.

Steere, B. F. (1988). Becoming an effective classroom manager: A resource for teachers. Albany, NY: SUNY Press. ISBN 0-88706-620-8.

Sternberg, R. J. (1985) Beyond IQ: A triarchic theory of human intelligence. New York: Cambridge University Press.

Sternberg, R. J. (1996) Successful intelligence. New York: Simon & Schuster.

The science of Health Newsletter. (January 2005) We Can Put an End to All Disease on This Planet. Retrieved from http://customers.hbci.com/~wenonah/news.htm

Tony Robbins (2016-01-21), Science of Achievement & Art of Fulfillment | Tony Robbins, retrieved 2017-07-18

Tony Robbins' True Love. Oprah.com. Retrieved 2017-07-03.

Tony Robbins: An Awakened Giant Within... Life & Lessons. One Life Success. 1 May 2014. Archived from the original on 20 July 2014. Retrieved 11 August 2015.

Topping, K.J., & Bremner, W.G. (1998). Promoting social competence: Practice and resources guide. Edinburgh: Scottish Office Education and Industry Department.

White, J. (1998) Do Howard Gardner's multiple intelligences add up? London: Institute of Education, University of London.

Williams, W. M., Blythe, T., White, N., Li, J., Sternberg, R. J., & Gardner, H. (1996). Practical intelligence for school. New York: HarperCollins College Publishers.

Awaken you wonderful we

Part XII: The Art of Happiness: Emotional Management and Meditation

Chapter 51: Mastering the mind by mastering the emotion

> Good state of mind is a powerful medicine
>
> The smile is the signs that we are really happy.
>
> Love is powerful medicine
>
> Smile and good acts, compassion are powerful medicine also
>
> All these can heal in an indirect way.

An amazing realization: investigators at Ohio State University were researching the effects of diet-induced atherosclerosis in rabbits. The researchers were able to induce atherosclerosis by feeding rabbits high-cholesterol diets, but one group inexplicably had 60 percent less atherosclerosis. The experimenters were baffled and tried to find the responsible factor. Nothing they tried proved to be it–not diet, not room temperature, not anything they could change and measure. Finally, they discovered that the particular researcher in charge of that group really liked rabbits. She would talk to them, pet them, give them lots of love. Other experimenters just put the food in the cages of rabbits. Sure enough, in every case, the rabbits that had been loved had at least 60 percent less incidence of atherosclerosis than those that were not shown affection. Atherosclerosis, by the way, is statistically the disease that kills the most Americans.

Love and compassion are necessary to us all and can even affect research. Caring and loving feelings can reach out and affect diseases and create healing–even when you are experimentally trying to induce illness.

*Quality of mind, thinking and belief will determine the way that e*very cell in your body regenerates. What is remaining? It is not cells, body, organs but the accumulation of state of mind, of consciousness. The human body replaces 98% of all it's atoms in one year. You make a new liver every six weeks, a new skin once a month, a new skeleton once every three months, and in less than a year, you replace your entire body down to the last atom!

Healing from inside: change the self, not environment: the compound of 60000 thoughts a day to weeks, months, years, and decades. Your inner dialog is continually emitting signals to your cells. Just a thought releases a flood of hormones, chemicals, and chemical messengers. All medical books give detail of these characters and the effects of these chemicals based on scientific researches, just mindful living, we can know the correlation. "As within so without" so we can detect from outside to see what is happening in the body. By knowing, we can figure the effecting way of correcting. Chopra says that whenever you react to anything, whether it's a traffic jam, criticism from your boss, a love note, or even the rainy weather, be aware of the signals being generated within yourself. Instead of reacting externally, concentrate on your internal reactions that will produce happy, healthy chemicals: these are healing chemicals.

For mastering the mind, mastering life, and mastering the self, the best way is to mastering emotion (irrational mind). There are four fundamentals we should know about emotional management.

Firstly, I have always questioned Aristotle's statement about anger:

Anybody can become angry - that is easy, but to be angry with the right person and to the right degree and at the right time and for the right purpose, and in the right way - that is not within everybody's power and is not easy. **Aristotle**

I always wondered to clarify the word right to understand this point.

Secondly, let go of the next definition of emotional management or self-management to understand the word right

Emotional management is the art of using emotion to achieve desired goals in a happy and effective way. I want to clarify the keywords here are art, emotion and desired goals, happy and effective way.

Thirdly, facts or stimulus to the individual creates a response. There is a silent pause before the response. We should take advantages of this silence pause. Imagine the situation: you, your child and your obsessed objects like flowerpots, expensive phones or precious wine. If your child accidentally breaks your items, how will you do? Can you remember your previous experiences have a pattern like this? If you surf through the pages of newspapers or observe around, you will see varieties of scripts that people may react crucially with their beloved people in unwanted situations. The way of responding will lead to different results or even tragedies in life. Most of them do not know the causes they create with negative emotion. It is not the environment or stimulus from the environment determines your life. It is the way you perceive, think and feel with the stimulus from the environment; and the way you react to the stimulus. The feeling, thinking and action you have when contact with the environment will determine your destiny mental life, physical life, spiritual life, and social life. Quality of a meal does not come from the food on the table, but the quality of the meal comes from the emotion and attitude of people enjoy the food. Unfortunately, most people, parents create so many negative causes on the life of children and the surrounding people.

Fourthly, the difference between the ordinary people and the successful ones can be summarized in the table:

Table 37: Differences between ordinary people and successful people

Criteria	Successful person	Ordinary people
1. Values, belief, attitude	Have clear values and belief	Most do not have or fuzzy
2. Goals, visions	Have short and long terms	Most do not have or fuzzy
3. The mission of life	Have clear mission	Most do not have, fuzzy
4. The action is driven by	Goals, long vision and principles	Irrational, emotions and without purpose
5. Pause between stimulating and responding	Pause for contemplating results with compassion and love	No pause, quick and immediately take action, rarely contemplating

Fact about the human being, people usually only work or act when they think they are right when doing it. People are angry, scolded and repressed come from the result of they think it is the right thing, they should do it, and it is the right way. Some people even beat brothers, friends, wife, children, and coworkers with the thinking that this is the right thing to do. Our subsequent actions and choices will always show consistency with the previous conclusion. Hasty people always cling to their own opinion and try to protect it. We may fall into the illusion of assumptions, expectations, and emotions.

The destiny of people is the accumulation of decisions they made, no matter these are small or big decisions. The decisions come from the emotion at the time of making decisions. Emotion people have in each situation is influenced by the feeling just before they approach the situation. If people are happy then they will look at things in the direction of fun, positive. They may have much more fun emotions. If they are upset, angry, they tend to see things with annoyance. The potential of the brain will make their negative emotion increase. They may create a stress situation if they do not pay attention to their feelings. The second things influence people's emotion is the angle they choose to look at things, the points they focus looking on thin, and the essence of situations. One situation comes from the combination of countless facts. Unfortunately, the quick-tempered people will quickly and shallowly grasp on several facts then quickly jump to the conclusion. They may blindly shut their mind and stubbornly attached to the conclusion. The third things influenced people's emotion is their greedy expectation. If they have an unwanted perception of the situation, their perceptions are worse than their expectation, they will be upset, angry, even get mad at their beloved ones.

In each time of making decisions, we collect data on cost and data of benefit. If the cost is more than the benefit then we do not make the decision. On the other hand, if the cost is lower than the benefit that we will make the decision to move forward. For example, to decide to enroll a college education or MBA course, people always measure the cost and the benefit of the decision to participate or not participate in studies. In buying a jacket, people always make calculate the cost and the benefit in mind. In purchasing a house, a luxury car or an expensive leather bag, people always have calculated the cost and the benefit in their mind. Cost and effect also have an influence on contract or start up a business. People spend hours to measure the cost and the benefit before each decision. If the cost is over the benefit of taking action, we will not take action. If the cost is smaller than the benefit, we will make the decision to take action and ready to bear the cost. Cost includes all the things and fee we think we will lose in taking action. The benefit includes all things and money we assume we will get in taking action. Unfortunately, cost and benefit are the assumptions of most people; these are the relative values. With hasty people, the data on cost and benefit usually be distorted by strong emotion. The data getting from the situation may vary a lot. The varieties of data we collect from situation depend mainly on the dots in mind, the ability to control the mind. The facts depend on our feeling, the angle we look at things and our expectations. When we feel sure about the data we collected, clear about cost and benefit, we will feel sure to make the decision. We will think this is the right decision.

In dealing with failures, pressing situations with huge loses in life and in business, most people like I, you, your spouse Warren Buffet, Steve Jobs, President Lincoln, and the president will make the different decision. The differences come from different feelings because we all have different belief systems, the pattern of thinking, perspective, set of values and principles. Astonishingly, we all think our decisions are the right decisions. The more we understand common principles, set of values, big visions, and understanding, the more effective we are.

> We are so different in the pattern of thinking, belief, mind, and brain that all seven billion people in the world, all identical twins in the world, there is no two individuals have the same fingerprint. So how we can jealously compare, compete and judge others.

The individual has own personal belief system, individual use it to see in the world, to interpret things they contact. This paradigm is like glasses of individual wearing. Through each lens, people perceive meaning and emotions from the environment. Energy or emotion comes from focusing on the mind. By focusing on richness, focus mind on the things we have: legs, arms, eyes, health, friends, weathers, family, parents, properties, the country we live in, our job and so on. These are the things that billions of people desire to have one of these things we have. When focusing on the things we have, we will live with a grateful mind. We are grateful for many things. Millions of things we inherit, we use but we do not have to build like phone, technology, television, cars, churches, pagodas, and knowledge; which are the result of passion, effort, and sacrifice of billion people. I am grateful for the valuable knowledge of all humankind accumulates in thousands of years have been put a single book. With a grateful attitude, we will make serving actions with joy and happiness. The more we are grateful, the less we expect from our action. With gratitude and contentment, we will know how rich we are, how lucky we are.

> We feel sad, angry or depressed because we do not get things we want, we do not get the things we expect. The best way to bring for us happiness is by reducing the want by getting objective understanding, then taking responsibility to maximize our ability to create wanted changes in the world.

We feel sad, angry or depressed because we do not get things we want, we do not get the things we expect. The best way to bring for us happiness is by reducing the want by getting objective understanding, then taking responsibility to maximize abilities to create wanted changes in the world. The fuel for this process comes from the imagination of the mind. The powerful mind has the ability of imagination; with a vivid imagination, the mind cannot distinguish the reality with the imagination. So when focus on grateful things, grateful moments and proud events we need to make it as vivid as possible with senses, sound, smell, and feeling. This process of imagination mobilizes every part of the brain to relive a happy feeling. We need to relive happy moments. The mind thinks that we have to get the things we want so it active the happy chemicals. Just by focusing the mind on imagination to visions and proud moments, we can create a happy state of mind. The brain in a happy state mobilizes a lot of hormones, chemicals to create powerful energy for our body to take action, to serve and to give. The more actions we take the closer to the success we are. Only five to ten minutes of focusing the mind on the grateful state each day, we can control our feeling and we can master our mind.

> "I had the blues because I had no shoes until, upon the street, I met a man who had no feet."
>
> **Denis Waitley**

Unfortunately, most people fall to a negative feeling or depressed state because of comparing with others. They often focus on the things they do not have but other people have. Moreover, they have so many needs and desires that even they live in richness and abundance but their mind still scans for the desired things that they do not have. Miserable people focus on lack. The more lacking focus, the more miserable they feel. Then the mind activates the stress state because of their obsessed desires are not satisfied. Greedy people see others with envy and angry eyes. Their unconscious mind of and the unconscious mind of people may detect the irritating signals all day, even they may live in richness. The mind actives the stress chemical in the body; it makes people feel stress, anger, misery in the life of abundance. This is the reason why many famous people seem to be successful in life and career but still think of suicide, affected depression, and addict drugs. They are more miserable than most of us can imagine. It is the focus of the uncontrolled mind makes them feel miserable and get stress.

To enjoy richness, we have to control the focus of the mind. We need to do gratitude exercise five to ten minutes every day. The more grateful we are, the richer and happier we become. We can put the body in the state of high emotion and high energy just by focusing the mind. In the book Man's search for the meaning of Viktor Frankl, the author has given a lot of stories about how powerful the mind can be. The human mind can create a happy state even in the worst circumstance of living. With this peak emotion, the peak of energy, people can easily make peak performance. The happy state of mind fuels the energy to pull us into taking action.

On the other hand, to take massive action, some people need to push into taking action. By focusing the mind on the tragedy caused by procrastination, bad habits, bad thought accumulating with time. The tragedy like broke, divorces, illness, diseases, severe pain put on them and their kids, they may feel miserable caused by their wrong habits. Surfing on the media, newspaper, tabloid we can see millions of the misery tragedies, with the game if then, we can use these tragedies to scare us to death. With the time of contemplation, we can see the results from our habits. Sometimes, we need to be scared to death by others' misfortune, just by imagining that these tragedies can fall on us, we can experience pain enough that it will push us into taking action. We need to be pushed into changing, push into acting to move out of comfort zone. The imaginative tragedies make us feel stressed and frightened, and our unconscious mind will memorize feeling and patterns these tragedies; the subconscious mind will send us gut signals if we fall into the traps of these tragedies. It will send us the urge to take action to stay away from misery.

With gratitude and imagination, we can create enough energy to take action from our mind. We have taken the first step to control our mind.

Emotional is like energy, it is transmissible. When you go home from work and join to the dining table. If you eat under stress, the stress chemicals are stimulated, adrenalin, norepinephrine, and cortisone secreted into your body unconsciously, it makes you feel chill, alert and irritated. You will overreact with little stimulation. Other members are also annoying from the work; they are more sensible and uncomfortable when seeing your negative expression and your actions. All subconscious minds alerted, if the alertness is not reduced, the conflict or argument might happen.

Every family member will fall into extreme stress. People will argue over others, skip meals or loss of appetite. This is the script we may meet every day. Our small babies are the most hurtful people with the stress in the family.

> "A crust eaten in peace is better than a banquet partaken in anxiety."
>
> **Aesop**

The story of the father went home late in the evening, although he was very tired, but before he entered home, he took off his jacket and hung up the robe at the door, shaking himself three times to change his state. Entering his home with a different state: vivacious, agile and fun. Neighbors questioned why he has such a habit before entering the house, the actions: put off the jacket, shaking body then change the entire state of mind. He said he do this because he wants to put off negative things from work, put off the fatigue and stress he had all day, then shaking the body to get in a new state of mind. He said he knew how his emotion would affect his children, and he knows what his children really need from him.

To deal with negative emotion, some experts teach that we should neglect or suppress negative emotions. I think this is not a good idea because the negative emotions are still inside us. When in a stressful situation, the hidden things have the chance to jump out with worse consequences. We need to have new approaches to destroy the negative emotion. Negative emotions arise when our expectation not matched by the condition. It means too much need with expectation and an unsatisfied condition can create negative emotion and stress. By reducing needs, removing expectations, or gaining the ability to change the circumstance, we can destroy negative emotion. And by looking deep to the negative emotion to understand it, understanding helps us control the emotion. Enlighten people understand life, themselves, others and emotion so that they can control emotion since emotion is weak.

Some powerful techniques to control emotions

A. The first way is to remove the personal assumption

Coming in with knowing nothing, without assumptions, we will try to find the views of others, freely swap the positions of partners to create understanding and sympathy for others.

You have to step out of yourself, immerse yourself in someone else's position to know and live with their perspective and emotions. Having a feeling of sympathy and understand others' point of views before judging.

By swapping positions: putting on shoes' of other people and walk for two miles to have empathy before making conclusions or judging others. Changing perspective leads to the change of mindset that creates empathy. When we get angry with someone, if we understand their pain, their loss, and their difficulty, our emotions will change. We will more open to communicating for deeper understanding; for creating the depth of listening and questioning so that we have compassion for others. We understand better the needs, intentions, and motives of the other people.

> "When I am getting ready to reason with a man, I spend one-third of my time thinking about myself and what I am going to say and two-thirds of him and what he is going to say."
>
> **Abraham Lincoln**
>
> "The struggle of my life created empathy - I could relate to pain, being abandoned, having people not love me."
>
> **Oprah Winfrey**

B. The second way is the power of time.

Over time, the level of anger will be subsidized, or the emotions will decrease its energy. When we are angry, we make a lot of irrational action. Once anger has gone we will make more rational decisions. This is the reason why experts recommend that when in anger, we need to stop before reaction; getting out of the situation when we know we are angry or upset. When calm down we can come back. There is an old saying can prevent us from regretting:

"**Do not promise when you are happy,**

Do not take action when you are angry."

To destroy negative emotions, to get into the peaceful state of mind; we need to understand more about the nature of life, the complexity of life. Accept that we are small and ignorant creatures. Think of the famous teaching of Socrates I know that I am intelligent because I know that I know nothing. Knowing we know nothing, we will have an open mind to absorb ideas, ignoring all our assumptions we will look more deeply at the situation, looking for data, referencing all angles. We will pick up the right information, real facts from the event. People with a lot of assumptions and prejudices, instead of picking up the objective information, their mind only pick up distorted information, which reinforces our previous assumptions.

C. The third way to control emotion can find in Buddha's and Confucius teaching.

The misery in life can be prevented by followed the teaching of Buddha: three things make us miserable in life are our desires, our anger, and our ignorance. Reducing desires and expectations, we will get real information instead of distorted information; realizing the appearance and development of anger, we can control the anger instead of letting anger control us. Accepting our ignorance, we will open to new ideas. We can practice the detachment with wrong opinions, carefully with forming the conclusion.

> People usually evaluate themselves and their actions according to their purposes; adversely, they often evaluate other people and others' actions according to their behaviors.

People usually evaluate themselves and their actions according to their purposes; adversely, they often evaluate other people and others' actions according to their behaviors. This is how we justify for ourselves, justify our angry emotion, easily blame others for our problems and rarely accept responsibility. If continues, conflict with anger and stress will dominate the relationships. By awakening and swapping positions, we can break the trap of shallow thinking and wrong conclusions. When evaluating the actions of an individual, look for three things in the teaching of Confucius Look at the means, which a man employs; consider his motives, and observe his pleasures. A man simply cannot conceal himself!

Injustice, when investigating a case, people investing in the means, the motives and the actions by answer three important questions

- What happened?

- How did it happen?

- Why did it happen?

Only get enough right answers for the three questions, the course of justice will pass judgment on someone. In the investigation of the judgment, the motives are much more important than the action. The motives can be viewed as evidence to reduce or increase the sentence. This is the way to create just judgment from good justices. This is the way of approaching the problem of the kind and smart ones. They get the right clues for the important questions before giving any judgment. They can prevent themselves from falling into the trap of irrational thinking, the trap of emotion, and psychological traps.

The scenario or a pattern of conflict, misery we see every day, Ha, a seven-year-old girl, wanted to help her mother to prepare for dinner before her mother comes home from work. She was very excited about the idea, she runs out quickly from the table full of toys. After washing vegetable, she moved the bowls, forks, and chopsticks from the basket to the rack. While moving, unfortunately, she broke a beautiful plate, which her mother loved the most. Ha was frightened shaking. At that moment her mother returned, she just exasperated from the work, seeing her broken plate, messy home. The mother was angry, scolding and beating Ha then knocking her into her room without saying a word. Ha was very frightened, painful and disappointed. Even worse, her mother was very annoyed angry and stressful, with a little of shame for beating her beloved child. Her anger could be more serious if her husband went home with some unwanted news or unwanted things.

This scenario, the injustice we encounter every day, in many families, in works place and even in our own family. Hope that before angry with anyone, especially with children, the dependent individuals, we need to pause and switch the position to have a deeper look at their purpose or motives. Take time to think or separate ourselves into the situation. Do not dive too much into the anger, awake with our tempting but hurting action. When taking time to look deep inside the wrong behaviors of other people, we may be touched with their noble purposes.

This may reveal the noble purposes of great men in their actions. The stories of the calmness and retreat of great men who encountered crucial events, that they acted differently or contradictory compare with most of the ordinary people. The ordinary people blamed a bad reputation for them because of action. They were bearing a bad reputation until the next generation of hundred years later can understand and clarify their noble purpose. Rarely great men on the world get support from all other ordinary people. Perhaps there is a big difference in the way of perceiving ideas because of the difference in understanding the above three questions. Great men perfecting the noble purpose before employ any actions and methods of actions; their actions are driven by vision, noble purpose and long-term gain, they are glad to welcome short-term pain. Ordinary men perfecting the action and method of action before choosing a suitable purpose; their actions driven by the praise and recognition of other people, by emotion, the ego and with short-term gain. The great men listen to the emotion, calm the irritating, and let the mind calm to look deeper into the situation, they got the different point of views with most of us then they act in a different, even shameful ways. They have controlled their mind, their emotion and their actions directly to noble purposes. Most of us do not get this high state of mind so we need to train a lot to understand them or at least do not harm or prevent them from taking action.

In daily interactions, we need to find the answers to these three questions too. We need a quiet and still mind to get real facts to make a better judgment; we need to understand the motives for empathy. We need to understand the way of action, not just go deep to know what and how. With understanding, we can control our mind to get the best result of the interaction in life. With understanding, we can create interdependent living; we can multiply the power of each separate individual. We can resolve all conflict and prevent useless stress in our life. This is the biggest present we can give to our spouses, children, family members and all other people around us.

D. The fourth way to control emotion is by taking action.

Doing physical exercises, participating in gymnastics, jumping, cheering, singing out loud, playing with kids, celebrating with the victory are the acts create energy. Massive action, especial massive action with joy, stimulates the brain to create chemicals of happiness. In a happy state, we will feel more joy, less pain, more open to opinions. We take more actions of love, caring, and generosity. The happy state makes us feel more confident and powerful than stress state so that we tend to take more challenges, accepting more unwanted things and looking to the bright side of problems. The bodies of happy people push out toxic chemicals and activate the process of healing. Happy people associating with laughing, a lot of muscles combine together to create the laugh. In reverse, laughing stimulates the happy state; it is like the conditioned response between the mind and body. Many laughter yoga clubs found all over the world to help people have more joy and happiness in daily life.

Individuals do not control their mind can be easily stimulated by tiny things. Subconscious mind detects unwanted things very quickly it sends the signal to the mind to arouse a stress state. Just seeing a small part of the action or a part of the way of action taken, the shallow mind very sensitive to these unwanted things, the mind will be stimulated. Without realizing and taming it down, the mind will agitate more aggressively, and stop looking deeper into the motive of action. A sequence of wrong events or wrong action has taken place; this is the first stage of misery in life. This is the scriptural pattern of conflict in life, in the family, and in society; where there is no understanding, no empathy, less sharing, less love people will find a lot of annoying and stressful signals. This can be called hell on earth. Individuals in these place hunger for love, connection and significance.

The emotion has been exploiting skillfully in business. Sale men, shopping centers, and luxury products are the masters at creating and increasing the emotion of prospects and customers. By telling attracting stories, creating noble emotions, noble images, and noble purposes, they make customers think that happy mean possessing luxury products and pain with not possessing the luxury products. When emotion goes up because of satisfying customers deepen needs, customers will passionate the luxury products. Customers are moved from not interested in the products to a keen desire of possessing the product unconsciously. With the obsessed desire of possessing the product, customers' mind will collect data to support the happiness relating to possessing products. Moreover, their mind tends to ignore the opposite information. At peak emotion, people easily take a credit card to buy expensive products; people make the decision by emotion. Peak emotion makes people blind in the calculation of real cost and real benefit in buying the product; peak emotion is the multiplier and divider with the varieties in the calculation of cost and benefit before making the decision. The luxury brands master at seducing emotions. Rarely an individual wake up and buy a five thousand dollar bag. In order to have a moment of paying big money for a luxury bag, the image of possessing the product with extreme happiness has been infused to the individual's mind the long time before; moreover, on the way look at the luxury product, lot of happy and noble feelings has been put vividly in the mind of the prospects. Most people including you and me do not have the ability to resist the temptation of satisfying obsessed desire when in high emotion. We will fail if we do not practice to control the mind and desire. This is our weakness that we need to know; this is our ignorance. Shopping and having more can reduce stress for a short time with irrational and emotional individuals, who usually driven by emotion. In fact, individuals who have been led by emotion in one area tend to be led in other areas. The indicators of our weakness in controlling emotion often appear in many decisions we have made. If we do not aware of this weakness, we can create misery in our life, our family and our society unconsciously. Adversely, we use self-talk, the stories, and wrong assumptions to justify our wrong behaviors; we consciously think we are right.

Great men can control emotion and resist the temptation; they have the deepest look at themselves and at objects of thought, with throughout understanding. They got wisdom in knowing others and they got the enlightenment in knowing themselves. How peaceful, how tranquil, how happy and how motivated we got when watching, hearing the great men, Mother Teresa, great monks, Buddha, Benjamin Franklin, and Abraham Lincoln walk, act and talk. On the other hand, how annoyed, how nauseous, how terrible and how depressed we got when watching, hearing rich, stingy and jealous men walk, act and talk. It may be good luck for people near caring, loving and generous individuals; and the bad luck for people near selfish, jealous and stingy individuals. There might be no difference in names of action they take, but there is the biggest difference in how much love, how much consideration, how much caring, how much empathy, how much pain and how much joy they put in the actions. If people pay attention to the invisible in actions, they not only can reduce misery, pain, and stress in life but also they can create warm, happiness, and the satisfaction of deepening needs inside for all relating individuals. This is an effective way of eradicating mental diseases, mental problems and other problems in family, school, and society. It is useless if we use anti-depressive medications to treat patients with depression without removing the sources of stress. The failure of treating patients with depression is mainly caused by patients are still living in a stressful environment. A large number of stress chemicals running throughout the body of patients antagonize all the effects of the medications.

To succeed in combating the self to create happiness, we need persistence in personal development, sharpen the skills. The process of personal development associates with changing oneself, and changing the attitude form demanding to serve. We cannot develop ourselves with the concept of self-help; we can only develop ourselves with the concept of helping others, Mother Teresa is an example. Owning for personal development, we can develop ourselves big enough to have talent and courage to create changes with changeable things in the environment to meet our needs. Moreover, with the process training and practicing, we gain wisdom and enlightenment to correct ourselves by reducing unnecessary needs, limiting the useless desires, controlling the anger, knowing our ignorance. With wisdom and enlightenment, we happily open to new idea and opinions; we can get a better understanding of other people. Understanding creates compassion and love. Persisting in practicing, we may develop ourselves big enough that we can gain peace and stillness of mind in chaos; we may gladly accept the unchangeable problems or the facts of life in our environment. Change is inevitable to gain happiness and peace of mind.

The best advice for the successful but unhappy individual is taking a course in meditation or managing oneself. After months or years of practicing, they may gain big changes inside and get a different belief system. It is like the process of changing from dark, timid lenses to bright lenses to view the environment. Previously, with dark and timid lenses, they only see misery, upset and injustice from the environment; the perception of life makes them angry and stressful, which leads to endless problems and diseases for themselves. After months or years of training oneself, they get the bright lenses to view the world, they see joy, gratefulness, and generosity from the same environment; the new perception of life makes them grateful and happy, which leads to endless wealth and wonderment in life. Life gets better not because of changes in the environment, but because of people changing themselves. Interestingly, by changing themselves, people become big enough that they can create the changes they want to see in the world.

References:
Jeanne Garbarino on November 15, 2011. Cholesterol and Controversy: Past, present, and Future. Retrieved from https://blogs.scientificamerican.com/guest-blog/cholesterol-confusion-and-why-we-should-rethink-our-approach-to-statin-therapy/

The science of Health Newsletter. (January 2005) We Can Put an End to All Disease on This Planet. Retrieved from http://customers.hbci.com/~wenonah/news.htm

Dr. Elaine (February 23, 2016). Mind Body Spirit Mind Body. Retrieved from http://drelaine.com/are-you-giving-your-heart-the-most-critical-nutrient-it-needs/

Annie B. Bond. (April 10, 2005). The Healing Power of Love – A True Story Retrieved from https://www.care2.com/greenliving/healing-power-of-love-true-story.html

ANewDayANewMe. (n.d). Oprah: Deepak Chopra. Good Thoughts Can Heal. Bad Thoughts May Kill! Retrieved from http://www.anewdayanewme.com/oprah-deepak-chopra-good-thoughts-can-heal-bad-thoughts-may-kill/

Chapter 52: The role of meditation to have a healthy, happy life

Practicing meditation regularly, people will have less emotional behaviors; they will reduce most of their greed and anger. Practicing meditation helps people gain the correct understanding of their body, feelings, perceptions, mental formations, and consciousness. Living with awareness, they have deep look at everything; they gain understanding. Understanding creates compassion and love. They can control emotion easily. Owning for practicing meditation, they can reach to state: the stillness of mind in the midst of changing world.

To practice meditation find a quiet place, sit on a chair with comfortable position, feet put straight on the ground; or we can sit on the floor, straight back, with our head, neck, and back aligned vertically. This allows the breath to flow most easily. Close the eyes slightly. For those who have dizziness hard to close their eyes can open their eyes and look down. We usually practice the sitting meditation either on a chair or on the floor. If choosing a chair, use one that has a straight back and that allows our feet to be flat on the floor. We sit away from the back of the chair so that your spine is self-supporting. If choosing to sit on the floor, sit on a firm, thick cushion to raise our buttocks off the floor four inches; thick cushion help us not falling backward; it can be a pillow folded over once or twice does nicely, or a meditation cushion. There are a number of cross-legged sitting postures and kneeling postures that some people use when they sit on the floor, choose the position that most comfortable for you. The main points to keep in mind your posture are to try to keep the back, neck, and head aligned in the vertical, to relax the shoulders in the picture.

Picture 1: sitting postures of meditation

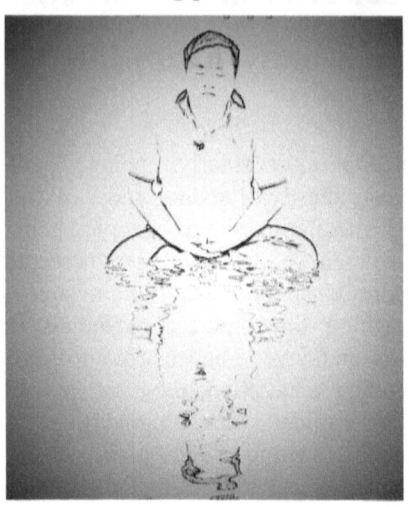

Before practicing meditation, people never thought about what was going on inside the body and mind. They rarely pay attention to the body, feeling, perception, mental formations, and consciousness, which appear and grow enough to make people follow their commands. With the habit of meditation, they realize all of these things still happen inside the mind are constantly changing things, they are aware of things going on and off; they get the better understanding so that they can know the time to stop, time to act and time to attach or detach. People can make a good decision whether or not to follow the commands, the conclusions, sensations, and feelings in the mind. They understand themselves better, and the understanding has given them more flexibility, freedom and peaceful mind.

Quality of life belong to the quality of the connection between beings, so do the connections of the neuron cells determine the power of the brain. All brain's parts active and work harmoniously during meditation. Mindfulness in meditation help the neo-cortex understands and establishes the connection to the limbic systems and other parts of the brain. Observing mind, body, breath, sensual signals and thinking but not chasing to the thoughts and feelings help us understand the mind, body, and life. During meditation, the cognitive mind start to observe the autonomic mind, the observation helps to create more bonds inside the brain. Owing to better quality and quantity of connection inside the brain, so that parts of the brain for the different function and billions of neurons become the identical brain. Good connections make the cognitive mind and autonomic mind work harmoniously. The more of practicing meditation, the more powerful the mind is. For any function of mind, all parts of the brain and neuron cells are synergic to fulfill the task. Scientists have measured that the brainwave of Tibetan meditation practitioners thinking of kindness is the highest human brain wave ever recorded; this brainwave is as high as the brain wave during seizure attack.

Meditation helps people live more mindfully, live close to the present, understand how mysterious life is so that they can sense the happy feelings. Meditation connects all the cognitive mind, intuitive mind, body, and environment together. Buddha connected to all other beings loved all other beings, and he contemplated to gain the highest understanding. Then all his life was to love, help, connect, give and teach needed people. His time may be the ignorant time of human beings but he had gained peace and stillness of his mind; he was the most content man ever. So that it is true to say Buddha is the happiest man ever.

A. Buddhism meditation

Thich Nhat Hanh told Buddha taught understanding gives rise to compassion and love, which in turn give rise to correct action. In order to love, it is first necessary to understand, so understanding is the key to liberation. In order to attain a clear understanding, it is necessary to live mindfully, making direct contact with life in the present moment, truly seeing what is taking place within and outside of oneself. "A person is a person who dwells in mindfulness. Life can only take place in the present moment. If we lose the present moment, we lose the life. He is aware of what is going on in the present moment, what is going on in his body, feelings, mind, and objects of mind. He knows how to look deeply at things in the present moment." Thich Nhat Hanh continued to recite the teachings of Buddha. If one makes good at present he need not care or looking for the future. Future is formed by the quality of present actions. So stop to pursuit the past, stop chasing to the future. Live closely and mindfully at present. Reading to this line, all you read one second before, one minute before and one hour before called the past. Do the moments perish? No, they all invisible embed in all parts, all cells of you. So if you live mindfully in present, you will gain the understanding to take advantage of the past and the future will take care of itself.

What is meant by "pursuing the past" and "losing yourself in the future"? To pursue the past means to lose yourself in thoughts about what you looked like in the past, what your feelings were then, what rank and position you held, what happiness or suffering you experienced then. Giving rise to such thoughts entangles you in the past. You may relieve the pain of the past, or regret the past that you forget that you are standing in the mysterious land. Losing yourself in the future means lose thoughts about the future, expectation and forget present. You imagine, hope, fear, or worry about the future, wondering what you will look like, what your feelings will be, whether you will have happiness or suffering. You may create some expectation in the future; you may be hurt or stressed of your expectation are not satisfied. Past and future only should use for your contemplation, for solitude but not for present living. Pursuing the past or losing in the future will distort your thinking, you may think you know everything or you only pick up the clues to prove your subjective judgments, assumptions or expectations. Your work, words, thinking will full of past and future events. At home, you will think at work, at work you will think and prepare for home or holiday. Staying with your children you may still relive the anger of the work, then, at work, you have to use the joy of playing with your children to bear the hardships of the work. Working like this you will never sense the joy of working, the invaluable of working. What a tragedy for the world when millions of people do not have a job, their desires may be having a job to feed the families, they may admire the neighbor workers. But they do not know that the workers and officers next door are tired and stressed because of the thinking have to work. Living with the success of the past or the victory of the future you will never see the mysterious around you at present. You will be slaved by desires and anxieties and lose the precious present. You will be exhausted from pursuing the past and future and losing of desires and anxieties because of the unwanted events in the past and future. Unfortunately, you may stressful and you will never really live. Mindfulness enables you to return to the present moment. You will lose your mindfulness and you will not be truly present for life.

> "Past and future only should use for your contemplation, for solitude but not for present living"

Mindfulness living makes you sense the joy, the wonder of living. Mindfulness living makes you understand life is so simple and life is full of paradoxes with intelligent people. When you live mindfully, you will remove all your assumptions and be open to new things. Mindfulness helps people know to detach with things, events, and phenomena. Art of selling has focused the mind of customers to live with the joy of the possessing in the future; the pain of not possessing; and the countless stories about what the product will make them feel. Customers will forget or do not pay much attention to the facts that they are trading in the present.

Mindful eating will make you sense the mystery of the foods, the delicious of the foods. Monks eat in mindfulness with simple foods. But un-mindful meal means when you eat you only focus on the unwanted things, unsatisfied desires, or any unwanted dishes on the table of delicious full dishes. Never angry, sad or greedy people satisfied with the food on their dishes. Eating and all other activities of human beings depend mostly on the state of mind. Greedy people will never satisfy with whatever food, whatever home, whatever living, whatever jobs; and their powerful brain will taking the order of anger mind to make them feel right. It is so funny that they do not understand the mind, they tend to things that it is the law of attraction, and they are the centers of attraction.

Does mindfulness help people from suffering the tragedy of living? Be aware in order to see both the suffering and the wonders of life. Thich Nhat Hanh said "Buddha teach being in touch with suffering does not mean to become lost in it. Being in touch with the wonders of life does not mean to lose ourselves in them either. Being in touch is to truly encounter life, to see it deeply. If we directly encounter life, we will understand its interdependent and impermanent nature. Thanks to that, we will no longer lose ourselves in desire, anger, and craving. We will dwell in freedom and liberation." To dwell in mindfulness means the practitioner remains aware of everything taking place in his body, feelings, mind, and objects of mind; these are the four establishments of mindfulness or awareness. The mysterious of meditation that rarely people know, sitting in meditation simply just need you aware of body, feelings, mind, and objects of mind. Aware then detach to see its changing. Meditation practitioners will understand the hidden philosophy in nature and all phenomena, the philosophy of kindness, unconditional love, and compassionate heart.

Practicing mindfulness strengthens the ability to look deeply into the heart of anything. When we look deeply into the heart of anything, it will reveal itself. This is the secret treasure of mindfulness. Meditation practitioners will awake that they and all creature beings are ones. The delusive mind makes them think that they are separate. Mindfulness in meditation leads to the realization of liberation and enlightenment. Anyone can gain these abilities of mind through meditation. This is the most effective way to gain long-lasting happiness.

Thich Nhat Hanh continued: "Buddha teach pay special attention to observing your breath. Meditate on your body, feelings, mental formations, consciousness, and objects of your consciousness. Look deeply in order to see the process of birth, growth, and fading of every phenomenon, from your own body, emotions, mind, and objects of your mind the happiness liberation brings is true unconditional happiness." Anyone can do and they will understand life is interdependent, timeless, egoless, and emptiness, "all in one and one in all". So that, mindful people will realize what is the most effective way of acting, ones can understand the philosophy of inaction of Lao Tzu, the philosophy of nonviolence of Gandhi, and the philosophy of kindness of Dalai Lama. These simple philosophies are true for all people; it is the root of all other science, education, business, and parenting and governing.

B. Simple mediation practices for busy people:

At home, you can sit cross legs on flat, on a small cushion under the bottom to avoid falling backward or sitting on the coach; where you can have enough quiet and uninterrupted time. Practice daily five to ten minutes in a quiet place. Straighten your body like a feeling of direct force pulls from the head to make upright; then let the body relax in the straight position. Practice some of these exercises of observing. There are people practice meditation for the first time, a lot of thoughts jump out and disappear. It is normal because this is the normal function of the mind. Do not worry, just identifying and naming the thoughts of past, future, positive, negative, nonsense, selfish. After recognizing and naming, thought cannot be self-sustaining, thoughts only sustain when we let ourselves breed and chase the thoughts. Just recognize and name the thoughts then come back to the observing. Practice each of these exercises from five to ten minutes. Whenever you want to stay focus, you can practice observing one of the following exercises.

Exercise one: Observe the relaxation of the whole body.

Stop the thinking process; observing the comfort, relaxation, and lightness of the body. Just breathing in and breathing out with the observing. Practice for at least three to five minutes.

Exercise two: Observe the breath.

Observe the breath in and out, inhalation and exhalation through the noses. Just recognize and observe the breath, do not try to control or adjust the breath. Observing, watching the breath, sensing the path of the breath. Feel the moving of the chest and abdomen when taking a breath. Practice for at least three to five minutes.

Exercise three: Count the breath during meditating

With the position of sitting for meditation, breathe in count one, breathe out count one; next breath, breathe in count two, breathe out count two. Then breathe in count three, breathe out count three. Do count less than five and do not count more than ten. When count to ten, we can count back from one. Practice for at least three to five minutes.

Exercise four: observe the lower abdomen

Observe the lower abdomen when breathing. Breathe in with the observation of moving of the lower abdomen and exhale the observation of moving lower abdomen. Watching the rising and falling of the lower abdomen. Practice for at least three to five minutes.

Exercise five: Observe the lower body in meditating

Observe the lower body when breathing. From the chest down, observe and sense the sensations of the hands, feet, and abdomen. Just observe the parts of the body; just realize the sensation of that lower part. Observe them as empty space cavity moving with the breath. We can feel joy with a sense of lightness and empty. Practice for at least three to five minutes.

If when you observe the body, thoughts appear, this is the normal function of the mind. Just realize the thoughts, do not follow thoughts. Come back to observe the breath. There are people practice meditation for t the, a lot of thinking jump out because of normal function of mind, do not worry, just identify and name the thought like past, future, positive, negative, nonsense, selfish. After naming, thinking cannot be self-sustaining. Just recognize and name the thoughts, then come back to observe the body and the breath. This is the characteristic of mind. Understanding the mind, we can control the power of the mind.

In this practicing of you can practice some of the following breathing techniques, each kind of breath you can do for several minutes. These breathing help you bring joy, happiness, and lightness for yourself, to some extent, it can help to heal your wounds, illnesses.

1. Breath in slowly and breath out with the feeling of happiness, just observing the breathing and feeling, do not try to control them.

2. Breath in slowly and breath out with smiling, just observing, do not try to control them.

3. Breath in with the feeling of lightness, the breath out with the feeling of coolness; just observe the breathing, and feeling of lightness and coolness.

4. Breath in with the feeling of warmness to the whole body, breath out with the feeling of warmness to the whole body, just observes the breath and feeling of warmness.

5. Breath with the feeling of gratitude, breath out with the feeling of joyfulness.

6. Breath in with the feeling of warmness in the body, breath out with the feeling of emptiness in the body.

7. Breath in with the feeling of joy, breath out feels lightness from letting go.

Exercise six: identify the thoughts that appear from the top of the head

It seems like there is a small brain at the top of the head to observe the thoughts appear in the head during meditating. Sitting in meditating position, just observe the thought appear in the head. Identifying and naming thoughts. Just identify, do not follow thoughts. Thoughts will appear and disappear constantly and out of our control. There are some people doing this exercise have a thousand thoughts in just ten minutes of meditating. With the time of practicing, the mind will reduce the habit of jumping around with thinking, and you will know the way to cut off thoughts, over time the mind will calm down. People practice meditation can gain the power of concentration.

> It is the mark of an educated mind to be able to entertain a thought without accepting it. **Aristotle**

Understanding gained by meditation, people can realize that we are wrong when totally believing, clinging to the old thought and protecting the old assumption. Clinging and attaching to previous emotions and assumptions is like covering the eyes with gray clouds. We consciously do not realize that our attachment to constantly changing things cause misery ourselves. With attachment to the previous assumption, we are blind to real facts, and good opinions; moreover, we anger to good but different opinions. Anger is another gray cloud covers our eyes. Many gray clouds of attachment and anger compound day by day into a thick black cloud. Because of attachment and anger, we ourselves make us like blind unconsciously. Looking back at our experiences, we will realize a lot of smart people became blind to the obvious truth when they were angry; their perceptions about facts have distorted. Detachment with any assumptions and detachment with any emotions are some of the ways that great scientists, entrepreneurs, politicians, and people use to do to get the real fact, real knowledge from experiments and events.

By practicing meditation, we can get a better understanding of our mind and our ignorance. We realize the problems we have are not the real problems, they the products of our expectation, our anger, and our ignorance. Understanding makes us more open to different opinions and ideas. We have to remove all assumptions before coming to the situation, we have to listen more, and create open conversations to get understanding. We need to contemplate to create the blueprint of our life first before taking massive actions. We need to find out our talents, strengths, love, and missions. With vivid vision, big goals, principles, values, compassion, serving heart, and persistence, individuals and organizations can achieve far more success than the ones without; these are not only the guiding stars but also the effective tools to direct our mind. Vision, goals, principles, values, compassion are the constants in the changing life; great men always remain constant to these. These are the effective tools for us to win over the self, the ego.

> "Things that I felt absolutely sure of but a few years ago, I do not believe now. This thought makes me see more clearly how foolish it would be to expect all men to agree with me."
>
> "It doesn't matter which side of the fence you get off on sometimes. What matters most is getting off."
>
> **Jim Rohn**

Practice meditation daily in a quiet place. When feelings of anger or negative emotions invade our mind, observe the thoughts and emotions from the top of your head to get a better understanding. Understanding will create compassion and love.

C. Mindfulness prevents us from making mistakes

Daniel Goleman cited a story in a rough neighborhood of New York City where there is a high rate of crimes: violence, robbery, murder. Most students have concentration problems and have witnessed or had relatives killed. Before class, students practiced an exercise of observing the movement of an object placed on the abdomen near the navel for five to ten minutes; this is one of the exercises of breathing in meditation. That daily ritual keeps the class environment calm and constructive and is empowering the children with self-control strategies early on. The class was fun, effective and little aggressive actions during the day. Researchers found that if teachers cut this exercise before class; the class was much more disordered and chaotic, and students were more irritated and aggressive. The scientific research evidence on the benefits of meditation is already compelling, and there are major studies underway.

We are usually anxious before an important interview or test; most of the time, the anxiety is out of controlled. We experience the symptoms of stress; which are the effects of overload stress hormones. We have many symptoms of stress in table 6: the most symptoms of stress that we can find in many patients. Even though, these symptoms may be worse if we still stimulate the mind with the thoughts or images of pain and failure from that event. The negative imagination can create far more fear and anxiety; we may think that we might fail, might make mistakes and might not do well. These thoughts in mind make us more afraid of a real event. The stress symptoms are obvious in the individuals who usually act according to emotion and irrational thinking. The thought itself makes us fall from anxiety to stress with symptoms of sweating, shaking, short breath, forgetting, pale, overreacting and high blood pressure. I see many senior healthy people come to a clinic to get the certification of health to go abroad to visit relatives; the results are good except the blood pressure is higher than the one they check at home. With little relaxation, some of them get high blood pressure near to the number they did at home. In practice, many physicians may see a lot of people have blood pressure rise when they see physicians in the white coat. Many patients are so afraid of injection that when they see a physician in white coat come only to check the blood pressure; most of the time the result may be higher than the patients do by themselves. This is proof that the unconscious mind controls us only with the imagination of the mind. The arousing of the mind can be calm down if we take the right understanding of the situation. In worse cases, if we breed the mind with lots of negative thoughts, the unconscious becoming stronger than the conscious mind. we may fall to extreme stress with a lot of wild actions, which can cause a lot of hurting and misery. When we are anxious, the good advice is to stop thinking, stop chasing the thoughts of past and future by direct the mind back to the body, back the mind to the present. Just by watching the breath, take control to make a deep breath, feel the breath, the sensation in the body, or just by counting the breath; these exercises direct the mind back to the body and cut the unwanted thoughts and make us calmer and less fear than before. When taking control of the mind, we focus the mind to present, we may direct the mind to focus on positive sides and positive figures of the event. Consciously looking to positive sides can make us confident to deal actively with the coming events. Our actions in a calm mind are more conscious and rational than the actions in stress.

Tragedy in the film starts with the knots: a character with power just only sees a small part of the unwanted action from another character, or he just gets distorted information; which he hates so much that he gets angry from perceiving. He makes series of mistakes like: without seeking more information to get the right understanding of the actions, without paying attention to the new emotions, skip reading the context, ignoring all opportunity to learn more about situations and stop digging to the purpose of the action. He hurries to draw out the wrong conclusion. Then he firmly clings to his conclusion and starts to make a series of following behaviors, which are supported by the conclusion. He creates the worst scenario of misunderstanding. These wrong actions cause terrible misery for good character because of misunderstanding. It is even worse than the individuals blindly immersed in bad and evil actions that cause injustice to good characters. During the film, these knots gradually dismantled.

Unfortunately, these tragedies appear all over the world, in countries and in families, because of the ignorance, we unconsciously create a lot of mistakes; the ignorant actions create extreme misery to our beloved people who are totally needed our love and support. Read stories in the newspaper or media we can see these kinds of tragedies in life. There are many successful people talked about the tragedies they got when they were young; fortunately, they bounce back better and get success in life. Oprah Winfrey, Tony Robbins, Steve Job are some of them.

In fact, our ignorance is unlimited; people have killed or created tragedies for many great men in history. Some of the western great men are Christ, Socrates, Galileo Galilei, and Abraham Lincoln. We cannot list all the misery of great caused by people's ignorance.

Unfortunately, ignorance is still in us, and billion other people. If we are not awake to train ourselves to become enlightened, we may create hundreds of ignorant behaviors each day, we may create suffering for relatives, ourselves and all other creatures. Nowadays, most of the wars, the act of terrorism, crimes, mental diseases, health problems, problems in family, schools, and society caused by the desire, anger, and ignorance of the people. Most of the victims and related people have ever experienced the stress symptoms, which listed in table three: the most symptoms of stress that we can find in many patients. Such a terrible, the actions caused misery for people are wearing noble masks of love, justice, peace, development, and sacrifice. Human beings are still be governed by the devil of ignorance. The masks not only make people feel at ease with the wrong actions and but also dull their gut feelings with wrong actions.

We need to practice more to gain wisdom and enlightenment. It is the best way we can do to help our beloved who are suffering. Outside intervention can only make people feel at ease with disease; it cannot eliminate the stress still arousing inside the victims. With enlightenment and wisdom, we can free ourselves and other people from the chains of ignorance.

D. People may be lead to crazy emotion if they lack mindfulness

The stories about the crazy state we can hear a lot from media like someone told that they did not understand what was wrong with them at the time of taking evil actions. They do not know why they do that crime, the action that they never thought of when they are in the normal state of mind. It is like there is a devil drove them to take crazy actions like beatings, stabbing, killing, and creating extreme hurt for others unconsciously.

Right understanding, they are just victims of uncontrolled peak emotions. They are so clingy to the expectation that they believe is true. The expectations were unsatisfied, they became angry. Stimulation of angry emotions made them uncomfortable with some signs. Combine with the chaotic environment, chaotic situation, or the chasing. The crowd, loud voice, loud music, shouting and chasing speed up the pulsating heartbeat, make emotion excited. Accumulation of time and many other unwanted things, their anger reached the peak of emotion. People will lose control of conscious mind when the emotion caused by unconscious my reach to peak. Most of the symptoms in the table two are so vigorous that we can easily realize like the heart rate is very high, the talking same as screaming, the hands are shaking, the pale skin, red face, stiff muscle. The conscious mind loses control of normal behaviors. The emotional brain completely dominates the whole body; on the other hand, the thinking brain is useless. It is like the animals in the extremely dangerous situation; there is no need for thinking, no need for other function put all the resources for fight and flight, put all resources for the irrational behaviors without paying attention for the damaging results. They act in extreme stress unconsciously like crazy men. The actions, at the normal state of mind they never ever think of, are taking.

Sadly, the fact is many parents become crazy with the unwanted actions of their small child. I cannot bear in the mind with the deep wounds, which are bearing by the fragile child trembling with crucial punishments by their crazy but loving parents. The stress distorts all perception from the facts, the distortion creating a more and more vicious circle of hurting.

Family tragedy happens when people fail to read emotional signals, fail to listen to nonverbal signals of themselves and other members. Not understanding or misunderstanding can create anger because they do not get the things they want. So that from small conflicts they do not handle well, they fall to anger, blindly blaming, insulting and shouting each other. They start to ignore the positive evidence, deny the explanation and refuse to cooperate to get understanding. They refuse all pieces of evidence contradicted with their conclusion; on the other hand, their unconscious mind works very efficiently in the situation of strong opinions and high emotions, the unconscious mind starts to scan unwanted things. So that small un-seemingly insignificant things now become the important things in conflict as long as it supports their conclusion, even the mind also call on the previous experiences to support their wrong conclusions. This is the reason for the advice that we should not reason with angry men. Their mind sees small un-seemingly insignificant things as seriously threatening. With distorted information, the calculation of cost and benefit of each decision become wrong and useless. They do not read their emotions and the emotions of the opposite person. The stress of conflicts so high that parents dare to make evil actions with the beloved child, which are not be done when they are in a normal state. Surfing the internet, newspaper, and magazines we see thousands of news of these tragedies and bad actions happen each day. The tragedy has the pattern, if we know it, we can prevent it. In medical, these tragedies created many terms of diseases.

From infants to adolescents or even adults are the victims of ignorant conflicts. Stress, lack of connection and lack of love and the ability of the individual are the ingredients make the quality of people living. If we make a test of the symptoms in table two the most symptoms of stress that we can find in many patients with the patients and people around the patients, we will get outstanding evidence of these causes.

Who let the emotions control so many times; they have been conditioned to the habit of responding in an irrational way. They always meet or create problem unconsciously with other people. Practicing meditation, reducing desires, anger, and ignorance, and forming the seven habits of highly effective people from Stephen Covey can help us not committing the wrong actions.

Mindful reading to emotional management

Read environment, read emotion, read the context, read gestures, read linguistic and non-verbal signs, and live in mindfulness. Read what you see, read what you hear, read what you feel. Be aware of the signs of emotion, emotions expressed through non-verbal signals. Some of the best ways are mute the TV, read the actor's feelings for at least ten minutes a day, start analysis scenario, realize the track of emotional development in actors. In the midst of the crowds, parks, or meetings, practice to read the emotions of people around, start with guessing and then finding the clues to sharpen your mind.

Always live in awareness to observe the body, feelings, perceptions, mental formations, and consciousness. Take quiet time to contemplate about the major things in your life. Spend time on major things, awake to do not spend major time on minor things.

Part XIII: Teaching of the Old

Chapter 53: The teachings of Buddha

The teachings of Buddha

1. Anger makes bigger ego, destroys the relationship: "In a controversy the instant we feel anger we have already ceased striving for the truth, and have begun striving for ourselves."

2. Contentment and faithfulness: "Health is the greatest gift, contentment the greatest wealth, faithfulness the best relationship."

3. Count nothing: "To live a pure unselfish life, one must count nothing as one's own in the midst of abundance."

4. Listen, peace available within: "Peace comes from within. Do not seek it without."

5. The long-lasting victory of the Self: "It is better to conquer yourself than to win a thousand battles. Then the victory is yours. It cannot be taken from you, not by angels or by demons, heaven or hell."

6. Love to cease hatred: "Hatred does not cease by hatred, but only by love; this is the eternal rule."

7. Peace and envy: "Do not overrate what you have received, nor envy others. He who envies others does not obtain peace of mind."

8. Real peace, letting go: "Those who are free of resentful thoughts surely find peace."

9. Root out lust, bitterness, and illusion: "He who gives away shall have a real gain. He who subdues himself shall be free; he shall cease to be a slave of passions. The righteous man casts off

evil, and by rooting out lust, bitterness, and illusion do we reach Nirvana."

10. The mind: "It is a man's own mind, not his enemy or foe that lures him to evil ways."

11. The Way, rarely people success by asking or praying, Buddha "I only point the way, you have to walk your path to save yourself"

12. What do you think of: "The mind is everything; what you think you become."

13. Life is full of misery, but if people train themselves with the teaching of Buddha, people can reach Nirvana in life.

Buddhism meditation by Thich Nhat Hanh and Zen masters

In science field, I am a pharmacist; in the science of personal development, I am a learner of many teachers, speakers, authors, singers, songwriters, poets, artists, educators, angel children, philosophers, and misery people. I am an atheist, but I am grateful and respectful to all religious leaders as the ordinary but enlighten people who have escaped the sensual world, the misery of the human world. So I gather a lot of their teaching to satisfy my curiosity about human behaviors, human religious rituals, human problems, human health, human wealth and the human mind. I develop owning for the advancement of Vietnamese society. I have once heard that Vietnam is the only countries that deserve to be a dragon and heaven on Asia and the world because of geographical advantages, philosophical advantages, and men's power advantages, but we do not. Keeping on searching, I awaken that not only Vietnam but also all other countries can become heavenly land for all people if they master the mind. Master the mind does not as hard as people usually think because the disabled people who master the mind can make the greatest contribution that rare people can think of. For example, Nick Vujicic, Stephen Hawking, and Helen Keller; and all other people who influence the human world are the ordinary people who have mastered the mind with some simple principles and virtues. The world full of intelligent men but fail or become the burdens of society because they are the slave of the mind with the desire to satisfied emotion, greed, and sensual feelings. It is the thinking of the people makes mastering the mind difficult. The thing that makes smart people fail because they do not understand that mind does not totally search for meaning, mind only search for satisfied feelings. All techniques in science achievement are to focus to create the force to pull and push people to worthwhile visions. It is helpful for people to make a good living but not a happy living. Even worse, blindly chasing to these can make people skip the most important things to them: present, living, love, connection, and family. Worst of all we may commit to mistakes to trade the precious, mysterious world to gain short-term pleasure for the mind. Chasing, hunting, taking, rewarding, punishing, and egocentric have pushed us too far to our core of living, ignoring the gut feeling. Many successful people start to lose their childish, lose the way of freely expressing emotion, their humor, their emotional life, their wild deepest need. The science of achievement, the science of living does not enough to make people happy but the art of living is. Science makes people gain knowledge and wisdom, but the art makes people awaken, enlighten and master the paradoxes of life.

Fortunately, the advantages of Vietnam help me understand the science and paradoxes of life in teachings of Buddhism, Taoism, Confucianism, the germ of sages, and Western philosophy. On the way of searching, Buddhism masters Thich Nhat Hanh, Thich Chan Quang show the way to crystallize all the knowledge I have to instruct the needed people. The masters teach me not only make meditation as simple as possible for all people but also put the philosophy of Buddhism as simple as possible for all people to benefit.

For the people who want to learn more about the meditation and practice it, below are the simple understandings that Thich Nhat Hanh has taught the teachings of Buddhism. The important things for the meditation practitioner to remember and practice for further advancement.

> **The four foundations of mindfulness are:**
> 1. Contemplation of the body,
> 2. Contemplation of feelings,
> 3. Contemplation of the mind,
> 4. Contemplation of mental phenomena-mental states and the arising and cessation of such states, along with the factors that produce such arising and cessation.

Firstly, the practitioner observes his body, his breath; the bodily postures, bodily actions, the parts of the body, the elements which compose the body such as water, air, dust, and heat; and the stages of a body's decay from the time it dies to when the bones turn to dust. While observing the body, the practitioner is aware of all details concerning the body.

For example, while breathing in, the practitioner knows he is breathing in; breathing out, he knows he is breathing out.

Breathing in and making the whole body calm and at peace, the practitioner knows he is breathing in and making his whole body calm and at peace. Breathing in and making the whole body in joy and happiness, the practitioner knows he is breathing in and making his whole body in joy and happiness.

Walking, sitting, talking, arguing, helping, and teaching, teaching, the practitioner knows he is walking, sitting, talking, arguing, helping, and teaching. The contemplation of the body is not realized only during the moments of sitting meditation but throughout the entire day.

Secondly, in the contemplation of feelings, the practitioner contemplates feelings as they arise, develop, and fade, feelings' characters, which are pleasant, unpleasant, or neutral. Feelings can have as their source either the body or the mind. When he feels pain from a foot, the practitioner is aware that he feels pain from a foot; when he is happy because he has received praise, the practitioner is aware that he is happy because he has received praise. The practitioner looks deeply in order to calm and quiet every feeling and mind to clearly see the sources giving rise to feelings. The contemplation of feelings does not take place only during the moments of sitting meditation. It is practiced throughout the day.

Thirdly, the masters continue, in the contemplation of mind, the practitioner contemplates the presence of his mental states. Craving, he knows he is craving; not craving, he knows he is not craving. Angry or drowsy, he knows he is angry or drowsy; not angry or drowsy, he knows he is not angry or drowsy. Centered or distracted, he knows he is centered or distracted. Whether he is open-minded, close-minded, blocked, concentrated, or enlightened, the practitioner knows at once. And if he is not experiencing any of those states, the practitioner also knows at once. The practitioner recognizes and is aware of every mental state which arises within him in the present moment as if there is a camera over his head record all thoughts appear and disappear. Knowing will make him mindfully live.

Fourthly, contemplation of mental phenomena, the masters continued the teaching of Buddha about the things that the practitioner should contemplate to gain mindfulness and enlightenment.

Contemplate the five skandhas, which comprise a person, body, feelings, perceptions, mental formations, and consciousness.

Contemplate the six sense organs and the six sense objects: the eyes and visible objects, ears and sound, nose and order, tongue and taste, body and touch, and mind and mental objects.

How to stop greed, hatred, and anger

Greed, hatred, and anger create misery in life. All raised from the ignorance. How to remove them, Buddha had pointed out the ways:

Firstly, understanding the Four Noble Truths means understanding life, and understanding the bearing of the physical body. The Four Noble Truths are

1. The existence of suffering

2. The causes of suffering

3. Liberation from suffering

4. The path that leads to liberation from suffering

Secondly, know that when greed, hatred, and anger comes.

Thirdly, practice the Noble Eightfold Paths to nurture the virtues, to gain the wisdom and enlightenment.

Fourthly, practice meditation, contemplation and live in mindfulness. Always contemplate the body, contemplate the feelings, contemplate the mind, and contemplation of mental phenomena.

The Noble Eightfold Path: eight right

1. Right view: our actions have consequences, right view, or understanding: the vision of the nature of reality, and the path of transformation.

2. Right or perfected emotion or aspiration, also translated as right thought or attitude. Liberating emotional intelligence in your life and acting from love and compassion. An informed heart and feeling mind are free to practice letting go.

3. Right Speech: clear, truthful, uplifting, and non-harmful communication.

4. Right Conduct: no killing or injuring, no taking what is not given.

5. Right Livelihood based on the correct action the ethical principle, only possessing what is essential to sustain life.

6. Right Effort or Diligence: guard against sensual thoughts, the concepts, states, aims at preventing unwholesome states that disrupt the mind. Consciously direct our life energy to the transformative path of creative and healing actions.

7. Right Mindfulness: never be absent-minded, being conscious of what one is doing; this, states, encourages the mindfulness about the impermanence of body, feeling and mind, as well as to experience the five aggregates, the five hindrances,

The Four Noble Truths and factors of awakening. Awareness and mindfulness of things, oneself, feelings, thought, people and reality.

8. Right Concentration: concentrate practicing meditation, culminating in the unification of the mind. Once the mind is uncluttered, it may then be concentrated to achieve whatever is desired. Right Concentration is turning the mind to focus on an object, such as a flower, or a lit candle, or a concept such as loving compassion. This forms the next part of the meditation process. Right concentration implies that we select worthy directions for the concentration of the mind, although everything in nature, beautiful and ugly, may be used for concentration. At deeper levels, no object or concept may be necessary for further development.

If you live right you will free from fear; your mind will find peace, happiness and at ease even in violence and chaos.

Sixteen breaths in Buddhism meditation taught by Thich Nhat Hanh

The masters continued the Buddha taught: "the method of the Full Awareness of Breathing if developed and practiced continuously, will bring great rewards and advantages. It will lead to success in practicing the Four Establishments of Mindfulness and the Seven Factors of Awakening, which will give rise to Understanding and Liberation.

These are the breaths that all people can practice to cope with stress and to enjoy the joy of life, happiness, love, and liberation. Practicing these breaths will up the level of mind and thinking. Practitioners will gain the four foundations of mindfulness by these sixteen breaths.

A. Contemplation of the body

1. The first breath: Breathing in a long breath, I aware I am breathing in a long breath. Breathing out a long breath, I aware I am breathing out a long breath.

2. The second breath: Breathing in a short breath, I aware I am breathing in a short breath. Breathing out a short breath, I aware I am breathing out a short breath.

These two breaths enable you to cut through unnecessary thinking, fear or regret, at the same time the breaths giving rise to mindfulness and enabling you to encounter life in the present moment. Forgetfulness and unwanted thinking is the absence of mindfulness. Breathing with awareness enables us to return to ourselves and to life. These breaths are very helpful for you to cope with stress and anger, to calm the mind and blood pressure down. Just by knowing or paying attention to the breath, the mind will calm and not chase to the unwanted thoughts or negative thoughts of past and future.

3. The third breath: Breathing in, I am aware of my whole body. Breathing out, I am aware of my whole body.

This breadth enables you to contemplate the body and be in direct contact with your own body. Awareness of the whole body and awareness of every part of the body changing like the endless streams in the body allows you to see the wondrous presence of your body, and the process of birth and death unfolding in your body. Breathing you will realize every part of the body is the masterpiece of nature.

4. The fourth breath: I am breathing in and making my whole body calm and peace. I am breathing out and making my whole body calm and peace.

This breath helps you realize calmness and peace in the body and arrive at a state in which mind, body, and breath are one harmonious reality. You may sense the feeling of calmness, peace, and emptiness. No words can express the experience of the meditator practicing the breath three and four.

These first four breaths, you are in the domain of the body, take your mind back to the body, you may sense the wondrous. Whenever you feel the negative feelings, practice these breaths will make you calm and control yourself.

B. Contemplation of feelings

5. The fifth breath: I am breathing in and feeling joyful. I am breathing out and feeling joyful.

6. The sixth breath: I am breathing in and feeling happy and smile. I am breathing out and feeling happy and smile.

With these two breaths, you come into the domain of feelings. These two breaths create peace and joy that can nourish the mind and body. Ceasing of dispersion and forgetfulness, you return to yourself, aware of the present moment. Happiness and joy available in you and will arise within you. You are the wonder of life to return to yourself you dwell on the wonders of life, able to taste the peace and joy mindfulness brings. Thanks to this encounter with the wonders of life, you are able to transform neutral feelings into pleasant feelings. These two breaths thus lead to pleasant feelings.

7. The seventh breath: I am breathing in and am aware of the feelings me. I am breathing out and am aware of the feelings in me.

8. The eighth breath: I am breathing in and making the feelings in me calm and at peace. I am breathing out and making the feelings in me calm and at peace.

These two breaths enable you to look deeply at all the feelings arising within you, whether they are pleasant, unpleasant, or neutral, and enable you to make those feelings calm and at peace. When you are aware of your feelings and can see deeply into their roots and nature, you can control them and make them calm and at peace, even though they may be unpleasant thoughts which arise from desire, anger, and jealousy. Just aware and make it calm and peace, you will live in mindfulness. You will sense the wonder of life. Practicing the breath of mediation you are calm, your child you huge will calm, and all people in the family will calm and at peace. All other indicators of your body will at ease inharmonious

C. Contemplation of the mind

With these four breaths, you cross into the third domain, which is the mind.

9. The ninth breath: I am breathing in and am aware of my mind. I am breathing out and am aware of my mind.

The ninth breath enables you to recognize all the states of the mind, such as perceptions, thinking, discrimination, happiness, sadness, and doubt. You observe and recognize these states in order to see deeply into the mind s activities.

10. The tenth breath: I am breathing in and making my mind happy and at peace; I am breathing out and making my mind happy and at peace.

11. The eleventh breath: I am breathing in and concentrating my mind. I am breathing out and concentrating my mind.

When the mind s activities are observed and recognized, you are able to concentrate your mind, making it quiet and at peace. Quite and peace come from recognizing and understanding then you just breathing and slowly making the mind at peace and concentration. This is brought about by the tenth and eleventh breaths.

12. The twelfth breath: I am breathing in and liberating my mind. I am breathing out and liberating my mind. With these four breaths, you cross into the third domain, which is the mind.

The twelfth breath enables you to release all obstacles of the mind. Thanks for illuminating your mind, you can see the roots of all mental formations, and thus overcome all obstacles. Strength, abilities, power, positive attitude and peace of mind are long-lasting because it comes from understanding when people pay attention to the body and mind, not from escaping or ignoring.

Some mental therapist help anxiety patients by helping them look into the painful or negative experience, during the treatment patients may be screaming and sweating when relived with the painful experiment. This technique just helps a little, but if the use the mindfulness breathing in meditation, they may be less painful and get better results.

D. Contemplation of mental phenomena- mental states

The practitioner will gain an understanding of mental states and the arising and cessation of such states, along with the factors that produce such arising and cessation. They are impermanent, appearing and disappearing constantly.

13. The thirteenth breath: I am breathing in and observing the impermanent nature of all dharmas. I am breathing out and observing the impermanent nature of all dharmas.

14. The fourteenth breath: I am breathing in and observing the fading of all dharmas. I am breathing out and observing the fading of all dharmas.

Understand the characters of mental phenomena you can contemplate on liberation, and letting go and forgiveness. When let go and forgive for people s mistake, the ones who are free are you. You will let go of all the unnecessary burdens, you will feel the joy of liberation, happiness, and lightness. You are free because of your forgiveness. You will enjoy the real joy, real happiness at present.

15. The fifteenth breath: I am breathing in and contemplating liberation. I am breathing out and contemplating liberation.

16. The sixteenth breath: I am breathing in and contemplating letting go. I am breathing out and contemplating letting go.

With these four breaths, the practitioner passes into the domain of objects of the mind and concentrates the mind in order to observe the true nature of all dharmas. Concentrating, observing all dharmas makes you have the understanding all dharmas. Follow the Eight Noble Paths and understand the dharmas, there is no space for fear, anxiety and negative feelings. You will be the master of the mind only when you understand the mind.

Understanding, mindfulness, letting go, and mastering the mind are some characters of enlightened one, they have attained liberation, joy, and happiness. They can live in peace and joy in the very midst of life.

Seven Factors of Enlightenment

"Master, there are many people who talk that they have the key to liberation, the key to happiness for all or they are the enlightened ones. How to know that they are enlightened or not? The master replied, "by contemplating the Seven Factors of Enlightenment, do they have it or not?"

1. Mindfulness to recognize the dharma, do they live mindfully, do they act based on understanding?

2. Investigation of dharma and phenomena to find out the quality or nature of things. Do they gain real understanding?

3. Energy or determination in action.

4. Joy or rapture in daily life: Do they have smile, happy feelings and enjoying all things?

5. Relaxation, ease or tranquility of mind and body.

6. Concentration with clear awareness; a calm, one-pointed state of concentration of mind;

Letting go or equanimity, to be fully aware of all phenomena without being lustful or averse towards them, do they forgive and forget other mistakes to lighten their burdens? Do they have unconditioned love, unconditional support, guiding without interfering? Unconditional love comes from understanding is different from blind love.

Chapter 60: Understand the teaching of the old, great men

All in one, one in all

Children are in the family,

The family is in children

The family is in the nation,

The nation is in children

There is no separation.

****

When can we realize our real problem?
What makes people stressed? What make adults and children fall into serious stress? The answer is the problem in modern society.

> "Confusion of goals and perfection of means seems, in my opinion, to characterize our age." **Albert Einstein**

> "Failure is the result of major in minor things and minor in major things." **Jim Rohn**

In daily life, people try hard to perfect the tools but rarely any of them understand why they should do it. When they spent the time to do but do not know the purpose of actions, do not know why things need to be finished. Lacking purposes, they waste time and energy on minor stuff. They like to do minor things at the major time. Running out of time so they have to do major things in minor time. They get exhausted but do not achieve any worthwhile things. They work ineffectively, over time, they become angry and stressful with the conditional they made. If list down every day all the thoughts they have, the emotions they have, the belief they have, the words they talk, they ways of using time and other resources; the action and reaction they take; the experienced people reading these lists can see that most people have the pattern that leads to failure. Most people in our modern society have patterns of failure in many areas of life like financial management, personnel management, family management, health management, career management, and emotional management. The individuals with a pattern of failure will get endless problems. Most people with the pattern of failure become anger and stress with the results and problems they created. Even worse, because of anger and stress, they unconsciously create stress for their beloved, their children, their spouse, their friends, their relatives, and related people. They have blindly conditioned the negative responses in their beloved. They are creators and the receiver of the misery for themselves and their beloved.

People only care to feed the bodies, feeding the sensual feelings and casually feeding desires. They do not care to feed the mind, feeding the soul, and feeding the spiritual life. They do not care to satisfy the desire of love and connection to their beloved. They do not care to satisfy the six basic needs of other people. Reading the advice of Mother Teresa, we will know that the people around us are hungry for many intangible things. We can help them by satisfying their hunger.

Mother Teresa taught:

- "Being unwanted, unloved, uncared for, forgotten by everybody, I think that is a much greater hunger, much greater poverty than the person who has nothing to eat."

- "Let us not be satisfied with just giving money. Money is not enough, money can be got, but they need your hearts to love them. So, spread your love everywhere you go."

- "Love begins by taking care of the closest ones - the ones at home."

- "Even the rich are hungry for love, for being cared for, for being wanted, for having someone to call their own."

- "The miracle is not that we do this work, but that we are happy to do it."

- "If we have no peace, it is because we have forgotten that we belong to each other."

How can we eliminate autism, depression, diseases, health problems and many social problems in our society? These are the problems or misery in modern society. Buddha showed the real causes of the misery of people 2500 years ago. The causes are lust, hatred, and delusion. The most effective way is to satisfy or support the satisfaction the hunger of the basics needs of human beings: for love, being cared for, being wanted by people by connection and love.

Masters teach:

"Human beings are not as special as they think.

Human beings are not as smart as they think."

Looking at the way of allocating all social resources, the way rich countries allocate their money, smart people do not sure about the fate of human beings.

Any Chief financial officers of any organization see this allocation of money, and resources they will have the strong gut feelings about the destination of the organization. If we still do the ways we used to do, we will end in misery and extinct sooner than we think. Any women who control the spending of money seeing the pattern of distribution of the wealthy in any family will have the gut feelings of sooner things will happen. Perhaps because of lacking the vital few, lacking trust, people are spending on weapons with the hope of keeping the peace.

Table 38: Discretionary spending 2015 of America

Subjects	Cost	Percentage
Military	**$ 596.5 Billion**	**54%**
Government	$ 72.9 Billion	6%
Education	$ 70 billion	6%
Medicare & health	$ 66 billion	6%
Veteran's benefits	$ 65.3 billion	6%
Housing & community	$ 63.2 billion	6%
International affairs	$ 40.9 billion	4%
Energy & Environment	$ 39.1 Billion	3%
Science	$ 29.7 Billion	3%
Social security, unemployment & labor	$ 29.1 billion	3%
Transportation	$26.3 billion	2%
Food and Agriculture	$ 13.1 billion	1%
Total	$ 1.110 billion	

Source: https://en.wikipedia.org wiki/2015_United_States_federal_budget

Global spending on health will expect to increase to $18280 billion worldwide by 2040. The money spend on finds good feelings for the people, they may forget that they have the abilities of self-healing and the abilities to heal for their friends, spouses, relatives, and children. If we do not awake, we will end up all money for useless possessions, robots, plastic world, weapons, wars, and medication; which brings the illusion of safety, significance, relaxation, certainty, development, and contribution.

Let see to have a relative meaning of global spending on health in 2040. The GDP of 2016 of United States is $ 18569 billion; the European Union is $ 16408 billion; China is $ 11218 billion; Japan is $4938 billion; Germany is $ 3,466 billion; the United Kingdom is $ 2629 billion, and France is $ 2463 billion.

Chapter 54: Gods and religions have taught us.

Many religions have precepts similar to this teaching of the Savior. The accompanying table lists several.

Table 39: Core teaching of some religions

Judaism	What is hateful to you, do not to your fellowmen. That is the entire Law; all the rest is commentary.
Buddhism	Hurt not others in ways that you yourself would find hurtful.
Confucianism	Surely it is the maxim of loving-kindness: Do not unto others that you would not have them do unto you.
Islam	No one of you is a believer until he desires for his brother that which he desires for himself.
Taoism	The Way that can be told of is not an unvarying way; The names that can be named are not unvarying names. It was from the Nameless that Heaven and Earth sprang; Mastering yourself to follow Tao was true power. I have three things to teach: compassion, simplicity, and patience.

Lao Tzu taught mastering others is the strength. Buddha 2500 years ago taught about how to end misery in life. Misery in life created by human beings; it appears in every aspect of life with the name of diseases, problem, and sufferings. In the teaching of Buddha, people suffer misery because of their lust, hatred, and ignorance.

Lustful people are so greedy for many things; they have a lot of needs. They want to possess many things, they want everything to meets their expectation to have feelings of happiness. They come to life with many wants, needs, expectations. They are obsessed with possessing many things to have happy feelings. After possessing new things, they get bored with the news thing very quickly, and they start to want to have other things. Greedy people always find that they lack many things even they may live in abundance. Lustful people with a lot of desires wants and expectations are the weakest people; they will easily become disappointed with many unwanted things; they easily anger if the condition does not meet their expectations. Easily become disappointed and angry, they constantly active the process of creating the stress chemicals, their body is constantly flushed with stress chemicals. Greedy people never experience real joy and happiness. They are the people have many obvious symptoms of stress described in table three: the most symptoms of stress that we can find in many patients. If they live in abundance, greedy people are the weakest people, their happiness belongs to other people, belong to outside condition; which is constantly changing. Their unconscious mind works all day to protects her greed. They never feel the moment of peace, the moment of stillness in mind. They are the victim of their lust.

> Having one car to meet your basic need can create happiness, but having five supercars to meet greed can create misery. Warren Buffet and Headed Buffet are the examples.
>
> Satisfying the basic need creates joy and happiness, but satisfying greed is the first step to hell. Hell means there will be ceaseless of pain and suffering. Greedy people are the victims of their and the creators of

problems around them.

When do not get things they want, greedy people become anger and stress. Their anger and stress make them feel uncomfortable; they tend to overreact to many normal things. Their greed, anger, and stress make them hate many things; these are like dark clouds covering their eyes. They only feel irritation, anger, and hatred in many things come to their life. The mind is always arousing with the thought of the future, the experiences in the past. They are rarely present to enjoy life. The thick dark clouds covering their eyes make them blink with many beautiful things next to them, or precious things under their feet. The thick dark cloud may blind the eyes, deafen the ears, dull the taste and blunt the thinking; they may make unconscious behaviors; their behaviors are controlled by the negative emotion, by the greed and the hatred. Most of the time, these behavior causes wounds, stress and make hurt to other people. They themselves are not only the victim of their lust and hatred but also they are the creators of the misery, problems, and diseases for their relatives and their society. Unfortunately, they rarely realize the situation to stop their lust and hatred.

The root of lust and hatred come from their ignorance. From the ignorance create a lot of the wrong delusions, and delusion makes them blind to the condition. The more ignorant people are, the better delusion makes them feel. Delusion blinds people's eyes, ears, tastes, thinking so that they do not have any concern about the misery they create for themselves and other people. Even worse, delusion makes people misunderstand that their wrong behaviors are good actions, the actions of justice. Their ignorance may delude them to make crucial actions, create destructive weapons, kill a hundred people, create extreme stress for others, destroy the environment and destroy human being without any hesitation. The history of the world was full of tragedies caused by ignorant people. The people with lust, hatred, and ignorance have conditioned with crucial responses by themselves or the condition of living.

We, the people of modern society still have the lust, hatred and ignorance; which may cause many diseases, problems and misery in the family and society.

How do we can stop making wrongs behaviors? By reducing the needs to the basic needs and noble needs; by controlling the emotion, controlling the anger as soon as possible; by destroying ignorance, removing delusion; step by step, we can reduce the misery in our society. With the poor, the disabled, the miserable people they have very few needs, few desires but they are still very miserable. The solution for them is keeping the basic needs, develop themselves to become strong and smart enough that they can create the wanted changes in the condition of living, which satisfy their basic needs. I will discuss how to overcome lust, hatred, and ignorance in the next sections.

These teaching of the old help us understand the characters of our potential mind. When we gain the right understanding, we will know how to master the mind and stay away from its traps.

Will human being be extinct or where they will go?

According to Buddha, all we suffer is from our hatred, anger, and ignorance.

According to Socrates, we suffer because we lost human virtues, natural virtues.

According to Benjamin Franklin, all our suffering comes from a lack of virtue, and from the discontent mind.

Please teach us to understand deeper, please show us the way, we will practice to save ourselves.

Chapter 55: The teaching of Lao Tzu, Aesop, and Socrates

Reading the teaching of Lao Tzu and Buddha, I know that great achievement and happiness comes from the action without expectation, action without condition, or unconditional love. Positive emotion, enthusiasm, energy belong to attitude, that why a positive attitude can be understood that taking action vigorously and selflessly without expectation. Positive people take little material but gain the most for the mind and brain. I want to brow the teaching of Lao Tzu to summarize some of the principles. His teachings are so profound that we can inherit to understand our stupid, to correct our mistakes. It is time to stop our ignorance; it is time to correct our mistakes. Only a few basics principles to follow to have a happy life, so that happiness comes from putting heart into actions that follow the moral and virtue, from understanding and acting; happiness does not come from knowing, studying and abundance living without taking action. People who master the science of achievement and success in career, but still violating the virtue, the principles in the art of happiness, also get stress in life.

Te Tao Ching

There is the effortless way in the teaching of the Lao Tzu from Te-Tao Ching, all he taught is the paradoxes of life. In history, some dictators may use the paradoxes and power of rhetoric to seduces people to commit the war. Owning for education, we know to understand these paradoxes and use it to mater life.

1. Tao and Primal Virtue:

All things arise from Tao.
They are nourished by Virtue.
They are formed from matter.
They are shaped by the environment
Thus the ten thousand things all respect Tao and honor Virtue.

Respect of Tao and honor of Virtue are not demanded,
But they are in the nature of things.
Therefore all things arise from Tao
By Virtue, they are nourished,
Developed, cared for,
Sheltered, comforted,
Grown, and protected.
Creating without claiming,
Doing without taking credit,
Guiding without interfering,
This is Primal Virtue.
Lao Tzu, Tao Te Ching

2. Rule a nation with justice.

Wage war with surprise moves.
Become a master of the universe without striving.
How do I know that this is so?
Because of:
The more laws and restrictions there are,
The poorer people become.
The sharper men's weapons,
The more trouble in the land.
The more ingenious and clever men are,
The more strange things happen.
The more rules and regulations,
The more thieves and robbers.
Therefore the sage says:
I take no action and people are reformed.
I enjoy peace and people become honest.
I do nothing and people become rich.
I have no desires and people return to the good and simple life.
Lao Tzu, Tao Te Ching

3. Practice non-action.

Work without doing.
Taste the tasteless.
Magnify the small, increase the few.
Reward bitterness with care.

Awaken you wonderful we

See simplicity in the complicated.
Achieve greatness in little things.
In the universe, the difficult things are done as if they are easy.
Great acts are made up of small deeds.
The sage does not attempt anything big,
And thus achieved greatness.
Easy promises make for little trust.
Taking things lightly results in great difficulty.
Because the sage always confronts difficulties,
He never experiences them.
Lao Tzu, Tao Te Ching

4. Peace is easily maintained;

Trouble is easily overcome before it starts.
The brittle is easily shattered;
The small is easily scattered.
Deal with it before it happens.
Set things in order before there is confusion.
A tree as great as a man's embrace springs up from a small shoot;
A terrace nine stories high begins with a pile of earth;
A journey of a thousand miles starts with one footstep.
He who acts defeats his own purpose;
Try to change it, ruin it.
Try to hold it, lose it.
The sage does not act, and so is not defeated.
He does not grasp and therefore does not lose.
People usually fail when they are on the verge of success.
So give as much care to the end as to the beginning;
Then there will be no failure.
Therefore, the sage seeks freedom from desire.
He does not collect precious things.
He learns not to hold on to ideas.
He brings men back to what they have lost.
He helps the ten thousand things find their own nature,
But refrains from action.

Lao Tzu, Tao Te Ching
5. The good

A good soldier is not violent.
A good fighter is not angry.
A good winner is not vengeful
A good employer is humble.
This is the Virtue of not striving.
This is the ability to deal with people.

Lao Tzu, Tao Te Ching
6. Paradoxes of more

Too many colors blind the eye.
Too many words deafen the ear.
Too many flavors dull the taste.
Racing and hunting madden the mind.
Precious things lead one astray.
Greed will destroy them.
I have three things to teach
Simplicity, patience, and compassion
Simplicity, patience, and compassion
These three are your greatest treasures.
Simple in actions and thoughts, you return to the source of being.
Patient with both friends and enemies,
You accord with the way things are.
Compassionate toward yourself,
You reconcile all beings in the world.

Lao Tzu, Tao Te Ching
7. Knowledge and humility

Knowing others is wisdom;
Knowing the self is enlightenment.
Mastering others is the strength;
Mastering yourself is true power.
He who knows he has enough is rich.
Perseverance is a sign of willpower.
He who stays where he is enduring.
To die but not to perish is to be eternally present.

Lao Tzu, Tao Te Ching

8. Ridiculous aimless

Stop thinking, and end your problems.
What difference between yes and no?
What difference between success and failure?
Must you value what others value,
Avoid what others avoid
Fight what others fight
Die what others die?
How ridiculous!
Other people are excited,
As though they were at a parade.
I alone don't care,
I alone am expressionless,
Like an infant before it can smile.
Other people have what they need;
I alone possess nothing. I alone drift about,
like someone without a home.
I am an idiot, my mind is so empty. Other people are bright;
I alone am dark.
Other people are sharp;
I alone am dull. Other people have the purpose;
I alone don't know.
I drift like a wave on the ocean,
I blow as aimless as the wind.
I am different from ordinary people.
I drink from the Great Mother's breasts.

Lao Tzu, Tao Te Ching

9. Embracing Tao, embracing love

Embracing Tao, you become embraced. Supple, breathing gently, you become reborn. Clearing your vision, you become clear. Nurturing your beloved, you become impartial. Opening your heart, you become accepted. Accepting the World, you embrace Tao. Bearing and nurturing, Creating but not owning, Giving demanding, Guiding without interfering, This is love.

Lao Tzu, Tao Te Ching

Awaken you wonderful we

10. Unknown primal

Close your mouth, block off your senses, blunt your sharpness, untie your knots, soften your glare, settle your dust. This is the primal identity.

Lao Tzu, Tao Te Ching

11. Desire and peace

When there is no desire, All things are at peace. Hope and fear are both phantoms
That arises from thinking of the self.
When we don't see the self as self,
What do we have to fear?

Lao Tzu, Tao Te Ching

12. Paradoxes of in and out, visible and invisible

True words aren't eloquent;
Eloquent words aren't true.
Wise men don't need to prove their point; Men who need to prove their point aren't wise.
The Master has no possessions.
The more he does for others, The happier he is.
The more he gives to others, The wealthier he is.

Lao Tzu, Tao Te Ching

13. Look inside the heart

My teachings are easy to understand
And easy to put into practice.
Yet your intellect will never grasp them,
And if you try to practice them, you'll fail.
My teachings are older than the world.
How can you grasp their meaning?
If you want to know me,
Look inside your heart.

Lao Tzu, Tao Te Ching

14. Aimless and purposeless

A good traveler has no fixed plans
And is not intent upon arriving.
A good artist lets his intuition

Lead him wherever it wants.
A good scientist has freed himself from concepts
And keeps his mind open to what is.
Thus the Master is available to all people
And doesn't reject anyone.
He is ready to use all situations
And doesn't waste anything.
This is called embodying the light.
What is a good man but a bad man's teacher?
What is a bad man but a good man's job?
If you don't understand this, you will get lost,
In grief and joy,
losing and gaining,
past and future.
However intelligent you are!
It is a great secret.
He who stands on tiptoe
Doesn't stand firm.
He who rushes ahead
Doesn't go far.
He who tries to shine
Dims his own light.

Lao Tzu, Tao Te Ching

15. Non-desire, unlearn, but Tao

He who defines himself
Can't know who he really is.
He who has power over others
Can't empower himself.
He who clings to his work
Will create nothing that endures.
If you want to accord with the Tao,
Just do your job, then let go.
Rushing into action, you fail.
Trying to grasp things, you lose them.
Forcing a project to completion,
You ruined what was almost ripe.
Therefore the Master takes action

Awaken you wonderful we

By letting things take their course.
He remains as calm at the end
As at the beginning.
He has nothing,
Thus has nothing to lose.
What he desires is non-desire;
What he learns is to unlearn.
He simply reminds people
Of who they have always been.
He cares about nothing but the Tao.
Thus he can care for all things.
Not-knowing is true knowledge.
Presuming to know is a disease.
First, realize that you are sick;
Then you can move toward health.
Lao Tzu, Tao Te Ching

16. What to improve, what to change?

Do you want to improve the world?
I don't think it can be done.
The world is sacred.
It can't be improved.
If you tamper with it, you'll ruin it.
If you treat it like an object, you'll lose it.
There is a time for being ahead,
A time for being behind;
A time for being in motion,
A time for being at rest;
A time for being vigorous,
A time for being exhausted;
A time for being safe,
A time for being in danger.
The Master sees things as they are,
without trying to control them.
She lets them go their own way,
And resides at the center of the circle.
A great nation is like a great man
When he makes a mistake, he realizes it.

Having realized it, he admits it.
Having admitted it, he corrects it.
He considers those who point out his faults
As his most benevolent teachers.
He thinks of his enemy
As the shadow that he himself casts.
Failure is an opportunity.
If you blame someone else,
There is no end to the blame.
Therefore the Master
Fulfill her own obligations
And corrects her own mistakes.
She does what she needs to do
And demands nothing of others.
Lao Tzu, Tao Te Ching

17. Paradoxes of true

True perfection seems imperfect,
Yet it is perfectly itself.
True fullness seems empty,
Yet it is fully present.
True straightness seems crooked.
True wisdom seems foolish.
True art seems artless.
Lao Tzu, Tao Te Ching

18. Learn from children

He who is in harmony with the Tao
Is like a newborn child.
Its bones are soft, its muscles are weak,
But its grip is powerful.
It can scream its head off all day,
Yet it never becomes hoarse,
So complete is its harmony.
The Master's power is like this.
He lets all things come and go
Effortlessly, without desire.
He never expects results;
Thus he is never disappointed.

He is never disappointed;
Thus his spirit never grows old.
Lao Tzu, Tao Te Ching

19. The gate of mystery

The Tao that can be told is not the eternal Tao.
The name that can be named is not the eternal name.
The nameless is the beginning of heaven and earth.
The named is the mother of ten thousand things.
Ever desireless, one can see the mystery.
Ever desiring, one can see the manifestations.
These two spring from the same source but differ in name;
this appears as darkness.
Darkness within darkness.
The gate to all mystery.
Without opening your door,
You can open your heart to the world.
Without looking out your window,
You can see the essence of the Tao.
The more you know,
The less you understand.
The Master arrives without leaving,
Sees the light without looking,
Achieves without doing a thing.
Lao Tzu, Tao Te Ching

20. Paradoxes are everywhere

Thus it is said:
The path into the light seems dark,
The path forward seems to go back,
The direct path seems long,
True power seems weak,
True purity seems tarnished,
True steadfastness seems changeable,
True clarity seems obscure,
The greatest is seems unsophisticated,
The greatest love seems indifferent,
The greatest wisdom seems childish.

Awaken you wonderful we

The Tao is nowhere to be found.
Yet it nourishes and completes all things.
Lao Tzu, Tao Te Ching

21. Intelligence versus enlightenment

Have done with learning,
And you will have no more vexation.
Intelligence versus enlightenment is
How great is the difference between eh and o?
What is the distinction between good and evil?
Must I fear what others fear?
What abysmal nonsense this is!
All men are joyous and beaming,
As though feasting upon a sacrificial ox,
As though mounting the Spring Terrace;
I alone am placid and give no sign,
Like a babe which has not yet smiled.
I alone am forlorn as one who has no home to return to.
All men have enough and to spare:
I alone appear to possess nothing.
What a fool I am!
What a muddled mind I have!
All men are bright, bright:
I alone am dim, dim.
All men are sharp, sharp:
I alone am a mum, mum!
Bland like the ocean,
Aimless like the wafting gale
All men settle down in their grooves:
I alone am stubborn and remain outside.
But wherein I am most different from others is
In knowing to take sustenance from my Mother!
Lao Tzu, Tao Te Ching

22. Out of sensory threshold

Look, and it can't be seen.
Listen, and it can't be heard.
Reach, and it can't be grasped
How intelligent men know the world?

Lao Tzu, Tao Te Ching

23. Balancing of a great way

The great Way is easy,
Yet people prefer the side paths.
Be aware when things are out of balance.
Simplicity without a name
Is free from all external aim.
With no desire, at rest and still,
All things go right as of their will.
So the un-wanting soul
Sees what's hidden, mysteriously
And the ever-wanting soul
Sees only what it wants, sensually

Lao Tzu, Tao Te Ching

24. Greatness Tao is from present to forgotten

When the greatness of Tao is present,
The action arises from one's own heart.
When the greatness of Tao is absent,
The action comes from the rules of kindness and justice.
If you need rules to be kind and just,
If you have to act virtuous,
This is a sure sign that virtue is absent.
The more lack of virtues, the more useless law, and rules created.
Chaos, destruction, fighting, diseases,
And extinction begins to flourish.
Dying and scarifying is honored
Values becoming upside down.
Countless efforts and ideas,
Intelligence and solutions turn to speed the extinction.
Or become useless because of the wrong roots.
Thus, we see the great hypocrisy.
Only when does the family lose its harmony
People soon do hear of dutiful sons.
Only when the state is in chaos do we hear of loyal ministers.

Awaken you wonderful we

Lao Tzu, Tao Te Ching
25. The master's way

The gentlest thing in the world
Overcomes the hardest thing in the world.
That which has no substance
Enters where there is no space.
This shows the value of non-action.
Teaching without words,
Performing without actions:
That is the Master's way.

Lao Tzu, Tao Te Ching
26. Great Tao is forgotten

When the great Tao is forgotten,
Goodness and piety appear.
When the body's intelligence declines,
Cleverness and knowledge step forth.
When there is no peace in the family,
Filial piety begins.
When the country falls into chaos,
Patriotism is born.

Lao Tzu, Tao Te Ching
27. Follow the Tao

If you want to become whole, let yourself be partial.
If you want to become straight, let yourself be crooked.
If you want to become full, let yourself be empty.
If you want to be reborn, let yourself die as go to sleep every evening.
If you want to be given everything, give everything up.

Lao Tzu, Tao Te Ching
28. Interdependent, inter-beings world

When people see some things as beautiful,
Other things become ugly.
When people see some things as good,
Other things become bad.
Being and non-being create each other.
Difficult and easy support each other.

Long and short define each other.
High and low depend on each other.
Before and after follow each other.

Lao Tzu, Tao Te Ching

29. The act of the master

Understanding the forming of forests
Nature and heavenly earth
Therefore the Master
Acts without doing anything
And teaches without saying anything.
Things arise and she lets them come;
Things disappear and she lets them go.
She has but doesn't possess,
Acts but doesn't expect.
When her work is done, she forgets it.
That is why it lasts forever.

Lao Tzu, Tao Te Ching

30. Bellows Tao

The Tao doesn't take sides;
It gives birth to both good and evil.
The Master doesn't take sides;
She welcomes both saints and sinners.
The Tao is like a bellows:
It is empty yet infinitely capable.
The more you use it, the more it produces;
The more you talk about it, the less you understand.

Lao Tzu, Tao Te Ching

31. In harmony with Tao

In harmony with the Tao,
The sky is clear and spacious,
The earth is solid and full,
All creatures flourish together,
Content with the way they are,
Endlessly repeating themselves,
Endlessly renewed.
When man interferes with the Tao

The sky becomes filthy,
The earth becomes depleted,
The equilibrium crumbles,
Creatures become extinct.
Whoever is planted in the Tao
Will not be rooted up.
Whoever embraces the Tao
Will not slip away.
Her name will be held in honor
From generation to generation.
Let the Tao be present in your life
And you will become genuine.
Let it be present in your family
And your family will flourish.
Let it be present in your country
And your country will be an example
To all countries in the world.
Let it be present in the universe
And the universe will sing.
How do I know this is true?
By looking inside myself.
Lao Tzu, Tao Te Ching

32. Paradoxes of Tao benefit enlightened ones

Intelligent ones say that my teaching is nonsense.
Other sage calls it lofty but impractical.
But to those who have looked inside themselves,
This nonsense makes perfect sense.
And to those who put it into practice,
This loftiness has roots that go deep
They are enlightened ones.
Lao Tzu, Tao Te Ching

Lao Tzu Quotes:

1. Art of living, Lao Tzu:"Manifest plainness, embrace simplicity, reduce selfishness, have few desires."

2. Bait, Lao Tzu: "Let him keep his mouth open, and spend his breath in the promotion of his affairs, and all his life there will be no safety for him."

3. Better few, Lao Tzu: "There are few in the world who attain to the teaching without words, and the advantage arising from non-action."

4. Changing world, Lao Tzu: "A violent wind does not last for a whole morning; a sudden rain does not last for the whole day."

5. Contentment, abundance, Lao Tzu: "Be content with what you have; rejoice in the way things are. When you realize there is nothing lacking, the whole world belongs to you."

6. Contentment, Lao Tzu: "The sufficiency of contentment is an enduring and unchanging sufficiency."

7. Contentment, Lao Tzu: "When you are content to be simply yourself and don't compare or compete, everyone will respect you."

8. Contentment, Lao Tzu: "When you are content to be simply yourself and don't compare or compete, everybody will respect you."

9. Courage, Lao Tzu: "A man with outward courage dares to die; a man with inner courage dares to live."

10. Disease of knowing, Lao Tzu: "To know and yet think we do not know is the highest attainment; not to know and yet think we do know is a disease."

11. Engagement, condition, and Tao, Lao Tzu: "She who has the attributes of the Tao regards only the conditions of the engagement, while he who has not those attributes of the Tao regards only the conditions favorable to himself."

12. Excellence water, Lao Tzu: "The excellence of water appears in its benefiting all things, and in its occupying, without striving to the contrary, the low place which all men dislike."

13. Getting and losing, Lao Tzu: "The getting that favor leads to losing it because of the apprehension, and the losing it leads to the fear of greater calamity: this is what is meant by saying that favor and disgrace would seem to be feared."

14. Give and take, Lao Tzu: "The heart that gives, gathers."

15. Giving or trading, Lao Tzu: "If we could renounce our benevolence and discard our righteousness, the people would again become filial and kindly."

16. Good for people, Lao Tzu: "If we could renounce our sageness and discard our wisdom, it would be better for the people a hundredfold."

17. Humble and great, Lao Tzu: "A skillful soldier is not violent, an able fighter does not rage, a mighty conqueror does not give battle, a great commander is a humble man. Humble means no desire, no anger and still in mind with understanding."

18. Illusive luxury, Lao Tzu: "When things in the vegetable world have displayed their luxuriant growth, we see each of them return to its root."

19. Impermanent, Lao Tzu: "If you realize that all things change, there is nothing you will try to hold on to."

20. Intelligence and virtues, Lao Tzu: "All difficult things in the world are sure to arise from a previous state in which they were easy, and all great things from one in which they were small. So what is the difference between productivity and effectiveness? What is the difference between intelligence and virtues?"

21. Know to stop, Lao Tzu: "If you keep sharpening a point that has been sharpened, the point cannot long preserve its sharpness."

22. Knowledge, wisdom and enlightenment, Lao Tzu: "Ordinary man hates solitude but likes studying and accumulating knowledge, striving he may gain knowledge and wisdom. But the Master makes use of it, embracing his aloneness, realizing he is

one with the whole universe, effortless he may gain enlightenment."

23. Love, the golden rule, Lao Tzu: "Therefore he who would administer the kingdom, honoring it as he honors his own person, may be employed to govern it. And he who would administer it with the love which he bears to his own person may be entrusted with it."

24. Nature of things, Lao Tzu: "Let movement go on, and the condition of rest will gradually arise."

25. Non-desire, Lao Tzu: "With no desire, at rest and still, All things go right as of their will."

26. The paradox of more, Lao Tzu: "Too much brightness blinds the eyes. Too much sound deafens the ears. Too much flavor ruins the tongue. Chasing desires to excess turns your mind towards madness and valuing precious things impairs good judgment."

27. Paradox, Lao Tzu: "So it is that some things are increased by being diminished, and others are diminished by being increased."

28. Patience, Lao Tzu: "Trying to understand is like straining through muddy water. Have the patience to wait! Be still and allow the mud to settle."

29. Peace, Lao Tzu: "Be simply yourself and don't compare or compete. You will find peace."

30. Powerful love, Lao Tzu: "Love is of all passions the strongest, for it attacks simultaneously the head, the heart and the senses."

31. Rich and satisfaction, Lao Tzu: "From self-complacency, and therefore he acquires superiority. He who is satisfied with his lot is rich; therefore, the sage seeks to satisfy the craving of the belly, and not the insatiable longing of the eyes."

32. Safety and inner peace, Lao Tzu: "To find safety and inner peace: the first is gentleness; the second is economy; and the third is shrinking from taking precedence of others."

33. Showing, desiring and safety, Lao Tzu: "Not to show them what is likely to excite their desires is the way to keep their minds from disorder. When gold and jade fill the hall, their possessor cannot keep them safe."

34. Stillness, Lao Tzu: "Stillness is the ruler of movement."

35. Subtle, wonder, Lao Tzu: "Where the mystery, is the deepest, is the gate of all that is subtle and wonderful."

36. Supreme water, Lao Tzu: "The supreme good is like water, which nourishes all things without trying to. It is content with the low places that people disdain. Thus, it is like the Tao. In dwelling, live close to the ground. In thinking, keep to the simple. In conflict, be fair and generous. In governing, do not try to control. In work, do what you enjoy. In family life, be completely present. When you are content to be simply yourself and don't compare or compete, everybody will respect you."

37. The Tao's way, Lao Tzu: "To bear and not to own; to act and not lay claim; to do the work and let it go: for just letting it go is what makes it stay."

38. To know, Lao Tzu: "To avoid disappointment, know what is sufficient. To avoid trouble, know when to stop. If you are able to do this, you will last a long time."

39. Virtue, disorder, Lao Tzu: "When virtue is lost, benevolence appears, when benevolence is lost right conduct appears, when right conduct is lost, expedience appears. Expediency is the mere shadow of right and truth; it is the beginning of disorder."

The teaching of Aesop

1. Gratitude is the sign of noble souls.

2. We would often be sorry if our wishes were gratified.

3. He that is discontented in one place will seldom be happy in another.

4. The smaller the mind the greater the conceit.

The teaching of Socrates

1. True wisdom comes to each of us when we realize how little we understand about life, ourselves, and the world.

2. Wisdom begins in wonder.

3. I know that I am intelligent because I know that I know nothing.

4. I am the wisest man alive, for I know one thing, and that is that I know nothing.

5. He is richest who is content with the least, for content is the wealth of nature.

Happiness comes from the virtues, happiness does not come from intelligence. Until you master the paradoxes of life, you will get real happiness, real wealth and real health. How do you understand the paradoxes? By curiosity and endless questioning, by removing the known things and all assumptions, opening to a new view, new possibilities, using heart, mind and gut feeling, you will soon master the paradoxes.

Ho'oponopono techniques and the combination to calm the mind

For fear and negative emotion, thinking, read this 5 times, and then staring as high as possible at a point on ceilings or sky, keep that for 10 seconds (count from one to ten) then slowly relax and close the eyes and read several times:

I love you
I am sorry
Please forgive me

> Thank you!
> **When needed, just staring the eyes for 10 seconds or just relex and read the phrase several times.**

Chapter 56: Teaching of Benjamin Franklin

1. A house is not a home unless it contains food and fire for the mind as well as the body.

2. Content makes poor men rich; discontent makes rich men poor.

3. Energy and persistence conquer all things.

4. If a man could have half of his wishes, he would double his troubles.

5. If you would be loved, love, and be loveable.

6. It is easier to prevent bad habits than to break them.

7. It is the eye of other people that ruin us. If I were blind I would want, neither fine clothes, nor fine houses, nor fine furniture.

8. It is the working man who is the happy man. It is the idle man who is a miserable man.

9. It would be a good blessing for the staffs if their leaders and manager follow the virtues.

10. Many a man thinks he is buying pleasure when he is really selling himself to it.

11. The discontented man finds no easy chair.

12. The doorstep to the temple of wisdom is a knowledge of our own ignorance.

13. The worst wheel of the cart makes the most noise.

14. There are two ways of being happy: We must either diminish our wants or augment our means - either may do - the result is the same and it is for each man to decide for himself and to do that which happens to be easier.

15. Who is wise? He who learns from everyone. Who is powerful? He that governs his passions. Who is rich? He that is content. Who is that? Nobody.

Thirteen virtues

During childhood, Benjamin Franklin was an ordinary boy with a lot of problems. Failure and pressures had taught him a lot of lessons about people and the importance of virtues. He had trained himself with thirteen virtues, In 1726, at the age of 20, Benjamin Franklin created a system to develop his character. In his autobiography, his thirteen virtues as:

1. Temperance. Eat not to dullness; drink not to elevation

2. Silence. Speak not but what may benefit others or yourself; avoid trifling conversation.

3. Order. Let all your things have their places; let each part of your business have its time.

4. Resolution. Resolve to perform what you ought; perform without fail what you resolve.

5. Frugality. Make no expense but to do good to others or yourself, waste nothing.

6. Industry. Lose no time; be always employ in something useful; cut off all unnecessary actions.

7. Sincerity. Use no hurtful deceit; think innocently and justly, and, if you speak, speak accordingly.

8. Justice. Wrong none by doing injuries, or omitting the benefits that are your duty.

9. Moderation. Avoid extremes; forbear resenting injuries so much as you think they deserve.

10. Cleanliness. Tolerate no uncleanliness in body, clothes, or habitation.

11. Tranquility. Be not disturbed at trifles, or at accidents common or unavoidable.

12. Chastity. Rarely use venery but for health or offspring, never to dullness, weakness, or the injury of your own or another's peace or reputation.

13. Humility. Imitate Jesus and Socrates.

These thirteen virtues had guided his daily life. Benjamin Franklin was an ordinary man but with noble purposes, selfless actions and guided with virtues.

To find your own happiness, I highly recommend the reader form their own virtues and principle to guide the mind and behaviors every day. Readers can practice one virtue a week, at the end of the day they can check what they do right with the virtues and what will they do differently. Readers will be astonished by the achievement with the guiding of virtues. It would be a good bless for million people if their leaders follow the virtues.

Understanding the vital role of the state of mind, it would be a great bless for you, your mind, your health, your longevity, and your brain if you follow the virtues. You will not see but you will feel the accumulation of small changes insides. Your mind will feel the safety, importance, significant, love, connection, growth, and contribution owning for the virtues. Your potential mind will be in a good state to serve you.

Chapter 57: Educators taught about the miracle of mind, principles, and lifelong learning

The United States Constitution

The United States Constitution is the document has the most influence on the development of the United States. There are six basic principles of government to govern the government and the acts of government in the most effective way. Before any crisis or adjustment in-laws, politicians have to look up the principles and instruction of the Constitution. The principles in the constitution also help to prevent the dictators and corrupt men who want to borrow the power of countries, an organization to make private profits. American may perish if they violate the universal principles in the constitution. Any organizations will also develop if they follow the universal principles of the constitution.

Six basic principles of government are

Firstly, Popular Sovereignty: Popular Sovereignty is defined as "a doctrine in political theory that government is created by and subject to the will of the people." This simply means that the citizens of the country are in charge of the government and how it is run. People are allowed to vote for who represents them in a government position. Then the person who was elected represents the people of their area and their opinions.

Secondly, the Limited Government defines how much power the government can have, which is decided on how much the people give them. This is why people vote on how much taxes are, people decide how much money the government can take from them. All problems are decided by a majority of the population.

Thirdly, Separation of Powers: the separation of powers allows the government to be separated into different groups. This allows them all to focus on one job only. This also makes it so one group not to have all the power. They are separated into the Legislative, Executive and Judicial. The Legislative is in charge of making laws; the executive is in charge of enforcing the laws; the judge decides on the punishments for those who break the law.

Fourthly, Checks and Balances: the system of checks and balances was designed to keep one branch of the government from getting to much power. If one branch has more than the other groups, the others either help to decrease the powers of that group or build themselves up so they are on the same level.

Fifthly, Judicial Review: Judicial review allows the Judicial Branch to decide on punishments that government officials deserve. If the President broke the law the Judicial review allows for a court to decide what consequences the president deserves to have. No government official is above the law of the citizens.

Sixthly, Federalism: Federalism is the idea of splitting political power between a large group and smaller groups. In the case of the United States, there is state government and a national (or federal) government. The state government is in charge of a small portion of people who live in their state, and the national government controls everyone who lives in the nation.

Organizations, companies, families, and joint stock companies should follow these principles for sustainable development.

The teaching of Stephen Covey: seven habits of highly effective people

Seven habits of highly successful people of Stephen Covey help people from dependence to independence to interdependence. The best way to gain success is following the principles.

First Independence

The First Three Habits surround moving from dependence to independence

1 - Be Proactive

Talks about the concept of Circle of Influence and Circle of Concern, work from the center of your influence and constantly work to expand it. Habit one: you are the programmer! Grow and stay humble.

2 - Begin with the End in Mind

Envision what you want in the future so you can work and plan towards it. Understand how people make decisions in their life. To be effective you need to act based on principles, important things and constantly review your mission statement. Habit two says: you are the programmer.

3 - Put First Things First

What is important and what is urgent? Priority should be given in the following order: Important and urgent; important and not urgent; not important and urgent; not important and not urgent.

Habit three says: write your program. Keep personal integrity: what you say to fit what you do.

Interdependence

The next three habits talk about Interdependence or working with others.

4 - Think Win-Win

Genuine feelings for mutually beneficial solutions or agreements in your relationships, value and respect people by understanding a "win" for all is ultimately a better long-term resolution than if only one person in the situation had gotten his way.

Think Win-Win isn't about being nice, nor is it a quick-fix technique. It is a character-based code for human interaction and collaboration. Do you like to lose in any relationship or any contracts? If no, other people want the same things as you. The best solution to strengthen the relationship is the win-win solution.

5 - Seek First to Understand, Then to be Understood

Use empathic listening to genuinely understand a person, which compels them to reciprocate the listening and take an open mind to be influenced by you. This creates an atmosphere of caring, and positive problem-solving. Gradually, it will build trust and the feeling of safety in people.

The order is important: ethos, pathos, logos - your character, and your relationships, and then the logic of your presentation.

6 - Synergize

Combine the strengths of people through positive teamwork, so as to achieve goals that no one could have done alone.

7 - Sharpen the Saw

The final habit is that of continuous improvements in both the personal and interpersonal spheres of influence.

Balance and renew your resources, energy, and health to create a sustainable, long-term, effective lifestyle. It primarily emphasizes exercise for physical renewal, good prayer: meditation, yoga, etc.; and good reading for mental renewal. It also mentions service to society for spiritual renewal.

Continuous improvements or lifelong learning create "Upward spiral". The Upward Spiral model consists of three parts: learn, commit, and do. Each set of three parts upgrade people to a new level. According to Covey, one must be increasingly educating the conscience in order to grow and develop on the upward spiral. The idea of renewal by education will propel one along the path of personal freedom, security, wisdom, and power.

Earl Nightingale: teaching the thinking

The strangest secret of Earl Nightingale: "You will become what you think about most of the time."

Formal education failed at teaching students to have "Actual Thought." If people think well in their life, they can gain massive progress in almost every aspect of life. Sharpen the mind means to sharpen the thinking. Mr. Nightingale suggested that put aside just an hour a day for thinking. Sit down with a cup of coffee or tea and a sheet of paper and just write down the thoughts. The opportunity to write down things thought of that could make life better and more efficient. In all years of schooling, no teacher had ever asked to do that. Following his advice, thinking becomes better substantially.

Brainstorming for a paper: "don't worry about other stuff right now, just think about yourself, your future, your problems, your solutions and jot it down no matter how ridiculous answers are." The results were incredible.

One hour a day of thinking with a piece of paper: write down the problem or the question on the top of the paper then brainstorm to write at least 20 to 30 answers for your problems. One week you will have at least one hundred answers for your problems. You will find that some of the answers you have are the invaluable answers that you may never think of. The more you do, the better your answer is.

After mastering the brainstorming for the good answers, you can sit with other people to have better solutions to the problems you have. When people participate to give the answers, they will engage in the activities.

Some examples:

- Sit down with your wife/husband/partner/boyfriend or girlfriend and think about how you can make the relationship better, stronger or just plain more fun.

- Sit down, talk with your child and ask him to think about how you can be a better parent to them and how they can be a better kid to you. Just writing the solution and make no judgment.

- Do some thinking with members of your family: spouse, brothers, and sisters.

- Try to hammer out some thoughts with a co-worker or even with your boss when you do that, your organization will become the ideas machines.

Brainstorm needs letting go, forget ego. Participants need to have a feeling of safety, motivation, and inspiration. People only get the best from the creativities when the creativities satisfied their need for safety and other basic needs.

After brainstorming, pick up just one good idea - easy to do and bring the most effectiveness - to carry it out. You will be astonished by the results you get after months or years of doing this. You can jot down the answers or ideas on your notebook every time you meet. After a thousand hours of thinking, you may become the master of thinking.

Jim Rohn's quotes: twenty of his greatest life-changing thoughts and personal development

1. "Don't wish it was easier, wish you were better. Don't wish for fewer problems, wish for more skills. Don't wish for fewer challenges, wish for more wisdom."

2. "How sad to see a father with money and no joy. The man studied economics, but never studied happiness."

3. "Days are expensive. When you spend a day you have one less day to spend. So make sure you spend each one wisely."

4. "Discipline is the bridge between goals and accomplishment."

5. "Failure is not a single, cataclysmic event. You don't fail overnight. Instead, failure is a few errors in judgment, repeated every day."

6. "If you don't design your own life plan, chances are you'll fall into someone else's plan. And guess what they have planned for you? Not much."

7. "The worst thing one can do is not to try, to be aware of what one wants and not give in to it, to spend years in silent hurt wondering if something could have materialized - never knowing."

8. "Motivation is what gets you started. Habit is what keeps you going."

9. "You must take personal responsibility. You cannot change the circumstances, the seasons, or the wind, but you can change yourself. That is something you have charge of."

10. "Learn how to be happy with what you have while you pursue all that you want."

11. "You are the average of the five people you spend the most time with."

12. "Take care of your body. It's the only place you have to live."

13. "The walls we build around us to keep sadness out also keeps out the joy."

14. "Asking is the beginning of receiving. I ask for all kinds of things. Make sure you don't go to the ocean with a teaspoon. At least take a bucket so the kids won't laugh at you."

15. "Get around people who have something of value to share with you. Their impact will continue to have a significant effect on your life long after they have departed."

16. "Formal education will make you a living; self-education will make you a fortune."

17. "Make rest a necessity, not an objective. Only rest long enough to gather strength."

18. "Effective communication is 20% what you know and 80% how you feel about what you know."

19. "No one else 'makes us angry.' We make ourselves angry when we surrender control of our attitude."

20. "You must either modify your dreams or magnify your skills."

Chapter 58: Teaching of Dalai Lama

1. "A lack of transparency results in distrust and a deep sense of insecurity."

2. "All major religious traditions carry basically the same message; that is love, compassion and forgiveness the important thing is they should be part of our daily lives."

3. "All religions try to benefit people, with the same basic message of the need for love and compassion, for justice and honesty, for contentment."

4. "Appearance is something absolute, but the reality is not that way - everything is interdependent, not absolute. The new view is very helpful to maintain a peace of mind because the main destroyer of a peaceful mind is anger."

5. "As a human being, anger is a part of our mind. Irritation also part of our mind. But you can do - anger comes then goes. Never keep in your sort of your inner world then create a lot of suspicions, a lot of distrust, a lot of negative things, more worry."

6. "Be kind whenever possible. It is always possible."

7. "Because of lack of moral principle, human life becomes worthless. Moral principle, truthfulness, is a key factor. If we lose that, then there is no future."

8. "Calm mind brings inner strength and self-confidence, so that's very important for good health."

9. "Death means to change our clothes. Clothes become old, then time to come change. So this body becomes old, and then the time comes, take the young body."

10. "Disagreement is something normal."

11. "Even an animal, if you show genuine affection, gradually trust develops. If you always showing bad face and beating, how can you develop a friendship?"

12. "Even when a person has all of life's comforts - good food, good shelter, a companion - he or she can still become unhappy when encountering a tragic situation."

13. "Even when we have physical hardships, we can be very happy."

14. "Happiness is not something ready-made. It comes from your own actions."

15. "Home is where you feel at home and are treated well."

16. "I always believe the rule by king or official leader is outdated. Now we must catch up with the modern world."

17. "I am just one human being."

18. "I find hope in the darkest of days, and focus on the brightest. I do not judge the universe."

19. "I have always had this view about the modern education system: we pay attention to brain development, but the development of warm-heartedness we take for granted."

20. "If some people have the belief or view that the Dalai Lama has some miracle power, that's total nonsense."

21. "If you can, help others; if you cannot do that, at least do not harm them."

22. "If you have a particular faith or religion; that is good. But you can survive without it."

23. "If you want others to be happy, practice compassion. If you want to be happy, practice compassion."

24. "In order to carry a positive action, we must develop here a positive vision."

25. "In the practice of tolerance, one's enemy is the best teacher."

26. "It is necessary to help others, not only in our prayers but in our daily lives. If we find we cannot help others, the least we can do is to desist from harming them."

27. "It is very important to generate a good attitude, a good heart, as much as possible. From this, happiness in both the short term and the long term for both yourself and others will come."

28. "Logically, harmony must come from the heart. Harmony very much based on trust. As soon as use force creates fear. Fear and trust cannot go together."

29. "Look at situations from all angles, and you will become more open."

30. "Love and compassion are necessities, not luxuries. Without them, humanity cannot survive."

31. "More compassionate mind, more sense of concern for other's well-being, is the source of happiness."

32. "My faith helps me overcome such negative emotions and find my equilibrium."

33. "When you practice gratefulness, there is a sense of respect toward others."

34. "Where ignorance is our master, there is no possibility of real peace."

35. "Whether one believes in a religion or not, and whether one believes in rebirth or not, there isn't anyone who doesn't appreciate kindness and compassion."

36. "Whether you call it Buddhism or another religion, self-discipline, that's important, self-discipline with awareness of consequences."

37. "The world belongs to humanity, not this leader, that leader or that king or prince or religious leader. The world belongs to humanity."

Chapter 59: Teaching of educators about education

Do you want to have parents, partners, teachers, and managers have good characters of successful people? The characters are not only humbleness, humor, patience, encouraging, kindness, respectfulness, enthusiastic, positive attitude, smile, and open-mindedness. But Characters also need good traits: major in major things, minor in minor things, guide without interference, learn from their people, engage in people, high expectations about your potential, provide warm and safe environment, allow mistakes as lessons, focus on why then trust in your creative in what and how, understand the different styles of people, let others shine, little or no greed and anger, and lifelong improvement.

For a long time, people misunderstand the concept of characters or a good attitude. The best understanding of the attitude and characters are the conditioned responses of the people. Before each event or situation happened to people, their pattern of thinking in the mind will create countless changes as responses; these responses will suit the term in the index of characters and attitude. If people have the negative attitude or negative characters before any events happen to them, they will have negative responses in their body: thinking, chemicals, changes, and behaviors in brain and body; unfortunately, they suffer the most of their negative attitude. Countless unwanted events and tragedy put on the positive people, they understand that they cannot change the event but they have the abilities to control and correct the responses inside their mind, brain, and body to fit with their values and visions despite how worst the tragedy. The compound of countless responses will determine the destiny of people measured in health, wealth, state of mind and surrounding people's lives. Men with strong characters and positive attitude benefit the most from life.

Revising the formal education from the educators

How men turn wild, enthusiastic, funny, flexible, energetic, curious, imaginative, and humorous children into rigid educated ones?

Watching movies, we will understand better the law of cause and effect. One year of real life is compressed into several minutes in movies; one life of the individual is reduced to one hour of watching. Watching movies, I realize that the students, staffs, soldiers or brothers who are mistreated one time will become the powerful people in the next time. Crucially punished young boys will become the soldiers or generals in ten or twenty years later. The young children with scars because of the punishment in nursery school will become the officers, managers or presidents of the countries.

They have changed, abusers have died but the events happened to them still available and constant in energy in the world that other people do not know. But the deep emotion, fear, and frightfulness still embed into mind, body, genes and thinking as self-talk of the victims. All of these invisible things will have affection for the attitude and characters of people. What the world will be if they meet enough phenomena and become intelligent men in power positions. Understanding life will make us more careful in treating other people whoever they are.

In the power positions, what is most important in the world between their characters or their intelligence?

All the process of formal education, all the tests, all examine, all the recruitment policies, and all the paper tests in the world mainly judge students and candidates by their intelligence? What will happen to the human world if we still mistreat the young, misjudge the young, and make countless mistakes in recruitment, rewards and punishment, and promotion? The most painful and tricky men know all the defects of our temporary systems, and they will defeat the good ones in taking the power positions. The greed, anger, pain, and indifferent mind will push them overcomes countless pain and suffering to get the position.

According to statisticians, some of the possibilities may happen:

- Corrupt men become the president and generals of powerful countries. They like the game of thrones, rewards and punishment, the art of seducing the mind, and art of killing. Will the world have world war III?

- the Greedy man is mixing an expensive chemical to make the solution for a batch of intravenous infusion medicine to distribute over the world. He is angry because his boss has just shouted at him. He also needs some money for his purposes, he now the way to fob a small part of the chemical to take $ 1000 that no one knows. If he fobs the expensive chemical, how much will the company and world lose? Ten million dollar, ten lives, or collapse of a giant company, no one will know exactly, it depends on how late they discover the corrupt act. Massive loses will take place if he tries to hide a screw in the engine of an airplane, or a screw in the engine of the spaceship or he manages the database of clients of a big bank of America.

- A man now takes the responsibility of operating nuclear power, or a nuclear bomb to keep the peace of the world. He was a good man when taking the responsibility but countless unwanted phenomena happened to him make him make relives all his pain and suffering, gradually he become a hurtful, greedy and angry man. Will the world in peaceful?

- How about the greedy, angry man work as a philosopher, will the world live in peace; will the next generations live in happiness?

Understand the importance of characters, and state of mind, many successful organizations try all to recruit good staffs and create the joyful, challenging, inspiring and supporting environment, for the staffs in a good state of mind to make the creative contribution for the organizations. Unfortunately, there are only a few organizations and families like this. There are still millions of families, schools, organizations, and governments are too stubborn to the old paradigms of treating with people. They do not know that the immeasurable influence of an ordinary man can make to the whole world because of the giant leaps in technologies. This is the time of mind, inspiration, art, and characters; it is no more the time of muscles, seducing, manipulating and threatening with rewards and punishment anymore. It is time for all people in the world to forget the old paradigm of education and adopting the new ones. Education should forget remembering, repetition, and useless examinations, certifications and degree orientation. Education should shift to nourish the good characters as great men have, serving heart, selfless purposes, abilities of thinking, problem-solving, the abilities of mastering mind, emotion, and lifelong learning to gain pearls of wisdom and enlightenment. The study should no longer boring, watching, dictating and suffering but the study has to become the process with exciting, engaging, thinking and enjoying. Observe the thinking, feeling and behaving of children and society before and after school, school seasons we will under the qualities of education.

Do you think what is most important for a leader in a powerful position? Especially in leading people to overcome disasters with the death of children?

What is the most important for a therapist to reduce the anxiety of a patient, to cure the stress of a schoolgirl or to treat hysteria of a group? Do you think ill people like intelligence with vague words, statistic, meaningless words or kind heart, warm brace, silently listening, warm hugs, and kind words from a peaceful mind?

What about teaching and playing with children? What do you think kids want from the teachers? Does formal education equip competent people for society?

How about parents, what do you think children need the most when they are in crisis? Do you think children with a fearful fragile heart like scouting, screaming about parents' miseries, pointing the mistake, beating for a lesson, or teaching with meaningless words? Or do you think a fearful fragile soul need love, connection, significance and support from their parents by listening, understanding, kissing, warm hugs, touching hand and shoulders, inspiring and trusting them to solve their problems? What are the most important things children want from parents when they meet the crisis?

Do you think that the children want the feeling of safety, motivating, and inspiring when they naked in their parents? Or they have to use most of their energy and mind to make covers for all their mistakes, all their pains, hurts to stay strongly and safely with their parents. Sadly, with the stressed children and stressed people, home is not home to mind and heart, home with them is the only home with food and place for the body. In the home, their mind and body have to stretch out to find safety and significance when they stay. In other words, the home may become another battlefield for heart and mind; they even have to pretend to hide their strong needs of love, significance, connection with their beloved ones. Over time, it is the lacking of positive attitude, virtues, and characters of people make others feel stress and the victim of stress diseases.

Going to school with the hope of finding the solution to their problems, the more they find, the more they get stuck with their problems. They may get hundreds of science books with countless facts, and hundred complicated answers that cannot solve their problems. Even worse, the culture of competing, showing, boasting of the intelligent mind makes hurt to the fragile but kind mind. Some parents said they do not know any strange in the behaviors of their suicidal child.

They will never see, even they think they are smart that the education equips for them. Smart does not help them see and feel the stress that their child has, they have to use the heart, to feel, to sense the nonverbal signals, and they have to listen to their gut feelings that are there something wrong there.

Stress does not care about social status, economic, houses, luxury possession. Stress happens to all who have the living style that lack of love from parents, relatives, and diverse nature; lack of connection with parents, relatives, and diverse environment. Lacking love and connection leads them to lack of abilities to deal with problems they have. They will become more and more stressed. The quality of love, connection, support, compassion, motivation, and inspiration comes from the kind loving heart; all are the products of belong characters. Intelligence and tricks do not build trust and peace of mind but characters and the kind heart does. Especially, in the specialized modern world, the need for characters of individuals becomes the most important factors to judge individuals.

Living with kind spouse, the partners and children feel so much safe and happy that they can put off all the masks and tool to sleep peacefully in naked because of trust and safety established. Whatever happened, characters and trust make them feel safe to focus to solve problems.

However, abundant living with a greedy and angry spouse the partner and children never find safe and happy that they have to wear a lot of masks to cover the weakness and faults. They have to use reasons to find an agreement to find safety. Sadly for them, they live, eat, sleep in abundance but in stressed mind. Constantly in the stress state, the level of constant preparation in their body to cope with the situation they have at home may be at the same level of stress of a wild animal chasing by a lion. Some have to find the medication and drugs to relieve their stress. Things are even worse with the greedy and angry partner's health.

Philosophy of the brain is seen as the software with the computer. The computer world has changed unimaginably in capacity and power. Memory cards have changed substantially, from floppy disk to 128 Mb memory card in 2007, and 128 Gb memory card in 2017. To catch with the changing world, after launching products, technology companies have to remove all their old knowledge and start to think differently to create new products. The life cycle of knowledge in the technology world is reducing substantially. To succeed in life we have to accept changing the mindset or old concepts of the world, possibilities, and impossibilities to adapt to the changing world. We cannot measure the capacity of the brain, but if observe closely the product of the brain, the capacity of our brain has developed far more than the development of the technology world. Can you imagine that the powerful computers of 2017 have to run by the operating systems of MS-DOS, or Windows 95, or Windows 98, or Windows Server 2003, or Window Vista, or Windows XP and run the Microsoft Office 2000, or Microsoft 2003 to create a document? How much power, resources, and potentialities will people lose if they use the old software for a new computer?

Unfortunately, the teachers and formal education still use the mindset, concepts of hundreds of years ago to teach modern children. How much have brain potential, resources, and energy of humankind lost because of the wrong way of education? Education is forming children and citizens. All the facts, events, problems, diseases, and natural disasters that human beings have been suffering have relation with education and hidden philosophy. We are nothing special; we are only the visible illumination of the hidden world. To change the world, to correct the problems, the most effective way is to start from the invisible world, and use warm heart, love, and kindness to sense the characters of children then educate them.

Because of the wrong mindsets and wrong philosophy in education, the countless effort becomes useless. How useless the meetings, seminars, and conference for correcting and revolutionizing the educations by correcting what to teach and how to teach when they never correcting and revolutionizing the old teachers and old administers. It will be great for children, students, and society if formal education changes the mindset of teachers to focus on:

- Focus on students, the needs of students and satisfy these needs.

- Focus on the cooperation of students and teachers instead of competition.

- Focus on why we should teach instead of what to teach.

- Focus on the characters, imagination, and curiosity of students instead of abilities to remember and citing.

- Focus on leadership characters.

- Focus on the seven habits of highly successful people described by Stephen Covey.

- And focus on interesting in studying, joyful in studying, happiness in studying, satisfying individuals' needs in schooling.

School should become inspiring, energetic, humorous, and safe places for all people to come. To do these, the school should study the teaching methods of some training programs where people may pay the fee equal the fee of half-year studying in college just for five-day-course of training. In one training, thousands of people jumping, repeating, singing, dancing, smiling, thinking, doing exercises, planning, visualizing, asking themselves the most important questions, shouting, screaming, hand-shaking, embracing, hugging, crying, bursting into tears in the programs, they may be awakened. No one want to skip just one hour of training, they have to trade a lot of precious things to have time and money for just a several-day course. And best of all they may change from inside, the changes are powerful enough that one to five years after the training they are still discipline to study, work and taking actions to create the changes they want. Astonishingly, the participants are successful men and women in the organization and society. Before participating, they all set up the goals and purposes of the study.

Studying does not mainly come from formal education as most people think. Children are formed the most by their families. Families have the biggest influence on the development of children. My teacher said, if the mother goes to study extra skill and knowledge, three generations of the family will benefit from studying the husband, the children an, the grandchildren. People are wrong to think the mother does not help them anything in solving problems because they do not know that understanding makes the mother has the right act, call, talk, stay away, support, silence and guide on time is the different factors of the generations.

If we want to change, we have to give to create changes. If we want to have a good life at present and in the future, we have to treat others, kids, and children well. The quality of our behaviors at present will determine the state of mind, the quality of our lives at present and in the future. Do not wait then blame others to make it. I want to borrow the teachings of the educators to make all people have the right understanding of education. Hoping that all people in society and the world awake about their vital roles to give hands to education.

By formal education with the techniques of conditioning, the mind with wrong rewards and punishments, the teachers and formal education have traded all the treasures of the children into the rubbishy knowledge of yes or no, right or wrong. What expensive trading! Does wrong formal education only affect the children or the youth? No, it does not. In fact, it affects the whole generation, the whole society, and the whole world. It is time for all teachers, educators, meditation practitioners, artists, philosophers, leaders, and politicians to think about the wrong of education and the way to fix it to save all, our children, and our world.

To find the answer for our problems, brainstorm to find the answer, ask the right person to find the answer, read the right book to find the answer, and ask the right person to have the answer. Best of all, find the instructions of successful people via their quotes.

Below are the invaluable suggestions of educators.

1. A child has the character of God: "When I approach a child, he inspires in me two sentiments; tenderness for what he is, and respect for what he may become. **Louis Pasteur**

2. The aim of education: equip self-education: "Self-education is, I firmly believe, the only kind of education there is." **Isaac Asimov**

3. All people on earth grew from ignorant children: "A child's life is like a piece of paper on which every person leaves a mark." **Chinese Proverb**

4. Art of knowing and acting is more important than remembering and IQ: "An education isn't how much you have committed to memory, or even how much you know. It's being able to differentiate between what you do know and what you don't. It's knowing where to go to find out what you need to know, and it's knowing how to use the information you get." **William Feather**

5. Art of teaching for parents and teachers: "True teaching is one that not teaches knowledge but stimulates children to gain it." **Jill Eggleton**

6. Art of teaching: "Teachers should guide without dictating, and participate without dominating" **C. B. Neblette**

7. The atrocity of former education: "The biggest atrocity of all is to indoctrinate our children into a system that does not value their creative expression, nor encourage their unique abilities." **Benjamin Greene**

8. Awaken schooling wonderful society: "Schooling confuses teaching with learning, grade advancement with education, a diploma with competence, and fluency with the ability to say something new." **Wendy Priesnitz**

9. Awakening education: "The supreme end of education is expert discernment in all things--the power to tell the good from the bad, the genuine from the counterfeit, and to prefer the good and the genuine to the bad and the counterfeit." **Samuel Johnson**

10. Back to why and purposes, trainers and educators, parents and teachers: "Training teaches how. Education teaches why." **Nido Qubein**

11. Be careful in treating with any individual: "Every individual matter. Every individual has a role to play. Every individual makes a difference." **Jane Goodall**

12. Best achievement of education is seeking wisdom and understanding, not remembering and accumulating facts: "The best educated human being is the one who understands most about the life in which he is placed." **Helen Keller**

13. Best homework: thinking homework: "I like a teacher who gives you something to take home to think about besides homework." **Edith Ann**

14. The best investment is in the self, head or mind: "If a man empties his purse into his head, no man can take it away from him. An investment in knowledge always pays the best interest." **Ben Franklin**

15. The best people live with constant standards, not on changing emotion: "The quality of a leader is reflected in the standards they set for themselves. **Ray Kroc**

16. The best reflection of ourselves: the language we use: "Our language is the reflection of ourselves. A language is an exact reflection of the character and growth of its speakers." **Cesar Chavez**

17. Best teachers, best parents: "A teacher is one who makes himself progressively unnecessary." **Thomas Carruthers**

18. The best way of teaching: "Teaching is a strategic act of engagement." **James Bellanca**

19. Best way to prevent students and kids from the big shadow of assumption of parents and teachers: "The true teacher defends his pupils against his own personal influence." **Amos Bronson Alcott**

20. Blind love takes all the opportunity to cope with challenges and adversity. Reading this reminded me the way to breed the domestic chicken: "Just as we develop our physical muscles through overcoming opposition - such as lifting weights - we develop our character muscles by overcoming challenges and adversity." **Stephen Covey**

21. Cannot measure the major factors - attitude and virtues, teachers choose the easier way to measure the minor factors - reading, remembering… or IQ. The fact is IQ or degree has some relation with the attitude and virtues so that teachers may think they are right. Unfortunately, IQ and intelligence do not enough to judge the attitude and virtue of a person, let alone judging the abilities. Even worse, the results of judgment may be distorted by some bad purposes, wrong assumption or poor understanding of the judges. Worst of all the wrong judgment may affect the life of the students: "Because we cannot measure the things that have the most meaning, we give the most meaning to the things we can measure." **Fred Hargadon**

22. Capable of becoming and treating: "Treat people as if they were what they ought to be, and you help them to become what they are capable of becoming." **Goethe**

23. Challenges build character: "Character cannot be developed in ease and quiet. Only through experience of trial and suffering can the soul be strengthened, ambition inspired, and success achieved." **Helen Keller**

24. The character is remaining, not knowledge: "Education is what remains after one has forgotten what one has learned in school." **Albert Einstein**

25. The child needs flexible, trusted friend, not rigid teachers, parents: "If a child is to keep alive his inborn sense of wonder, he needs the companionship of at least one adult who can share it, rediscovering with him the joy, excitement, and mystery of the world we live in." **Rachel Carson**

26. Children love attention: "The greatest gift you can give another is the purity of your attention. **Richard Moss**

27. Children need love, connection, safety, example, inspiration, and touching moments to nourish the souls or drive 3.0: "Rewards and punishments are the lowest forms of education." **Chuang-Tzu**

28. Children will determine your happiness for your lifetime: "If you want happiness for a lifetime, help the next generation." **Chinese saying**

29. Concerning character, "Be more concerned with your character than your reputation, because your character is what you really are, while your reputation is merely what others think you are." **John Wooden**

30. Confession of character: opinion of the world: "People do not seem to realize that their opinion of the world is also a confession of character." **Ralph Waldo Emerson**

31. Correction and encouragement: "Correction does much, but encouragement does more." **Goethe**

32. Curiosity, does formal education protect it?, "Curiosity is a delicate little plant that, aside from stimulation, stands mainly in need of freedom.." **Albert Einstein**

33. Definitely, an eagle is the dummy in crowing: "The eagle never lost so much time as when he submitted to learn from the crow." **William Blake**

34. Different time, different understanding, and different point of view: "Don't limit a child to your own learning, for he was born in another time." **Rabbinical Saying**

35. The different way of learning, different intelligence: "Every student can learn. Just not on the same day or in the same way." **George Evans**

36. Distinguish is more important: "Education has produced a vast population able to read but unable to distinguish what is worth reading." **G.M. Trevelyan**

37. Do schools and families reward uncreative mind or creative mind? "The uncreative mind can spot wrong answers, but it takes a very creative mind to spot wrong questions." **Anthony Jay**

38. Do teachers respect students? "The secret of education is respecting the pupil." **Ralph Waldo Emerson**

39. Does education teach simplicity or complexity? "In character, in manner, in style, in all things, the supreme excellence is simplicity." **Henry Wadsworth Longfellow**

40. Does formal education create learners or parrots? "In a time of drastic change, it is the learners who inherit the future. The learned usually find themselves equipped to live in a world that no longer exists." **Eric Hoffer**

41. Does formal education encourage or discourage students, parents, and teachers? "Nine-tenths of education is the encouragement." **Anatole France**

42. Does formal education nourish these foundation stones: "The foundation stones for a balanced success are honesty, character, integrity, faith, love, and loyalty." **Zig Ziglar**

43. Does formal education teach dismal and fatuous notion? "We must reject that most dismal and fatuous notion that education is a preparation for life." **Northrop Frye**

44. Does formal education value mistakes and correction? "Anyone who has never made a mistake has never tried anything new." **Albert Einstein**

45. Does learning have self-motivation for the genius mind? "Perhaps the greatest joy is learning how to motivate yourself." **Floyd Maxwell**

46. Does schooling encourage or teach self-education? "Self-education is the only possible education; the rest is mere veneer laid on the surface of a child's nature." **Charlotte Mason**

47. Does schooling nourish or diminish the natural desire? "All men by nature desire to know." **Aristotle**

48. Does your education satisfy the aim of action? "The great aim of education is not knowledge but action." **Herbert Spencer**

49. Educate leadership to get along with people: "I suppose leadership at one time meant muscles, but today it means getting along with people." **Mahatma Gandhi**

50. Educated children will be the masters of the society in the next decade: "If you are planning for a year, sow rice; if you are

planning for a decade, plant trees; if you are planning for a lifetime, educate people." **Chinese proverb**

51. Educating heart or character is more important than educating mind or intelligence: "Educating the mind without educating the heart is no education at all." **Aristotle**

52. Education creates abilities: Education is the ability to meet life's situations. **Dr. John G. Hibben**

53. Education involves all people, not only teachers: "Education is not something which the teacher does ...it is a natural process which develops spontaneously in the human being: parents, politicians, friends, teachers, grandparents, and every people." **Maria Montessori**

54. Education should teach to learn more, do more, fail more, act more, think more and dream more: "The greater danger for most of us is not that our aim is too high and we miss it, but that it is too low and we reach it." **Michelangelo**

55. Education, discipline mind to use its potential, not the accumulation of others: "The great end of education is to discipline rather than to furnish the mind; to train it to the use of its own powers, rather than fill it with the accumulation of others." **Tryon Edwards**

56. Education, take control of life: Education is not a form of entertainment, but a means of empowering people to take control of their lives. **Unknown**

57. Education: how to learn from the self: For the sole true end of education is simply this: to teach men how to learn for themselves; and whatever instruction fails to do this is effort spent in vain. **Dorothy L. Sayers**

58. Effective class: "In an effective classroom, students should not only know what they are doing, they should also know why and how." **Harry K. Wong**

59. Effective pursuing in school: "What we want is to see the child in pursuit of knowledge, and not knowledge in pursuit of the child." **George Bernard Shaw**

60. Encouragement and safety in schooling will create thousands of ideas and solutions." The best way to have a good idea is to have lots of ideas." **Linus Pauling**

61. Equality: All of us do not have equal talent, but all of us should have an equal opportunity to develop our talent. **John F. Kennedy**

62. Eye follow the attention of the mind: "People only see what they are prepared to see." **Ralph Waldo Emerson**

63. Fail of the formal teacher, "There is nothing in a caterpillar that tells you it's going to be a butterfly." **Buckminster Fuller**

64. Failure key, think to avoid it: "I don't know the key to success, but the key to failure is trying to please everybody." **Bill Cosby**

65. Failure of men with shouting "Pay attention", "No use to shout at them to pay attention. If the situations, the materials, the problems before the child do not interest him, his attention will slip off to what does interest him, and no amount of exhortation of threats will bring it back." **John Holt**

66. The fault of schooling: "My schooling not only failed to teach me what it professed to be teaching but prevented me from being educated to an extent which infuriates me when I think of

all I might have learned at home by myself." **George Bernard Shaw**

67. Find a good teacher, not only the intelligent ones: "Better than a thousand days of diligent study is one day with a great teacher." **Japanese Proverb**

68. Find the few: "Few things help an individual more than to place responsibility upon him and let him know that you trust him." **Booker T. Washington**

69. The first task of the teacher, "To stimulate life, leaving it then free to develop, to unfold, herein lies the first task of the teacher." **Maria Montessori**

70. Focusing on children, not teacher or method; "If a child can't learn the way we teach, maybe we should teach the way they learn." **Ignacio Estrada**

71. Free child to his companions: "If a man does not keep pace with his companions, perhaps it is because he hears a different drummer. Let him step to the music which he hears, however, measured or far away." **Thoreau**

72. Freedom, stimulation cure curiosity: "Curiosity is a delicate little plant that, aside from stimulation, stands mainly in need of freedom." **Albert Einstein**

73. From right understanding, accumulation on the way is always more valuable than results: "The discipline you learn and character you build from setting and achieving a goal can be more valuable than the achievement of the goal itself." **Bo Bennett**

74. Genius sees the potential: "To see things in the seed, that is genius." **Lao Tzu**

75. The gentle way can shake world: "In a gentle way, you can shake the world." **Mahatma Gandhi**

76. The goal of true education: intelligence plus character: "The function of education is to teach one to think intensively and to think critically. Intelligence plus character - that is the goal of true education." **Martin Luther King, Jr.**

77. Good character difficultly slowly formed: "Good character is not formed in a week or a month. It is created little by little, day by day. Protracted and patient effort is needed to develop good character." **Heraclitus**

78. Good educator build, the poor teacher like repairing: "It is easier to build strong children than to repair broken men." **Frederick Douglass**

79. Good leadership or effective means little or no emergency problems: "One of the tests of leadership is the ability to recognize a problem before it becomes an emergency." **Arnold Glasow**

80. Good news all physical disability and poor student: "It is not by muscle, speed, or physical dexterity that great things are achieved, but by reflection, the force of character, and judgment." **Marcus Tullius Cicero**

81. The grade of the real educator: "If I ran a school, I'd give the average grade to the ones who gave me all the right answers, for being good parrots. I'd give the top grades to those who made a lot of mistakes and told me about them, and then told me what they learned from them." **Buckminster Fuller**

82. Great character: "By constant self-discipline and self-control you can develop greatness of character." **Unknown**

83. Great leaders are inspiring leaders: "The greatest leader is not necessarily the one who does the greatest things. He is the one that gets the people to do the greatest things." **Ronald Reagan**

84. Greatest service is teaching the independent growing, not feeding: "To teach a man how he may learn to grow independently, and for himself, is perhaps the greatest service that one man can do another." **Benjamin Jowett**

85. Growing mind: "A man's mind, stretched by new ideas, may never return to its original dimension" **Oliver Wendell Holmes Jr.**

86. Guide without interfering: "Teachers should guide without dictating, and participate without dominating." **C. B. Neblette**

87. Guiding principles making great things: "Great ambition is the passion of a great character. Those endowed with it may perform very good or very bad acts. All depends on the principles which direct them." **Napoleon Bonaparte**

88. Hacking what? "Hack your education." Steve Hargadon

89. Help them find, inspire them find: You cannot teach a man anything; you can only help him to find it within himself. **Galileo**

90. How about when students talk, teachers? "When people talk, listen completely." **Ernest Hemingway**

91. How can read people? "One's appearance bespeaks dignity corresponding to the depth of his character. One's concentrated effort, serene attitude, taciturn air, courteous disposition, thoroughly polite bearing, gritted teeth with a piercing look - each of these reveals dignity. Such outward appearance, in short, comes from constant attentiveness and seriousness." **Yamamoto Tsunetomo**

92. How genius becomes stupid: "Everybody is a genius. But if you judge a fish by its ability to climb a tree, it will live its whole life believing that it is stupid." **Albert Einstein**

93. How to read a man: "A man's character may be learned from the adjectives which he habitually uses in conversation." **Mark Twain**

94. How to think is more important than what to remember, "The aim of education should be to teach us how to think, rather than what to think. To improve our minds, so as to enable us to think for ourselves, rather than to load the memory with thoughts of other men." **Bill Beattie**

95. Ignorant remembering of inert facts: "Nothing in education is so astonishing as the amount of ignorance it accumulates in the form of inert facts." **Henry Brooks Adams**

96. Illiteracy and not reading may be the same: "The man who does not read good books has no advantage over the man who can't read them." **Mark Twain**

97. Important of character: "Because power corrupts, society's demands for moral authority and character increase as the importance of the position increases." **John Adams**

98. Important question is what counts? "Teaching kids to count is fine, but teaching them what counts is best." **Bob Talbert**

99. Interdependent success: "It is only as we develop others that we permanently succeed." **Harvey S. Firestone**

100. Invisible learning: "That which we do not call education is more precious than that which we call so." **Ralph Waldo Emerson**

101. IQ is not intelligence but characters and enthusiasm is: "Intelligence is not to make no mistakes, but quickly to see how to make them good. **Bertolt Brecht**

102. It is the mark of an educated mind to be able to entertain a thought without accepting it." **Aristotle**

103. It is time to forget old education for the development of family, nation, world and human beings: "The aim of public education is not to spread enlightenment at all; it is simply to reduce as many individuals as possible to the same safe level, to breed a standard citizenry, to put down dissent and originality." **H.L. Mencken**

104. Job of educator: "The job of an educator is to teach students to see the vitality in themselves." **Joseph Campbell**

105. Key of society: "Be aware that young people have to be able to make their own mistakes, and that times change." **Gina Shapira**

106. Knowledge and character, "Knowledge will give you power, but character respect." **Bruce Lee**

107. Leader require character and moral, not degree or intellectual, "Leadership consists not in degrees of technique but in traits of character; it requires moral rather than athletic or intellectual effort, and it imposes on both leader and follower alike the burdens of self-restraint." **Lewis H. Lapham**

108. Leaning is fun; with fun every difficult thing can be learned. Nourish the fun, joy, eager and enthusiasm in every activity of children is the priority of parents, adults and teachers: "Children want to learn to the degree that they are unable to distinguish learning from fun. They keep this attitude until we adults convince them that learning is not fun." **Glenn Doman**

109. Learn from talking people: "I learned most, not from those who taught me but from those who talked with me." **St. Augustine**

110. Learn the value of religion: "Religion is meant to teach us true spiritual human character. It is meant for self-transformation. It is meant to transform anxiety into peace, arrogance into humility, envy into compassion, to awaken the pure soul in man and his love for the Source, which is God." **Radhanath Swami**

111. Learn to ask, teach asking questions: "A prudent question is one-half of wisdom." **Sir Francis Bacon**

112. Learn to learn, not learn to remembering, "Learning how to learn is life's most important skill." **Tony Buzan**

113. Learning and teaching: "By learning you will teach; by teaching you will learn." **Latin Proverb**

114. Learning from friends: "I pay the schoolmaster, but it is the schoolboys that educate my son." **Ralph Waldo Emerson**

115. Learning from history: "Human history becomes more and more a race between education and catastrophe." **H.G. Wells**

116. Learning is living: Education is not preparation for life; education is life itself. **John Dewey**

117. Learning is making fun: "Children want to learn to the degree that they are unable to distinguish learning from fun. They keep this attitude until we adults convince them that learning is not fun." **Glenn Doman**

118. Learning leadership: Leadership and learning are indispensable to each other. **John F. Kennedy**

119. Learning means understanding: "Life is a succession of lessons, which must be lived to be understood." **Ralph Waldo Emerson**

120. Let make education become the wings to life student, not the burden for their development: "The only thing that interferes with my learning is my education." **Albert Einstein**

121. Let see the repetition to know the character: "Winning takes talent, to repeat takes character." **John Wooden**

122. Let them go, do not interfere, perhaps one good thing for self-made billionaire like Warren Buffet, Bill Gate, Jack Ma is that their parents do not prevent, interfere their work. They may feel safe from behind to cope with the challenges from business: "Don't let what you cannot do interfere with what you can do." **John Wooden**

123. Lifelong learning: "Learning is not compulsory. Neither is survival." **Dr. W. Edwards Deming**

124. Lifelong legacy: "To encourage literature and the arts is a duty which every good citizen owes to his country." **George Washington**

125. Little key, heavy door: "A very little key will open a very heavy door." **Charles Dickens**

126. Looking for pleasure or attitude in all activities, "The test and the use of man's education is that he finds pleasure in the exercise of his mind." **Jacques Barzun**

127. Love understanding: "One never learns to understand truly anything but what one loves." **Goethe**

128. Love: "Children need love, especially when they do not deserve it." **Harold S. Hulbert**

129. Manmade stupid: "Men are born ignorant, not stupid; they are made stupid by education." **Bertrand Russell**

130. Marriage, contract, assumption, relationship, and position make boasters think they have power: "Nearly all men can stand adversity, but if you want to test a man's character, give him power." **Abraham Lincoln**

131. Master nature, connection to nature: "Earth and sky, woods and fields, lakes and rivers, the mountain and the sea, are excellent schoolmasters, and teach some of us more than we can ever learn from books." **John Lubbock**

132. Master, teacher, awakening: "A master can tell you what he expects of you. A teacher, though, awakens your own expectations." **Patricia Neal**

133. Mind is for use and formed from using, not to hide: "The more you use your mind, the more you'll have to use." **George A. Dorsey**

134. Mission service: "Teaching is not just a job. It is a human service and it must be thought of as a mission." **Dr. Ralph Tyler**

135. Most of schools are wrong: "Learning is not a spectator sport." **Anonymous**

136. Naive, no more classes: "It would be extremely naive to expect the dominant classes to develop a type of education that would enable subordinate classes to perceive social injustices critically." **Paulo Freire**

137. Need of society is changing: "School is the advertising agency which makes you believe that you need the society as it is." **Ivan Illich**

138. No knowledge under compulsion, "Knowledge, which is acquired under compulsion, obtains no hold on the mind." **Plato**

139. No, teachers and adults are dumber than their children are. In any subject, any skill children will master faster than adult and parents if children have joy and curiosity in learning: language, vehicle, smart devices, and new equipment: "I am beginning to suspect all elaborate and special systems of education. They seem to me to be built upon the supposition that every child is a kind of idiot who must be taught to think." **Anne Sullivan**

140. Noble teaching shaping the world: "Teaching is a very noble profession that shapes the character, caliber, and future of an individual. If the people remember me as a good teacher, that will be the biggest honor for me." **A. P. J. Abdul Kalam**

141. Noble teaching: Education is soul crafting. **Cornel West**

142. Not only school as most people think: "A child educated only at school is an uneducated child." **George Santayana**

143. Not weakness in IQ: "Weakness of attitude becomes weakness of character." **Albert Einstein**

144. Nourishing the strong desire is better than sharing: "The greatest good you can do for another is not just to share your riches, but to reveal to him his own." **Benjamin Disraeli**

145. Paradoxes of governing: "All who have meditated on the art of governing mankind have been convinced that the fate of empires depends on the education of youth." **Aristotle**

146. Parents, adults and teachers should know to add value to others: "To add value to others, one must first value others." **John Maxwell**

147. Parents, leaders, politician should learn from these successful teachers: "The greatest sign of success for a teacher is to be able to say, The children are now working as if I did not exist." **Maria Montessori**

148. Parents, leaders, teachers, educators should be the models, not empty talkers: "Children have more need of models than of critics." **Carolyn Coats**

149. Patience with nature, not intelligence: "The key to everything is patience. You get the chicken by hatching the egg -- not by smashing it." **Arnold Glasow**

150. Philosophers, religious leaders are the teachers of humankind: "A teacher affects eternity; no one can tell where his influence stops." **Henry Adams**

151. Planting continually asking question in students: "The one real object of education is to have a man in the condition of continually asking questions." **Bishop Mandell Creighton**

152. Power of sample: "Example isn't another way to teach, it is the only way to teach." **Albert Einstein**

153. Pretend to treat others as geniuses, pretend to treat oneself well, our illusive mind will think that it is true: "We are what we pretend to be, so we must be careful about what we pretend to be." **Kurt Vonnegut**

154. Price of great: "Great spirits have always encountered violent opposition from mediocre minds." **Albert Einstein**

155. Problems, suicidal, destructions, illnesses, and diseases may be the side effects of laggard education, especial in feudalism or autarchy: "Almost all education has a political motive: it aims at strengthening some group, national or religious

or even social, in the competition with other groups. It is this motive, in the main, which determines the subjects taught, the knowledge offered and the knowledge withheld, and also decides what mental habits the pupils are expected to acquire. Hardly anything is done to foster the inward growth of mind and spirit; in fact, those who have had the most education are very often atrophied in their mental and spiritual life." **Bertrand Russell**

156. Provide for learning: "I never teach my pupils. I only attempt to provide the conditions in which they can learn." **Albert Einstein**

157. Providing is more important than teaching: "I never teach my pupils. I only attempt to provide the conditions in which they can learn." **Albert Einstein**

158. Quality of responding and reacting: "Bad things do happen; how I respond to them defines my character and the quality of my life. I can choose to sit in perpetual sadness, immobilized by the gravity of my loss, or I can choose to rise from the pain and treasure the most precious gift I have - life itself." **Walter Anderson**

159. Questions of well-educated mind: "A well-educated mind will always have more questions than answers." **Helen Keller**

160. Real effective education: "Education is a better safeguard of liberty than a standing army."

The world needs great teachers; whoever has these ten characters:

1. Great Teachers Are Humble.

2. Great Teachers Are Patient

3. Great Teachers Are Kind and Show Respect.

4. Great Teachers Have Enthusiasm for Their Subject Matter.

5. Great Teachers Show Not Tell.

6. Great Teachers Learn from Their Students.

7. Great Teachers Are Positive; Great Teachers Smile

8. Great Teachers Engage their Students.

9. Great Teachers Have High Expectations.

10. Great Teachers Provide a Warm Environment and Allow Their Students to Make Mistakes.

Chapter 60: We are the creators of our lives and the creators of our children

"GOD IN US

WE ARE GOD

ALL ARE GOD"

****

We can make good or bad about our life and people's life. We have the same power as God has. One day, some of use may be seen as the Holy Spirits by our great-great-grandchildren. Please, awake the power and influence we have.

The journey of finding "Why"

There is an old story: a scholar wanted to find the key to success and failure in life.

One day they came to the village where famous for a lot of successful football players, he came to the village patriarch to find the answer. "How were football players born here?" "No, only babies" the patriarch replied

Another day he came to the village where famous for a lot of doctors and professors, he came to the village patriarch to find the answer. "How were doctors and professors born here?", "No, only babies" the patriarch replied

The other day, he comes to the village where famous for leaders, generals, and heroes; he came to the village patriarch to find the answer. "How were leaders, generals, and heroes born here?", "No, only babies" the patriarch replied

The other day, he comes to the village where well-known for criminals, murderers, and terrorists, he came to the village patriarch to find the answer. "Why are there so many bad people: criminals, murderers, terrorists born here?", "No, only babies" the patriarch peacefully replied.

Looking, watching and contemplating

1. Watching a strong girl screaming and running away when seeing a cockroach, I understand the power of character and the weakness of knowledge and intelligence.

2. Watching a healthy fainted when seeing someone is bleeding, I understand the power of things on his mind and the weakness of the strong muscles and assumed intelligence.

3. Watching a young, healthy man running away and left his friend behind when seeing the danger, I understand the power of characters is more important than the power of muscle and power of knowledge.

4. Watching a small dog bravely attack bigger dog to protect his owner, I understand the obsessed desires, and brave is more important than strong muscle and big muscles.

5. Understanding the fears, roots of fears, the drives, habits, and behaviors make me understand deeper about human beings, and the hidden of a powerful mind.

6. Watching a well-known manager scolding his staffs then taking home the properties of the company when no one seeing, I understand the importance of characters, virtues, and compassionate mind than ever before.

7. Watching a rich man wearing many luxury things, like praising, boasting then angrily scolding his staffs for a small error, I understand the power of character, intelligence, wealthy, healthy, and contentment.

8. Watching many handsome intelligent men misery because of losing money in gambling still try to find a way to play gambling, I understand what is the most important to a man.

9. Watching a successful manager like to accumulating, possessing, taking, making a big profit and celebrating, then taking drugs at home for sleep, quiet mind, and at ease, I understand what is the deeper needs of mind of beings and what is the real hunger of the rich.

10. Watching the joy of children play in nature, with natural objects: carrot, potato, flower, sand, rock, earth, tree, grass and fruit; and natural creatures: fish, chicken, dog, cat, duck, and so on. Then watching they play indifferently with plastic objects, emotionlessly playing in an artificial environment, artificial flower, bored with playing with intelligent robots, an intelligent robot shaped dog. I understand the vitality, sophistication of nature that human beings only understand very little. Children may jump, sing, dance, and smile with the dog, cat, and duck in water but they may never do that with the intelligent robots with dog-shaped, cat-shaped, and duck-shaped in luxury car, or shinning castle. We need to understand more our children's deepest needs. We need to understand the hunger of the children in wealthy and prosperous.

11. Watching the science document films, I understand that the most sophisticated technology and printing can only print the object shaped orange; they can never print out the real orange had the same in countless varieties for our children to eat. To have a real orange as soon as possible, scientists only have to figure out the way to speed up the process of making the fruit of orange trees. They will take a long time to understand what is nature really is let alone creating an apple had the same characters as the real apple? Not understanding, how they can create? At least, they can create an object that all sense of people cannot recognize the differences by all human senses; they cannot create the same object.

12. Living, studying, sleeping, working, and walking in the artificial boxes cuts all chances for people to get the connection with mysterious nature. They will be out of balance then creating more out of balance. This finding makes me awake to the problem of our society

13. Watching the tribes in the Amazon jungle, I think of the living of modern human ancestors. To have modern human beings as we are today, our ancestors have to study, do, think and create need changes inside out to adapt well to the slow changes of nature. Too much and to fast changes of nature means too big the problems, too much pressure can destroy the whole tribes, communities, and nations. So the needed temperate changes, temperate pressures have pushed our ancestors to study, do, think, create and invent. In another world, the needed temperate changes in nature and society have made human ancestors evolved to have strength, abilities, and power to live well. This is true for all of us: infants, kids, students, adults, employees, and the old also.

14. Watching a lot of successful men, women, well-fed children and who have the high standard of living have been taking a lot of medications, sedative medications, and painkiller medication to have temporary at easy and good feelings. Some of them even taking drugs, committing crimes, and committing suicide, I awake with what are really the hunger of modern people, the power of characters, ability, understanding and the real lacking of modern society. I understand the root of our society's problems: greed, anger and ignorance, and lack of characters.

15. Watching a successful father angrily scolding and crucially beating his children even they are screaming, crying and saying sorry so many times. Then the father turned back to the wife shouting that he has to sacrifice all his time, money, energy, and even his life for his children but they do not obey his advice, do not know his sacrificing and his suffering. I understand that the characters like love, compassion, talking for understanding, kind heart, open-minded and mastering the art of using golden rules are much more important than IQ, intelligence, wealth and powerful muscles.

16. Reading human history, human wars, I understand that pace of nature, the laws of life and the paradoxes of life that scientists hardly to put on the mathematic equation. History is not made by the enforcement of power but make by the virtues, characters of great men. When one society lacked virtues and goodness, chaos and witty start to dominate society until there are men with virtues, characters, and understanding taking responsibility to make changes.

17. Looking at large crowd and many people in the society hysterically running and screaming, blaming then getting ill, I understand the power of the mind and the destruction of not understanding.

18. Reading the autobiographies of great men, leaders and billionaires described since they were the babies, toddlers, youths and adults, many incidents have impacted their life. Then they train the mind and well governed the mind, they, the weak ordinary people, have made the changes and advancements in society. None of the great men said their success and understanding comes from their intelligence. They all value the persistence and characters.

19. Reading the list of life of billionaires, the autography of most influential people, the great president, and their education, I understand the useless value of formal education, the useless value of boasting degrees, and boasting certification. I am awakened with the value of lifelong learning, persistence, and humility. I understand intelligence, IQ or degree to some extent reflex the abilities, values, and virtues of integrity men: "as within so without". But with cheating men, they are the good tools to cover all their defects and weakness inside. Some bad men even like to accumulate degree and boast about it to make them temporary satisfy their needs and their greed. Do not listen to the sounding words, just close the eyes and feel the attitude, love, compassion, purposes, the pattern of speech, listen to greedy words, selfish words, you will not be cheated by them. They may be the slave of passions and sensual desires. They build thick covers, sounding words, sounding certificates, and aggressive strong emotions to hide and compensate for the weaknesses inside. Never taste the real happiness because of discontentment they constantly accumulate stuff to create thick, heavy, flashy and catchy covers. "Excessive outer to cover the weakness inside". All their words will reveal their weakness. In and out are not the same, they start the process of imbalance. Sensitive mind and sensitive brain will silently suffer the imbalance that people do not know if they do not mindful. Then the imbalanced mind will silently control the people to create countless bad cause for them, relatives and all other people described in the law of cause and effect.

20. The brain, with the weakest, soft, fragile nerve cells in the world, is the softest thing that controls the hardest cells, strongest cells, and whole body's organ. When brain and cells become much stiffer, and much more rigid, the process of self-destruction will begin. This maybe is the hidden paradoxes pattern of evolution of materials in the universe.

21. The changes in society are not from the power and intelligence of royal members, but from the characters and virtues of ordinary, weak men: Benjamin Franklin, Mother Teresa, Mahatma Gandhi, Abraham Lincoln, Socrates, and so on

22. Observing, watching all phenomena around make me understand that things are interdependent, inter-being, one in all and all in one, this because of that and that because of this. There is no separate self and separate being. Then I awaken that human beings are falling apart from their essence, virtues, and goodness.

23. Our children may become the victims and creators of the misery of lust, hatred, and ignorance. Because of the blind love of parents, ignorant parents support to satisfy the needs of their children quickly and unconditionally. After many time of quick satisfaction, the children become obsessed with happy feelings, they want to have more happy feelings without putting any efforts. Gradually, they become the greedy children. Because of greed and unsatisfying the greed, they may constantly fall into stress. They may become the victims of stress chemicals, the victims of living condition. To remove the greed and hatred, children need to study more, train more and practice more to gain the knowledge and essential skills. Knowledge can help children stay away from the traps of delusion and ignorance. With knowledge, skills, and patience, children can control the needs, can control the anger and control the behaviors to move forwards noble goals. Children can create joy and happiness for themselves by their ability like characters, skills, and patience. Unfortunately, to gain knowledge, patience and essential skills gained from the hard labors like studying, training and practicing is quite hard and

painful at first. Some parents love their children so blindly that they cannot stand seeing their children suffering pain in first working so that they interfere or jump in to help their children. Parents may unconsciously take all chances for their children to gain and develop essential skills, knowledge, patience and strong characters. Children with greed, hatred, and ignorance; and without knowledge, patience, and essential skills may suffer endless pain and stress at their later life. To some extent, the bad characters and the disadvantages of parents may be inherited by their children.

Let make the answer to table 29 below with the skilled children and unskilled children to see the burden of lacking essential skills and ignorance put on unskilled children. With curiosity, encouragement, passion and the feeling of safety from the trust, children may find flow state in solving their problem, this high state of mind will make the brain works most effectively to create the incredible results.

Table 40: The relation between abilities, problems, and stress

The daily activities	1. Hard/ pain/ stress 2. Easy/happy/pleased 3. Flow state in working	
	Unskilled children	Skillful children
1. Taking care of themselves		
2. Prepare books, clothes, drink for school		
3. Clean the house, wash dishes, helping parents		
4. Play with and take care of younger siblings		
5. Solving problems in class: poor results, fail the test, pressure of studying and connecting with the friend.		
6. Overcome the stress in family, school, and society.		
7. Joining to a new crowd of people		
8. Taking responsibility, initially solving problems at work		
9. Asking questions to find answers to their curiosity, raising the voice		
10. Fail in an important test that makes parents		

disappointed, feeling of shamefulness		
11. Fail in an important test that ruins all of their goals and noble purpose		
12. Raising voice, give an opinion on the subject they know in front of the crowd		
13. Fighting against the attacking of small, wild animals, bugs, and ugly worm		
14. Politely, asking the things they want to feel the relief.		
15. Accepting the unwanted things		

Peace, tranquil, stillness, intelligence belong to the mind, no one can take it from you; these can create lasting safety and happiness for you. You can live in the way you want. Moreover, fame, possession, admiration, praise belong to other people's opinion, anyone can take it from you; these are the things that constantly changing; which constantly create the feeling of stress, danger, and losses for you. You have to live in the way people want, not the way you want.

Giving, in the perception of greedy people is giving possession, losing possession, the wrong thinking makes them angry and unsafe. However, giving, in the essence of life is the creating life, creating abundance, creating chances for development; in return, it creates an abundance of spiritual and material life. Warren Buffet and Headed Buffet are the examples. Any thought, words, actions will put as a dots into the mind. We are the perception of the hologram created by countless dots.

The work of the potential mind is the answer to all laws of life, all principles of life. All laws explain the manifestation of mind and thinking about the environment. These laws will show the relation of mind and other conditions. The basic law is the law of cause and effect, from this law, its varieties create many other laws: laws of inside and outside, law of above and below, law of thinking and living, law of the mind and the condition of living, law of attraction, law of accumulation, and law of thinking, believing, behaving and acting. To have the right to understand these laws we need to use the Yin and Yan philosophy to have a deeper understanding of the essence of phenomena and the perception of the phenomena.

When the desires and needs are satisfied, tragedy may happen because these are selfish actions. Tragedy starts with the irrational emotion, negative thinking, negative feeling that people have after satisfying.

If people satisfy the basic needs, noble desires by following the core principles, miracles will happen to individuals because of selfless actions, selfless purposes. Miracles will happen to homes, miracles will happen to countries, and miracles will happen to the world.

Warren Buffet succeeds because he is so obsessed with his core principles. The principles help him to control the mind, to understand the mind and the environment; the principles also make him feel safe when taking actions despite the noisy crowd. His core principles appear in every action: buying, selling, accumulating, spending, taking and giving. He likes money; he takes money as if money is the rewards from the games of life, but he is not the slave of money. He is not the smartest people, he does not have the highest IQ, he does not use high technology machines to have the best decision, in fact, he use some simple tools, he observes the most, listen the most and think the most. The principles and understanding help him become the richest people in an astonishing way that we cannot imagine. Life is so fun with him. He is the example of the one who mastered the mind.

Chapter 61: Time to create heaven on earth

The heavenly earth has suffered enough by the ignorance of you, me and most of the human beings. There are enough pain and miseries caused by greedy, lust, hatred, anger and ignorance of human being. And human beings are suffering from the problems they have created. The illusion of faraway heaven makes people so blind that they have created countless problems on earth with the blind thought that they will be welcome in heaven.

How many percents of the population will come to heaven after death? No one can answer, even religious leaders.

What will happen if one million people in a population of seven billion people will go to heaven after death? Just imagine that we will still have the same thinking, belief, and ego as we are now praying or making worship when we live in heaven, next to God and Holy Spirits form our ancestors. We may live happily all day, not worrying, not doing, not laboring, just enjoying with the immense supply and protection from God and Holy Spirits. Oh no, we will make heaven become hell.

How do I say that? Please answer this question: what are the characters of God, Holy Spirits in heaven? Presume that they exist; will they have the characters as we usually think they have like other human beings as we usually see on the television or as the myths in the religious books? No, these assumptive characters in myths and films are not Holy Spirits because they still have greed, anger, and ignorance. If they have a small part of these ill characters, how fast will heaven become hell? Because with greed, they start to accumulate and possess all things: the bowls they use, the chairs they sit, the houses they sleep, the car they drive, the planet they live in, or even the whole universe. Million people come to heaven will be a big threat to their God and Holy Spirits unless they remove their greed, anger, and ignorance. If removing greed, anger, and ignorance, they can enjoy heaven on earth or they can reach Nirvana on earth. God or Goodness will never make human beings have the power to make others live in misery, never make human being have the power to destroy all other species.

From the wrong assumption about the existence of God and Holy Spirits, human beings have created countless miseries, tragedies, destructions and killing on the behalf of their God and Holy Spirits. Some even create hell from heavenly earth with blind thinking that on the behalf of their God, Holy Spirits or Heroes. Some people may convict killing, beating, sacrificing to worship their God and Holy Spirits.

Sometimes I wonder where was the God and Holy Spirits? Which sides they stand for in the battles during human wars: American civil car, civil wars, World War I, World War II and millions were between siblings, father and son, this family and that family, people of this commune and people of that commune, people of this region and people of that region, people of this religion and people of that religion, the black and the white, people of North America and people of South America, European American and Native American, the slavers and the owners; Napoleon Bonaparte and his enemies who defend their countries, the creators and the sufferers of tragedies.

Are there any people participated in the war, as warmongers and defenders, thought that they are against their common God and Holy Spirits? No, both sides have the belief that their God and Holy Spirits are on their side, so they dare to sacrifice, they do not afraid of dying and killing. Holding Holy objects, God's images in hand, they are ready to sacrifice to kill others. Even if the soldiers on both sides of war die, they may think these are the noblest death. We are in hands of Satan and gosh but we have the illusion that we are in hands God and Holy Spirits.

No, that is nonsense! Human beings have suffered enough from their illusion and ignorance. We should keep our God and Holy Spirits are the creators of our world. God and Holy Spirits are in our head, they create heaven on earth by our human hands. In one action, we create countless invisible phenomena for our society. If the created phenomena are good, we have given hand to create heaven on earth. If the created phenomena are bad, we have given hand to create hell on earth. The marks of good phenomena and bad phenomena, heaven and earth in our countless behaviors of human beings are embed in our brain, mind, spiritual health, mental health, physical appearance, energy, and fingerprint. The countless phenomena are the sources of their radiating energy; which are visible and invisible to the visual threshold; but they all caught by our conscious mind and unconscious mind of all people. All the illuminations of these phenomena operate with the law of cause and effect. Law of cause and effect apply to all people's behaviors now, from this moment into the future. All results, phenomena in the world are the results of cause and effect that human beings have created.

To know how precious we are, how precious our earth is, let see the finding from the scientists in nationalgeographic.com, Scientists analyzing data from NASA's Kepler Space Telescope report the closest thing yet to another Earth, a world in a habitable orbit around a red dwarf star are some 493 light-years away. It means that if we have aliens or move people to live there. The more scientist search on the living of aliens in space, the more they are disappointed with the finding of how lonely human beings are in the universe.

If there is the life on the planet that is 493 light years away, human beings use electromagnetic radiation - with the speed of light- to communicate with us on earth in 2017, the message takes 493 years to reach that planet and 493 more years to reach the earth. Only the aliens' great-great-grandchildren live in 2510 can receive the message we send to them: "Hi friend, Mr. Alien, I Am Stephen from earth. How are you? 2017_ dates of earth calendar."

Their great-great-grandchildren in 2510 received and replied, then until the year 3003 the message may reach to our great great great grandchildren live on earth: "Hi, Mr. Stephen. We are the great-great-grandchildren live in 2510 responding. Our great-great-grandparents had all died. We are their next seven generations, hope to see you soon!"

We are the creators of our world. In all activities, we may create heaven or hell on earth for ourselves and all people. Please become awaken! Please become enlightened for the sake of you, for the sake of our children and for the sake of the world.

> One life is too short to create and enjoy the miracles that the chance of being a being.
>
> How rare, how precious, how invaluable human beings are!

I want to end my word about religion with the quotes of human educators:

"There is no need for temples, no need for complicated philosophies. My brain and my heart are my temples; my philosophy is the kindness philosophy." **Dalai Lama**

"Your daily life is your temple and your religion. When you enter into it take with you your all." **Khalil Gibran**

"I believe in the fundamental truth of all great religions of the world." **Mahatma Gandhi**

"Rivers, ponds, lakes, and streams - they all have different names, but they all contain water. Just as religions do - they all contain truths." **Muhammad Ali**

"The major religions, Christianity, Judaism, Islam, they deny somehow that God has a feminine face. However, if you go to the holy texts, you see there is this feminine presence."

Paulo Coelho

"Religion is an illusion and it derives its strength from the fact that it falls in with our instinctual desires." **Sigmund Freud**

"The truths of religion are never so well understood as by those who have lost the power of reason." **Voltaire**

References:

2015 United States federal budget. (n.d.). In Wikipedia. Retrieved September 19, 2017, from https://en.wikipedia.org/wiki/2015_United_States_federal_budget

Absolute_(philosophy). (n.d.). In Wikipedia. Retrieved September 19, 2017, from https://en.wikipedia.org/wiki/Absolute_(philosophy)

Brodwin, Erin. (2017, April 10). 5 Life Skills Successful, Happy, and Healthy People Have in Common According to Science. Retrieved September 19, 2017, from https://www.inc.com/business-insider/life-skills-successful happy-healthy-people-have-in-common.html

Clear, James. (n.d.). Book Summary: The Compound Effect by Darren Hardy. Retrieved September 19, 2017, from http://jamesclear.com/book-summaries/the-compound-effect

Cleary, Thomas F., et al. The Essential Tao: an Initiation into the Heart of Taoism through the Authentic Tao Te Ching and the Inner Teachings of Chuang-Tzu. HarperSanFrancisco, 1993.

Collins, Jim. Good to Great. Harper Business, 2001.

Covey, S. (1989). The seven habits of highly effective people. New York: Simon and Schuster.

Daskal, Lolly. (n.d.). The 100 Best Leadership Quotes of All Time." Inc.com, Inc. Retrieved September 19, 2017, from https://www.inc.com/lolly-daskal/the-100-best-leadership quotes-of-all-time.html

Education Quotes. (n.d.). BrainyQuote.com. Retrieved September 19, 2017, from BrainyQuote.com Website: http://www.brainyquote.com/quotes/topics/topic_education.html

Fabregas, Marelisa. (n.d.). How to develop your character - Benjamin Franklin's Thirteen Virtues. Retrieved September 19, 2017, from https:// daringtolivefully.com/ben-franklin-thirteen-virtues

Favorite Authors. (n.d.). BrainyQuote.com. Retrieved September 19, 2017, from BrainyQuote.com Website: https://www.brainyquote.com/quotes/favorites. HTML

Franklin, Benjamin, and Louis P. Masur. The Autobiography of Benjamin Franklin. Bedford Books of St. Martin's Press, 1993.

FranklinCovey. (n.d.). The 7 Habits of Highly Effective People Signature Edition 4.0. Retrieved September 19, 2017, from https://www. franklincovey.com/Solutions/Leadership/7-habits-signature.html

Gankyil. (n.d.). In Wikipedia. Retrieved September 19, 2017, from https://en. wikipedia.org/wiki/Gankyil

George, Charles, and Linda George. The Dalai Lama. Lucent Books, 2010.

Get Motivation Motivation, Self Improvement, and Success Strategies." Jim Rohn Articles - Multiple Skills for the 21st Century. Retrieved September 19, from 2017, http://www.getmotivation.com/jimrohn/jrmultiple_skills.html

Gia Fu Feng. (n.d.). In Wikipedia. Retrieved September 19, 2017, from https://en. wikipedia.org/wiki/Gia-Fu_Feng

Gladwell, Malcolm. Blink: The Power of Thinking without Thinking. Penguin, 2006.

Gladwell, Malcolm. Outliers: The Story of Success. Back Bay Books, 2013.

Hanh, Thich Nhat. (2017, September 19). See the Universe in a Sunflower. Retrieved September 19, 2017, from https://www.lionsroar.com/see-the-universe-in-a-sunflower/

Hanh, Thich Nhat.(1987).Old path white clouds: Walking in the footsteps of the Buddha. Parallax press.

Hargadon, Steve. (n.d.). Great Educational Quotes. Retrieved September 19, 2017, from http://learningrevolution.com/page/great-educational-quotes

Hillin, Taryn. (2014, October 3). What The Cost Of Your Engagement Ring May Say About Your Marriage, The Huffington Post. Retrieved September 23, 2017, from http://www.huffingtonpost.com/2014/10/03/expensive-weddings-study_n_5929056.html

Hussain, Anum. (n.d.). 7 Habits of Highly Effective People [Book Summary]. HubSpot Blog. Retrieved September 19, 2017, from https://blog.hubspot.com/sales/habits-of-highlyeffectivepeople- summary

I Ching. (n.d.). In Wikipedia. Retrieved September 19, 2017, from https://en. wikipedia.org/wiki/I_Ching

Juma, Aly. (n.d.) The 13 Virtues of Life: Benjamin Franklin's Guide to Building Character. Retrieved September 19, 2017, from http://alyjuma.com/13-virtues/

Laozi, and Jonathan Star. Tao Te Ching: The New Translation from Tao Te Ching: the Definitive Edition. Jeremy P. Tarcher/Penguin, 2008.

Laozi, and Stephen Mitchell. Tao Te Ching. Frances Lincoln Ltd, 2015.

Laozi, et al. The Teachings of Lao-Tzu: the Tao Te Ching. St. Martin's Press.

Laozi. (n.d.). In Wikipedia. Retrieved September 19, 2017, from https://en. Wikipedia. org/wiki/Laozi

Leadership Quotes. (n.d.). BrainyQuote.com. Retrieved September 19, 2017, from BrainyQuote.com Web site: https://www. brainyquote.com/quotes/topics/topic_leadership.html

Marelisa. (2016, July 16). 45 Morsels of Wisdom From Earl Nightingale. Daring to Live Fully, Retrieved September 19, 2017, from https://daringtolivefully. com/earl-nightingale-quotes

Marketwatch. (2014, October 15). The Pricier the Ring, the Likelier the Divorce. New York Post. Retrieved September 23, 2017, from http://nypost.com/2014/10/15/the-pricier-the-ring-the-likelier-the-divorce/

Maxwell, John C. Developing the Leader within You Workbook. T. Nelson, 2001.

Maxwell, John C. The 21 Indispensable Qualities of a Leader: Becoming the Person Others Will Want to Follow. Magna Publishing Co., 2012.

Montenegro, Robert. (2014, October 9). Expensive Engagement Rings Linked to Higher Divorce Rates. Big Think. Retrieved September 23, 2017, http://bigthink.com/ideafeed/expensive-engagement-rings-linked-to-higher-divorce-rates

Nardin, Bo. (2015, July 24). 7 Life Lessons I Have Learnt from Jim Rohn Which Greatly Improved My Life. Lifehack, Lifehack. Retrieved September 19, 2017, from http://www.lifehack.org /274141/7-life-lessons-have-learnt-from-Jim-Rohn-which-greatly-improved-life

Nightingale, Earl." The Strangest Secret - Advantedge Article By Earl Nightingale." Nightingale Conant: World Leader in Success, Personal Development, and Motivation.

P21. (n.d.). Framework for 21st-century learning. Retrieved September 19, 2017, from http://www.p21.org/our-work/p21-framework

Paradox. (n.d.). In Wikipedia. Retrieved September 19, 2017, from https://en.wikipedia.org/wiki/Paradox

Peterson, Deb. (n.d.). Do You Practice the 5 Principles of Adult Learning When You Teach? ThoughtCo. Retrieved September 19, 2017, from https://www.thoughtco.com/principles-for-the-teacher-of-adults-31638

Qigong. (n.d.). In Wikipedia. Retrieved September 19, 2017, from https://en.wikipedia.org/wiki/Qigong

Ricard, Matthieu. Altruism: the Power of Compassion to Change Yourself and the World. ATLANTIC BOOKS, June 2016.

Robbins, Anthony. Awaken the Giant within How to Take Immediate Control of Your Mental, Emotional, Physical & Financial Destiny! Simon & Schuster Paperbacks, 2013.

Rohn, Jim (2017, March 3). Rohn: 7 Personality Traits of a Great Leader." SUCCESS. Retrieved September 19, 2017, from , http://www.success.com /article/Rohn-7-personality-traits-of-a-great-leader

Shapiro, Jordan. (2015, March 26)." This Year At The 'Davos of Education.' Plus, The 16 Most Critical 21st Century Skills." Forbes, Forbes Magazine. Retrieved September 19, 2017, from https://www.forbes.com /sites/jordanshapiro/2015/03/22/this-year-at-the-Davos-of-education-plus-the-16-most-critical-21st-century-skills/#18a2d64b3ff1

Six Basic Principles. (n.d.). The US Constitution. Retrieved September 22, 2017, from http://theconstitutionpolik6.weebly.com/6-basic-principles.html.

Tai chi. (n.d.). In Wikipedia. Retrieved September 19, 2017, from https://en.wikipedia.org/wiki/Tai_chi

Tao Te Ching Quotes. (n.d.). Goodreads. Retrieved September 19, 2017, from https://www.goodreads.com/work/quotes/100074-d-o-d-j-ng

Tao Te Ching. (n.d.). In Wikipedia. Retrieved September 19, 2017, from https://en. wikipedia.org/wiki/Tao_Te_Ching
Tao Yin. (n.d.). In Wikipedia. Retrieved September 19, 2017, from https://en. wikipedia.org/wiki/Tao_yin
Tao. (n.d.). In Wikipedia. Retrieved September 19, 2017, from https://en. wikipedia.org/wiki/Tao
Teach: Make a Difference. (n.d.). Teacher Personality. Retrieved September 19, 2017, from https://teach.com/who/great-teachers-have-personality/
Temple of the Five Immortals (Shiyan). (n.d.). In Wikipedia. Retrieved September 19, 2017, from https://en.wikipedia.org /wiki/Temple_of_the_Five_ Immortals_(Shiyan)
The 7 Habits of Highly Effective People(n.d.). In Wikipedia. Retrieved September 19, 2017, from https://en.wikipedia.org/wiki/The_7_Habits_of_Highly _Effective_People
Thirteen virtues. (n.d.). Retrieved September 19, 2017, from http://www. thirteenvirtues.com/
User, Super. (n.d.)." Ten Traits of a Great Teacher." Catholic Education Resource Center. Retrieved September 19, 2017, from http://www.catholiceducation.org/en/education/catholic-contributions/ten-traits-of-a-great-teacher.html
Wu Xing. (n.d.). In Wikipedia. Retrieved September 19, 2017, from https://en. wikipedia. org/wiki/Wu_Xing

Part XIV: Questions, answers, and some advice

Here are some useful piece pieces of advice about the techniques; which I usually give to the readers to answer their questions about how to help children with problems.

1. The ten effective ways to help children with problems

Firstly, you should seek advice from specialists before any intervention. They will guide you in the right way. Listen and ask questions to get understanding the basic elements of the instructions from a specialist before applying.

Secondly, you should embrace the child and dance, dance in the melodies of fine music with child, kidding the child to create the laughter. People only laugh when they feel safe, which is the same as the child. Laughing is the most important indicator of happiness. Persistence, compassion, unconditional love, creating peace for the child, making friend with the child are the keys when playing with a child. Remember what you do in your childhood you will have the compassion for your child.

Still, keep the logic thinking of adults will not help you when playing with your child. The infant from two months old can understand some sound of the environment, they can understand that parents are talking to them or not. Try to talk as much as possible to your children this month. Try to create meaningless sound, noise, and spell the vowel words to catch the attention of your infant. Try to make the child want to express, eager to express by "uh", "ah", raise or move the mouth and smile. Play, talk with your children to recognize as soon as possible the early problems in your infant. If there is any strange signal, unnatural responses or behavioral problems, no need for the intervention of experts, just quiet your mind: by meditating, helping, giving, and letting go, them embrace your child. Embrace the pain, fear, and irritation of your child with love, kindness, and peaceful mind until your child feels peaceful, at ease and smile in your hands. This job only is done well by parents, the love and consideration of parents; husband and wife have to increase as much unconditional love, unconditional support, caring, touching, smiling, kissing as possible to create a warm, happy, supportive environment to save the infant child, mother, and family.

Thirdly, increasing the amount of time for your child to listen to classical music, meditation music is very good for brains, help to calm down the arousing mind. Watching meaningful movies with interesting dialogue and watching humor scripts with good meaning will stimulate the mind of your child with a warm feeling, and the urge to talk. Abandon the wailing films, violent films, and crucial films; these film can infect the mind of your child with negative images, negative feeling, even some child also feel sorrow and imitate bad habit of characters. Care about feeding your mind and your child's mind.

Fourthly, give your child more chances to have more fun, excitement daily. Increase the time nature, other children, animals, and crowd. There are some costs of dirty, scratches, tire, sneezing, runny nose or event mind pain. In fact, no pain no gain. Focus on the huge gain in the future you will gladly welcome this short-term cost. This is the part of the thinking of self-made millionaires; they want their child to experience pain from labor to gain in the future. Some even anger with the safety of their lazy child, because they understand the real facts to create a successful life. They aim at the long-term gain, by principles and visions in the future. If blindly seeing, we see them as selfish parents, but with results in the future, we will realize that they are the smartest parents. They are the master of the art of using pain, gain, love, crucial action, detachment from the ego. When pushing your child to the crowd, if he has signs of insecurity. We should hug, temple his emotion, make him feel safe enough to take the risk of joining. Do not blindly shout at your child and criticize him, which make him feel more unsafe.

Fifthly, train yourself to have peace, happiness, love, especially unconditional love before spend most of your time with your child is the best thing you can do for your child. Your state of mind will translate to your child's mind in many mysterious ways.

Sixthly, the child will learn very fast if you make him have the feeling of love, safety, happiness with the skills, or knowledge you want for the child. How many languages the child can speak if his father is American, his mother is Japanese and they live in Vietnam. If getting enough support, your child can gain an admiring achievement. If you have the skill to influence people, you will create more joy for your child with hard work and study. Results depending on the feelings the child has when studying and working. Some children feel of joy, happiness with the studying; and feelings of pain, lose, hurt with gaming, wasting they will study all day without forcing from parents or teachers, and gain a large amount of knowledge from the studying with less labor. On the other hand, some children feel of pain, hurt with the studying; and feelings of joy, delight with gaming, wasting they only can bear one or two hours of studying with the extreme forcing from parents and teachers, they only gain little knowledge from the studying with the huge effort. This is the meaning of relativity; people feel an hour of joy is short as a minute, and an hour of pain as long as a day. We can sense the relativity from your chatting with nice, smart and person and your other chatting with the bossy, stingy, and angry person. It is not only because of you in the feelings you have, it is also the person with talk to. The person you talk to, beauty or handsome does not relate much to your feeling; all lye in the art of understanding your needs, the art of satisfying your need to create the senses of happiness and joy during the conversation; and the art of controlling temptation to speak, do the things that make you anger or stress. Please pay attention to the art of living when dealing with the child, especially the child you think is naughty. Creating the feeling of love, safety and joy for the staff are the main jobs of leaders and managers in the organization.

Seventhly, replace old habits, which associated with comfort for the child, need to thoroughly understand the real causes, then gradually direct the child to other useful habits by the funny process of touching rewards and touching punishment. If there is a child likes to tearing paper, throwing things, cutting the fabric or beating friends; the main reason is that the child misunderstands the action, he associates the action with joy, comfort and does not notice to the pain and the cost he makes. It is a good way that parents can get to understand the child, patiently observe the child to get real facts from the action then rendering the art of influencing to help the child.

Eighthly, increase the amount and quality of time for your children by talking, crawling, jumping, making noise, hugging and kissing your children with fun and joy. Make your children feel safe and joyful enough that the children start to smile, speak "Gugu gaga", or senseless words, it is fine because the child only talks when feeling safe and happy. You can mimic your child's words and actions with the smile to encourage them because these are the actions person in happiness. Sometimes embracing your child and dance with music can help a lot for both of you. Eliminate all things, which may deplete the quantity and quality of time you spend for your children. Remembering the needs, experiences from your childhood will create empathy for your children and make your actions more naturally. if you think that these silly actions can harm your reputation as a successful person, remove the doubt by reading the stories about Albert Einstein, Richard Branson, and many other happy people.

Ninthly, the parent can borrow punishment with nasty children. It is fine, but they should pay attention to avoid violent, crucial fines, they should punish in mindfully to have a better understanding and find out other effective solutions. Do not punish because of anger. Considering punishment is the opportunity to increase your emotional account in your children mind. Do not blindly punish your children to satisfy your anger, your ego. Blind punishment, violating the principles can deplete all your emotional bank account in your children. Always smile to break the tension if needed. The misery in life causes desire, anger, and ignorance. The ignorant child will have a lot of desires; if the desires are not satisfied, the child will be angry or stressful. Most of the rebellion of the child is the fruits of anger;

To some extent, the rebellion can help the child calm the stress. If pay attention, parents can understand the unsatisfied need. The punishment the rebellious child with is hard for parents and can stop the unwanted action temporarily. Most of the skillful parents use the unconditional love, patience and compassion remove the root of rebellion; they are skillful in teaching their child to remove the ignorance.

Tenthly, have notebooks to write these four things. Divide the notebooks into for parts, There will be invaluable advice and knowledge and inspiration when have time reviewing these notes. Do not lazy in writing. Do not trust your memory. Use narrative writing, make the writing clearly with 5WH: who, what, when, why and how.

A. The good things you do each day. You do to help others, the disable or anyone needed help. Each day does at least three good work, cherish hopes of good for your child to help him have the strength to overcome the problem. The parents of the autistic child can use the good work they do each day to talk to their child. The stories may stimulate the child mind, urge the child to want to talk.

B. Write down as much as possible the things you are grateful every day. Start to look at the bright side of the problem to write down. People feel wealthy and healthy with a grateful mind. These things may use to talk to your children.

C. Write down your events, thoughts, emotions and your actions; which are interesting and need to remember. Especially the thoughts, emotions you have in playing with your child. If busy, at least, jot down the facts, the thoughts, and feelings.

D. Write down in detail as possible about your children's development, personality and temperament. The actions, the emotions, and reaction appear before, during and after acting, and if interrupted from outside. These are invaluable knowledge about your children that create understanding. Understanding is very useful for intervention.

Completing these notes will create huge joy and happiness for you directly, your children and relatives indirectly.

2. Love is the verb, right understanding is unconditional love, how to get the right understanding?

Love is the action. It means when you love someone. You should put heart in the action you do for your lovers. Love is serving with heart. We have to learn the love of Jesus, Buddha, and Mother Teresa. They have real love; they love people without any expectation, which called unconditional love. When a man loves a woman, he has love in all actions like serving, caring, flirting, making a surprise, helping, motivating, sharing, respecting. Real love no need of return.

Mother Teresa did not demand anything when helping the one needed help. From caring, helping she gained the greatest joy and happiness than any bodies else. With love, everything was the marvel to her; she found joy and happiness in everything, the power of love so great that she created the greatest legacy with little resources. Love is action, a man in love find joy and happiness in any actions they do for their lover. He finds happiness in responsibility also. We can easily imagine a man in happiness in every action; he is dancing, jumping, smiling, cheering, singing, walking and opening too many things. The individual in love never thinks of doing any harm to the lover. The observer can easily see the pattern of happiness in the action of a man in love. Mother loves her child unconditionally; she can sacrifice her life to save her child in danger. Her love is immeasurable. A girl does not need to see ask advice to know if he loves her, just finding is the happiness in him staying stay with you when doing with you. He is controlled by the highest emotion so that he can do many silly things. If he loves you, play with you with too much consciousness, perhaps he does not love you enough.

If people in love but expect in return: "I serve her, I care for her, I give her flower. In return, I want her to do good to me. She does not do good to me, it makes me a little bit sad." Hold on, she does not do good back to you, and you said. You see, love with expecting is like exchanging. IT IS NOT LOVE AS YOU ILLUSIVELY THINK. Expecting can kill your love. With expectation, you do thing consciously, you are pulling out of the moment of taking action to the expectation: lack of mindfulness. It makes the action unnaturally. If you receive less than expectation, you can become angry, you can harm her.

The fact is, love with expectation mean "I love myself" not "I love her". It is a selfish love, greedy love. People misunderstand that they love themselves but they think they love others. Sometimes they think they do good action in love as a sacrifice. The greedy love can hurt for both. Love that is still clinging, giving but still looking forward to receiving, waiting for returning is the love of selfish person; it is not generous love to others, but the selfish love for themselves. The selfish love making people feel pain or hard in the action. When making the action of love instead of finding happiness as the unconditional love, they find pain, hard work or even misery. It looks like an exchanging in the relationship. With unconditional love or real love, people find happiness, joy and energy in action for both doer and receiver. On the other hand, with selfish love, to some extent, people find misery, pain and exhausted in action. Selfish love can create misery or stress for both people. So that if a girl read any signs caused by happiness chemical from a man when he thinks or dates with her, it means he likes or love her; because he is doing the things that he loves the most. The belief deep inside harmony with the outside action to create the action, he finds happiness. If a girl can find any signs of stress chemical from a man when he is dating or doing kind work to her, it means that he finds stress in action, deep belief inside contradict with outside activities. He has to use a conscious mind alone to take action, it is exhausted, overworked, sometimes can make him stress. The experienced people can see the pretending smile from him, or have the gut feelings when hearing he laughs.

People tell lie to have the stress signal also. Observe ordinary people telling lies, we can find the embarrassing behaviors in them. The unconscious mind detects the mind bad consequences from the lying, so it creates the signal of a little stress. People telling lie do not have eye contact, do not see direct eye to eye, the pupil shrinks, tension muscle, up the heartbeat, sweating and many other symptoms of stress, so that the words are not naturally. The degree of symptoms stress may vary a lot from people to people. The experienced individual can have the feeling of chill or gut feeling if he sees a man telling lies, which may lead to serious consequences, without any stress signal on the face, voice or gestures and without the signal of emotion. The experienced man will pay special attention to him.

Parents also need unconditional love for their children. The conditional love express: "parents love you so you need to do this", and "parents love you so you need to do that to make parents happy." to make your parents happy; otherwise, children will be fined, beaten, burned books, torn clothes if the children do not obey the order of parents and adults. Look closely, they are invisible braces that splint the arms and legs of their children. Selfish parents make children eat, work and study without any passion, no curiosity, and no excitement. They just follow the instructions of adults. Kids are like the puppets of their parents; parents use love, orders, rewards, punishments, and emotion to control the puppets. Sadly, in Vietnam, the kids have many splints from their adults like grandparents, parents, brothers, sisters, friends, and teachers; who are so blindly violating the basic need of freedom of the kids; the need of freedom they forget that they also ask for and complain all day at work, clubs, and in society because of lacking freedom.

We use love as splints to splint the two legs, the two hands and the behaviors of our children unconsciously. Interfere the kids' behaviors by their parents may create passive children; because parents dictate the children what to do and what not to do because of their love; kids rarely make anything by themselves so that they are very self-deprecatory, low self-esteem. Kids never have the sense of conquest, of victory to proud of, they get everything done by their parents. The blind love of parents take all the chance for hands, legs, eyes, ears, and head to do its job; parents repeatedly serving for their children to satisfy unwanted needs of their children; they unconsciously spoilt their children. Kids grow up in an environment where everything is ready-made by parents not only lack the skills but also have much more wants, desires than normal kids. When the desires are not satisfied, kids become angry with screaming, shouting, rebelling to ask for things they want. Time after time, parents with selfish love blindly create bad habits for their kids with too many desires, anger and ignorance; these are the causes of misery.

Lao Tzu taught "instructions without interference". We as parents should draw out the destinations, expectations, visions, with the principle and values, then use love and patience to encourage our children and let them do their own. Our love and support are good enough for the kids to feel safe to take more challenge in life. Our children will surprise us with their creativity and ingenuity. The temperaments like self-confidence, self-esteem, self-reliance, initiative and proud of victory created by the process of working. Do not love your children so blindly that make tired, harmful to children and related individuals.

Stephen Covey taught about how to heal the relationship in the family for a husband: "love her" "But I do not love her anymore" "Dear friend, you are wrong, love is a verb; love is action, not emotion. People are in love have passionate action for the one they love" "so if you have to love her to heal relationship, you have to take numerous action to care for her: making her surprised, taking care of her, picking her up, dating with her, taking care the children for her, helping her the housework. Many think you can do if you really want to relive the love. Do it unconditionally."

With children having problems need the unconditional love from their parents the most to repair the problems inside. They are need guiding without interfering with their parents when they have done the work, they feel proud and confident from inside. The children having the problem already have the problem so that parents should not expect too much from them. The unsatisfied expectation can make parents anger and hurt, which in return will hurt the children. Love your kids without condition; welcome all the good things and bad things to your children, celebrate with them, guiding without interfering, give support to make kids feel safe enough to take more action, to make changes and corrections if needed. Especially the children with the mental problem, who are in stress, need so much love, connection and support from parents to have the feeling of happiness. The happiness and the chemical of happiness secreting in the brain and body is the best cure for mental problems. When taking action of love, practice three things: simplicity, patience, and compassion.

3. Problem-solving skills: are you learning the root or learning tops? New view

Many people complain that they have a lot of work, backing home with many works. Flooding in work, study, and family, they do not have free time for themselves. They start learning problem-solving skills. Once applied, life seems easier and lighter than before. In fact, if looking back they are still busy or busier than before. What are the real solutions? What are the bottlenecks need removing?

Problem-solving skills are taught:

After hundreds of blah blah from the teachers, we realize the problems are outside. Problems from family is not ideally happy, sisters do not unite, conflicting all day, spoiled children; my spouse, my children, and my boss do not listen to me; the job is too hard, the price is too expensive, the price escalates, life is difficult due to political instability, politicians, government. Even worse, people blame for the million stars shined in the wrong ways from twenty to fifty years ago when they were born. We find endless sources for our problems from outside. Then we start solving rigidly with the 5WH technique, with a lot of efforts, resources put in to solve the problems. After a while, exhausted from the unsolved problems, or even problems getting bigger and bigger, we stuck to extreme stress. We are ineffective in solving problems. So what is the real problems?

This reminds me of cutting trees. The trees are like your problems; tree of problems in the family, in work and in society. We start to cut down the problem tree. A tree has three parts are roots, stem, and leaves. The ineffective ones carry the ax cut trees in the leaves, tops, and flowers. They can mobilize a lot of people into cutting down foliage, breaking down branches with hundreds of people, tens of years, billions of dollars. People take place hundreds of miscellaneous things around the problem tree with the hope of the tree will die. The tree is still there, although they mobilize a lot of wealth, resources and people. Many useless rewards and conferences have put forth. Useless rewards used for tiny and small achievement which are misunderstood that the milestone achievement.

The problem solved effectively when people cut the ax into the trunk or the root of the tree. One, two, three, four, and five minutes of cutting with about one hundred cuts, with only two people and the tree fall down.

"Oh you really do not need to do this fast, so quickly like that, this is where we get paid for; this is the source of our income. We are paid by time." Moreover, "you are less recognized, praised and less rewarded."

With the metaphorical image above, the skills learned above are important but not critical; it is equivalent to using axes to cut the leaves of the problem tree; it is hard but ineffective but ineffective people get the most rewards. It can call the paradox for effective and ineffective people.

The decisive factor in solving the problem is not the problem but the individuals who solve the problem. When looking at correlations of solving the problem, let compare the magnitude of the individual and the magnitude of the problem. Moving a ten kilograms stone is a big deal for a small child or a dwarf, but moving a ten kilograms stone is a small problem for an adult or an athlete. Another example is the fifth-grade problem is difficult for students in grade fourth but is a simple problem for students in grades sixth or seventh. Is the problem of reducing difficulty? No problem is still the same, is the problem solver that has matured over time. In the field of life, there are such problems as fatherhood, motherhood, husbandry, self-management, financial management, and spiritual management. Do you say that you are good at solving these problems? If yes, I do not believe much, look at the emotions, the mood of those around you relating to the problem. When I self-arrogate, I often remind myself "Vietnam is a developing country or actually poor country, I am an average member in the country, in society and in the industry; I live in an average apartment in Vietnam, having an average living, which means I have poor thinking in some extent. So please do not be angrily and aggressively defends my point of views - the view of poverty. Do not force others to follow my expectation".

"I am wrong, not only with wrong actions. The deepening roots of misery are my wrong thoughts; the wrong thoughts creates wrong assumptions; the wrong, assumption creates wrong expectation; the unsatisfied wrong expectation creates wrong emotion; the wrong, emotion creates wrong actions; the actions create misery and stress in life. Wrong things compound with wrong things unconsciously. So the most effective way is I need to learn more to remove my ignorance". This is my best reminder to help me from the action at the tempting moment.

Mastering or cutting off the root of the problem here is to enhance the individual's capacity or individuality. Make them bigger than the problems. Instead of complaining that there are too many things, too many problems need to solve; let identifying your small, your foolishness or your ignorance, which real things need to adjust. You need to do more, practice more, challenge more, accumulate more skills, gain more wisdom and achieve the enlightenment. According to many authors, identifying the right sources of the problem has helped solve fifty percent of the problem.

From the authors' teaching, we can find out how to cultivate the best in process of personal development. Here are some of the ways I collected:

First, Jim Rohn and Brian Tracy recommend have a learning library, lifelong learning, goal - setting, and university on the wheel.

Jim Rohn recommended a library of books, notebooks, and photos, to read, to think and to recite at least 30 minutes a day, several hours a week, one weekend at the end of the month and 2-3 weekend days of the end of the year. Work hard in creating a library, creating a diary. You will not remember the content of the lecture or interesting conference last week, last month or last year. Trust me, if you listened to an interesting lecture a year ago, you will not be able to remember ten percent of that message if you did not record or review in previous time. Please try! Do not trust your memory. Setting goals, when achieving goals, the goals are not important anymore but the person you become when achieving your goals.

Brian Tracy recommends spending at least 30 minutes a day to read the knowledge related to the skill you want to improve. Try to read a lot, one month read at least one to three books. After one year, you have a large amount of knowledge. He used the number of reading books to illustrate, to get the doctorate, learners have to read and study approximately fifty-five books. If you read and apply fifty-five books in the skill you want to improve, you are already a self-studied doctor. Interestingly, what you are self-motivated is much more effective than the motivation from the pressure from the environment. Learning because of wanting of desiring with the enthusiasm of passion, self-discipline is far more effective than the formal learning; because these are the vital ingredients creating great achievement.

In addition, Brian Tracy also mentions "university on the wheel", meaning that every day we move at least 2-3 hours, if in the car that we listen to audiobook, interesting ideas from books, conferences or teachings. One month we have approximately ninety hours of studying, after a year we have about one thousand hours of studying, which are equivalent to the number of credits in a year of studying in college. University on wheels, after nearly ten years of listening, people can have ten thousand hours of learning, they will become outliers. Read the "outliers" of Malcolm Gladwell to understand the concept of ten thousand hours.

Secondly, sources are western philosophy, oriental philosophy and street philosophy. Streets, crowds, life, nature is the place to practice, to contemplate and to apply what we learn and read. Life needs contemplation, testing, and adjustment. Always pay close attention to the PDCA in everything: planning, doing, checking and adjusting. Skillful in apply the lessons from Buddha, Jesus Christ, Mother Teresa, Confucius, Lao Tzu, Socrates, Plato and many other great men, who create the foundations of modern philosophy. Their teaching contains empathy, love, persistence, generosity, serving heart, dedication, simplicity, self - discipline, principle, virtues, compassion, humility; which are enduring values.

Thirdly, we can gain wisdom and enlightenment by practicing meditation. In a lot of teaching of Buddha; and the follower of Buddha are Dalai Lama, Thich Nhat Hanh, and Matthieu Ricard, people can easily practice and take the most advantage of meditation. People can create joy, happiness, and peace of mind from meditation. The scientists can control the focus of the mind, have a better view of themselves so that they will not fall into the trap of thinking.

Fourthly, Seth Godin, John C Maxwell, Daniel Goleman, Stephen Covey, Tony Robbin, Albert Einstein, Thich Nhat Hanh, and many other extraordinary authors. They mention EQ: emotional intelligence, PQ: passion intelligence, AQ: adapting intelligence and SQ: spiritual intelligence. These are the abilities to master one's emotions, to master the self; the ability to lead others, the ability to interact with people, environment to create the wanted changes. The individuals mastered AQ, EQ, PQ, SQ is the leaders in society. In addition, they also recommend that children and adults should remain the precious characters: endless curiosity; creativity, skillfully in asking the question; nourishing the imagination and keeping the spirit of the young child inside. These are the channels to keep the energy run smoothly between individuals and the environment. Use these channels people can stimulate the ideas directly to the unconscious mind, create happy emotion long before the conscious mind know what is happening. The smoother the energy, the better the body, family, and organization are. Parents can nourish these qualities in their children much more effective than the schools do. These qualities can be safe for the rigid of modern education. Pay attention to lead, learn and act so that you and others around you have these qualities of endless curiosity; creativity, skillfully in asking the question; nourishing the imagination, keeping the spirit of the young child inside, and the intelligence of AQ, PQ, SQ, EQ.

4. How do parents affect their children?

LETTER TO PARENTS

Dear parents,

Thank you very much for your love, your interest in the children in the family, here are some insights and suggestions on how to love children in the right way.

From the top educators, they all assert that children develop character in the first 6 years of life. Especially the first three years, the children are born as pieces of white paper, where adults who love children can draw on easily with the love, compassion, rewards, and punishment. Have you ever asked why developed countries have good welfares for children and mothers after giving birth? Understanding that the quality of living the small children create the good characters, which will shape the quality of the nation in future, advanced people consider the children not only belong to the parents, the children but also are the precious property of the nations. The parents, who are well educated about caring and loving children, know how to love their children in the right way. Unfortunate for the children in developing countries, adults do not know these understanding, so that the children are nourishing casually, carelessly or even crucially. It is not standard of living or the love of parents making the difference of living in the small children, but the understanding. It will be great for small children if their parents gain an understanding of loving the right way.

As a result, Vietnamese corporations have to hire the 1970s or 1980s children are invited to work with a salary of one hundred to two hundred million dongs per month (5000$ - 10000$ per month), to manage the 1970s and 1980s Vietnamese children. Vietnamese children like you and me and our friends with the salary of from three, five to ten million dong per month (from 100$ to 500 $ per month)

Have you ever measured how much our generation lost?

This is the visible loss in hundreds of visible losses, which we have to bear. Sadly, the hundreds of visible losses compare with the real losses are like the top of the iceberg to the iceberg. We can sense endless misery in daily life, in the newspaper, in media, which are the result of our ignorance, of misunderstanding lead to mistreating our children. With wrong interpretation, lack of understanding, we as the parents creating millions of loses for our children unconsciously without noticing. If we are not awake, our disadvantages and losses will become the disadvantage of our descendants. Most of the western children also bear the losses, if you look at the gaps of ordinary people with the successful ones you will see the losses. The ordinary people to some extent they are lacking some skills so that they are the products of the environment.

Teachers in developed countries, teach in nursery school and elementary school, need a higher degree than the teachers in high school, at least a master degree. They seem as educators, they educate children with ethic, virtue, and characters. On the other hand, teachers in high school seem like trainers, they train students with skills. The new kindergarten teachers properly called Educators because they are shaping the personality of a human being. In Vietnam, it is quite the reverse, so I hope you not only play the role of parents but also the role of educators.

There are two exercises and suggestions I would like you to practice with your children:

First, imagine you have a magic wand, you can swing and turn your children become anyone who they can become like politicians, entrepreneurs, educators, reformers, innovators, or the individuals you admire. What kind of characters do your children have? They can be some of these: confidence, independence, bravery, sharp thinking, creativity, humor, enthusiasm, charisma, great attitude, and the virtues of a leader. To have these characters, you are in the role of shaping: What is the specific work that you do daily, monthly and annually do for your children, when your children are one-year-old, two-years-old, three-years-old and so on until they become mature.

There is a fact I always remind ourselves: "there will be those born in 2012, or 2016, after thirty to forty years later, some of them will become the prime ministers, the presidents, the directors, the leaders, the composers, the musicians, and the successful people. On the other hand, some of them can also become guards, motorbike carriers, taxi drivers, transporters, dullards, criminals, and drug addicts.

Just slicing of our society to observe, there will be varieties kind of people like described in society, who born in the 1960s, 1970s, and 1980s were like angels. After time looking after, teaching and caring in the families and society, under the good ways of respecting, love, encouragement, praise, gradually raising the challenge, have the opportunity to communicate, experiencing and open their own eyes. Unconsciously, under wrong way being abusive, being crucial punished, insulting, poorly labeled, negative affirming and without respect. Our societies in countries all over the world with a lot of dark sides and bright sides are now the results. Do not just criticize the regime, society. I affirm that now is the best regime in Vietnam and the world. We gain the most advancement in the last three hundred years; there is no time in the past better than this time of the present. Most of the results are due to the family's identity, the influences of parents, relatives, environment and the way of using resources during the early stage of life of our children. Sometimes we do the good influences consciously, most of the time we make bad influences unconsciously.

Looking at our angels, I think there is nothing impossible with them. Things that they think impossible or cannot later in life are thoughts mainly forced by adults, accidentally or intentionally loaded in children's head. Adult use rewards and punishment make the coercion, the obligation, the prohibition, the blindly love, screaming and shouting with anger and the irrational reaction to gradually forming their beliefs. Our ways are quite different from that of parents living in the mansion, the millionaires, or billionaires, parents on the world.

Do not give trust in television and movies, mesmerizing movies, scandals, and negative news. Be wary of media and television, the main purpose of the television is to compete to get more viewers. The mind has characters attracted to negative news, not interested much with good news. Therefore, the negative stuff full of the media and television; it is easy to get and have the highest appeal. There will be no bright men, or positive people watch television all day. Their level of lucidity decreases as they exposure to cheap films and negative news on television. We can figure out that the top farmers, artists, lecturers, experts, speakers, professors, and politicians rarely spend time on television, especially with negative media. Negative television can be a resource of negative energy that infuses negative energy to all aspects of our lives unconsciously. We can sense the negative energy if we pay attention.

Second, you also have a role as subordinates and the employees in the company, you often have desires, feelings, and expectations from your superiors. Sometimes you also bear the shamefulness and anger from your ignorant managers. In fact, your children have the same desire, feelings, and expectations of you. Sometimes, your children also bear the shamefulness and anger from your ignorance. At work, you have the feelings of joy, excitement, enthusiasm or sadness and disappointment in the interaction with your managers, which lead to the quality of work; at home, sometimes your children have the same feelings, which lead to the quality of your children's life. Conflict is hard to avoid, but the role of the person in charge of the interaction can make the differences in the conflict. Your children expect you to pay attention to their emotions, needs, thoughts, and aspirations in solving the conflict; the good marks or bad marks you leave in solving the conflicts, which are high in emotion and attracted attention, can contribute the biggest influence to your children's life. Anything from emotions, thoughts, to beliefs you have created in your children, will form the characters of your children in the future.

Stay mindfulness to observe your motivations, thoughts, feelings, and expectation in every situation, review it every night; you will have a lot of ideas and right emotions to talk to your children. The quality of the conversation and interaction compound with time will make the big differences in your children. Be aware of the observation, and learn from your experiences to gain compassion, love, and patience to play with your children.

As you see the best present give to your child is your signs of progress every day. There will be happy children if they have the best parents, who become better every day, every month, and every year. Good parents lead to good brothers, good neighbors, good grandparents, and most important is the parents themselves. Good parents understand themselves, their children, and life enough that they can help their children with problems

Good parents have the habits of learning, reading, good characters and good habits described in the book "Seven habits of highly effective people" of Stephen Covey, of which child will observe and learn very quickly by imitation form their parents. Researchers show that children learn very quickly through imitation: the words, behaviors, gestures, or even curses from parents and environment, they learn very quickly with the process of rewards and punishments. They learn so quickly that three years old children have the amount of vocabulary that foreigners have to learn from five to ten years to get that amount of vocabulary. If parents are from two differences countries, their children can speak fluently two languages easily when they are five years old. In addition, children also have bad parental habits. Just by observing the small children and adults separately in a party, observers can easily match which children belong to which parents by the behaviors, habits, and tone of voice. In addition to learning through imitation, children are also excited to learn through all the five senses like holding objects, touching, biting and tasting by mouths; interesting sounds and light can attract the attention of children too. Children have an endless curiosity for learning and observing the environment if parents encourage and support them. Owing to the safe and interesting environment that parents give to children, with the enthusiasm, endless curiosity of the children, the children can learn many things in a very short time compared to the adults. Please meet the curiosity of children, welcome the discomfort you have. With the question that you do not know the answer, you can ask for help from other people or work with your children to find the answers, do not disappoint your children, do not interrupt the flow of energy in your children. The more energy flow in your children's body, the better, the healthier your children are. The small children have a lot of energy, energy need to nourish by actions; this is the reason why small children ask, talk, play, run, jump and study all day without tired. The more support of parents, the better the energy.

When the children suppressed by the environment, they start to suppress the energy, they do not ask, do not talk, do not run, do not jump, and do not study. The approximate illustration is a three years old child asks a hundred questions a day endlessly without tired. After threatening, denying, and punishing by the environment; the five years old child asks only ten questions a day; the ten years old child is so afraid to ask that only ask three questions a day. The students labeled as ignorant students in the class, never asked, or questioned how to solve the problem; they lose the important skills in life, going to school or work, they never dare to ask any question so they never get the right answers. The labeled ignorant students have the patterns of behaving the same as the patterns of the old, which seem like poor energy, they do not ask or question any unwanted things. We are as the parents need to relive the energy in these children with love, encouragement, funny actions, and joyful environment.

In nature, softness, weakness, eager to learn and curiosity are the indicators of life and development. Rigidity, conservatism, stiffness, refusing to learn and lack of curiosity are the indicators of death and recession. We can see these indicators in water and rock, small plants and the old plants, the young and the old. Einstein taught "curiosity and imagination are the save of traditional education." So please encourage and satisfy the curiosity of your children; and nourish the imagination with the fairy tales.

Do not work so hard but ineffective, just teach your children and form the good habits in family-like creativity, positive feedback, sharing, loving, supporting, open communicating, not attacking personal, and focusing on solving the problems. As parents, you need to create fun and excitement in the formation of these characters. Remember to enhance self-esteem and confidence in your children by making children feel important; always praise, encourage, appreciate your children. In interaction, pay attention to justice, respect, kindness, generosity, and love. Do not let your children experience feelings of fear and inferiority because of comparing. If you remember the past events solving your problems with your parents, you will understand and compassionate the thoughts, feelings, and desires of your children in a difficult time. Because the children have the same basic needs, thoughts, feelings, and desires as you when you were in childhood.

These are some of my ideas, thank you for listening, I hope that you will remind me when I break the rules, and I will not mind to remind you if you commit any mistake.

Few people realize in Vietnamese song:

"Parents are the shield,

Protect entire the child's life."

This deep-rooted insight is in stark contrast to the western way of teaching and caring for children. We need to remove for the children to have the chance to develop. In difficulty, children have chances to use the function of hands, legs, eyes, ears and all other senses, and the brain to think. If parents protect their children every day because they are afraid of their children can get hurt when doing and solving the problem, they accidentally take away all the chances to develop the children' ability.

You need to take time to contemplate on these views.

First is extremely cruel, extremely loving - the book title

Second is shallow looking catch the love, but looking deep, we can realize, To some extent, it is extreme cruelty; some parents love their children so blindly that their love destroys the characters of the children, they force children to adopt the things which they think are good for their children. Cursing and comparing in hope that children will do better, crucially forcing the children to eat a large number of foods at all cost, raising children as fatty as possible. This is the heartless love, selfish love; parents use violence in the mask of love to force the children the things parents want but do not care much about what the children want. Love that goes with crucial forcing without understanding the children can hurt the children the most.

The third is how to make your children have passion and love for learning, working and training. Passion and love are only gain through kind guidance, compassion, open-mindedness from parents to wake up responsibility and compassion in children. People with passion can create extraordinary results.

Excellent students like studying, working and training. In the mind of excellent students, they match studying, learning, and working with fun and excitement; moreover, they attach enjoying, useless playing, playing the game online, wasting time with the suffering and misery. If they play and waste time, they will sense the loss of time to reach their goals, they will sense the pain from missing the visions, they can feel the pain their parents will bear, and the misery their family will suffer. They can feel imaginative misery as strong as real misery. The pain bearing in future is far bigger than the joy of enjoying or playing the game. In the equation of cost and benefit in taking the decision, good students always have enough good clues to make good decisions. These students do not need strict management from their parents.

On the other hand, students with poor results are afraid of studying, thinking, working, and training. In their mind, they misconceive learning, studying, training with pain, fatigue, and exhaust. They conceive useless playing, playing the game, wasting time, and habit of destroying with fun and excitement. If they play and waste time, they will not sense any loss of time, they do not care much in finding, and pursuing the goals, they will not sense any pain from missing the blur visions, they can feel no pain even their parents have to bear in future. They feel the temporary joy and excitement of the playing, destroying, and wasting time. They are not familiar with the hard works needing effort, concentration, and contemplation; they feel extreme pain and boredom with studying, thinking, working and training. The temporary pain and joy collect from the present. In the equation of cost and benefit in taking a decision, bad students always have enough clues of temporary pain and joy, which are combining into bad decisions and bad actions. These bad students have a huge amount of energy that has been suppressed for years, it is like the flow of water; if being suppressed too much, even with thick, strong dam of rules; one day the energy can break out the dam with extreme power and making the children rebel unconsciously leaving the extreme wounds for everybody. These students do need management from their parents with love, compassion, patience, and understanding. These are vital elements to direct the wild energy to the useful routes. The parents skillful in parenting can create benefit changes in their rebelling children. Reading the stories of many successful men, we can see the turning point in their life owning for the love, compassion, considering, patience and understanding from the skillful people. The skillful people can be their parents, relatives, heroes or anyone they accidentally met.

Fourth is it leads a management perspective "management is an excessive act if the group is well-lead." In my point of view, this management perspective is also true for the family. The good leader is one of the explanations that some families gain outstanding achievement and happiness with leisure in action and less effort. On the other hand, the family with the bad leader, people work hard all day, tired without any comfort; gains no happiness, little achievement even putting the huge effort into action.

Fifth is in psychology, people often do or take action to make them feel comfortable and happy, and people avoid doing things that cause the feeling of pain or discomfort. To some extent, some bad habits like smoking cigarettes, drinking alcohol, addicting drugs, playing the game, or rebelling can satisfy some of the needs of the children, the satisfaction of needs can make children feel joyful or happy. These bad habits can help them to create a feeling of comfort so that when in stress, these kids want to find these bad habits to make them feel at ease. So that the effective way of quitting the addiction is having the support, compassion, and love from people around, which are helpful in creating supporting environment to prevent the stress, and the helping if needed when stress comes.

It would be great if you, your family, schools and your society could create the feeling of fun, excitement and meaningful in the studying and work for your children; and create the feelings of hatred, pain or regret in smoking, playing video games, addicting, wasting time and overeating. Unfortunately, the conscious or unconscious behaviors of Vietnamese parents make the children feel sick, tired and bored with working and studying. That is one of the reasons that many kids want to avoid working and studying and want to find the things that make them immediately feel joyful like watching television, playing the game online, playing gambling and rebelling. Understanding the motivators of actions, parents can think and observe to find the best way to change the bad habits in children to the good ones gradually, with little efforts but the most effective.

Sixth is when you learn and practice, you will gain understanding. On the process of learning and practicing, you will encounter with the concept of Pareto principle or the 80/20 principle, which is similar to "first thing first" of Stephen Covey, to find out and prioritize what is important first. In Jim Rohn teaching we can find this pattern: "successful people are major in major things and minor in minor things, and unsuccessful people are minor in major things and major in minor things.

These are my suggestions. I hope you can contemplate at a suitable time to help your children.

Let think how hard for parents of Mother Teresa, Mahatma Gandhi, Bill Gate, Steve Job, Warren Buffet, Mark Zuckerberg, many other self-made millionaires, activists, and the educators to raise their children to become self-made billionaires, self-made billionaires. When you find the right answers, you will understand the keys of advance education system of developed countries, the keys of mastery parents, the keys of leadership. Best of all, you have the chance to awaken that the highest art of action, simple is non-action.

5. I AM SORRY VICTIMS, WE ARE WRONG.

> **I love you**
>
> **I am sorry**
>
> **Please forgive me**
>
> **Thank you!**

Dear readers, fathers, mothers, teachers, educators, politicians and soldiers,

We are wrong; we need to change for our kids, our beloved ones, our people and ourselves.

When do all of us know and treat ADHD, Autism, Depression and Suicide, Homicide, Gunfire, autoimmune diseases, and all problems? And the hidden causes?

The world is spending half of it money: $ thousand billion on buying the weapon for finding safety, certainty or peace. Then they spend $ thousand billion on medicine, luxury products, cars, villas for find the feeling of significance, recognition, importance, and they spend other $ trillions on medication, drugs with the hope of sleeping well, relaxing, relieving, and enjoying the artificial comfort and happiness?

A stress moment can kill a student.

A stress moment can kill a banker

A stress moment can kill a CEO

A stress moment can kill a politician

They are strong but the severe stress moment can have an effect on all their life. It embeds in their brain, cells, organs that we do not consciously know but the subconscious mind know that moment: smell, sound, noise, invisible signal then create the conditioned responses to it. You see soldiers in the war ended 1950 are still under stress with any mild unwanted triggers.

Language, religions, accent, belief, behaviors, rituals, religions and funeral religions are the conditioned responses: you, your friend and partners have big differences in these: Will you dare to try to change with other people to enjoy their belief, rituals, and religions. Even the name of you and your dogs are results of Conditioned responses with languages. You like all of these because you have been conditioned, not because you like and chose these. The process of conditioning is so well and silently that you may illusively think you have the Ego,... You may die or sacrifice for the adopted assumption, belief, and religions. People are so ignorant that people in one family, community, region, district, class, city, countries are fighting for changing opinions.

Value of character: the kind of conditioned responses:

Discontented men react to good unwanted things discontentedly. "Discontented men may shout when seeing thorn in the bushes of roses."

Contented men have conditioned responses to response contentedly to any unwanted things, problems, and challenges. "Contented men happy, joyful and hope when seeing a rose in the bushes of thorns."

Value of character, the adjective of character: Discontented men react to good unwanted things discontentedly. Contented men have conditioned responses to response contentedly to any unwanted things, problems, and challenges. He is ADJECTIVE character means he conditioned ADJECTIVE responses or his responses to things adjectively.

Worst of all, he is intelligent but corrupt, means he finish well the corrupt works intelligent that no one until a hundred years later.

Seeing a girl with college education screaming and running away when seeing a cockroach I understand the useless of knowing or formal education. Seeing a small brave girl ready to fight with a thief, a dog to protect her friends and understand the value of characters.

But

They live in stress, eat in fear, sleep in anxiety, playing in the boring safe side, wear luxury clothes in discontentment, study with pressure, and sexing with contempt. They never find real joy and happiness.

Stress chemical: Adrenalin, noradrenalin, and cortisone. And happy chemicals: Endorphin, Dopamine, Serotonin, Oxytocin; these chemical secreted in the body according to the state of mind. If an individual changes the state of mind, they may change the chemical in the body. Chronic Stress people may get the serious side effect of Stress chemicals. List the effects, and side effects on the medical books we know the results of stress on the body.

Effects of Adrenalin: Sweating, Nausea and vomiting, Pale skin, Feeling short of breath, Dizziness, Weakness or tremors, Headache, Feeling of nervousness or anxiousness.

Effects of Norepinephrine: Pain, burning, Numbness, weakness, or cold, Slow or uneven heart rate, Trouble breathing, Vision, speech, or balance difficulties, Blue lips or fingernails, and Spotted skin.

Less serious side effects Cortisol: Acne, dry skin, or thinning skin, Bruising or discoloration of the skin, Insomnia, Mood changes, Increased sweating, Headache, Dizziness, Nausea, stomach pain.

Serious side effects cortisol: Vision problems, Swelling, Rapid weight gain, Shortness of breath, Severe depression or unusual thoughts or behaviors, Seizures, Bloody or tarry stools, Coughing up blood, Symptoms of pancreatitis: pain in your upper stomach that spreads to your back; nausea and vomiting; or fast heart rate.

Because of me, because of you I always enjoy these chemicals in eating, receiving, getting, giving, sleeping and enjoying.

In psychology, they overreact, want to be alone, and have abnormal behavior: it is the instinct of the weak in the stressful environment in the hope of find out safety for the self.

By observing, parents can know the early symptoms or pattern of stress, non-safety in children since they are one week, one month or two-month-old or three months old babies to predict the problems they will get: ADHD, Autism, depression or hysterical anxiety, so that you may know what, when and how to help your children mindfully. The family is the only place where the enemies sleep the same bed. But all will sleep with the stress hormones, very tired, terrible sleep: because they do not find trust or safety from the partner. It is devastating to both wife and husband. But the baby bears it all: the infant with the fragile, sensible brain. The immature brain is forming under stress.

"Because of you
I never stray too far from the sidewalk
Because of you
I learned to play on the safe side so I don't get hurt
Because of you
I find it hard to trust not only me but everyone around me
Because of you
I am afraid"

Kelly Clarkson: "because of you"
Happy kids are free to play, do, try, fail and have unconditioned support." They are safe to work"

Stressed kids are so fearful that they have to play in safe, learn in the clean, walk-in trail, and never fail. They have to bury the instinct nature: "They have to work to safe"

"All on one

One in all

Children are family

The family is a nation

A nation is a world"

Happiness chemicals:

Dopamine: get a goal, finish a task, and achieve a purpose, finish a job, win the lottery: gambling, betting. Get hits, like or good comment on Facebook, Get good grade. When you find a big bargain in a buying, your purple widen. Excessive dopamine can increase the heartbeat, ventricular arrhythmia, atrial fibrillation, ectopic heartbeats, Tachycardia, angina, palpitation, bradycardia, vasoconstriction, hypotension, hypertension, shaking or collapsing are listed on all pharmacology books.

When you are joyful or excited, you have Piloerection, Nausea, vomiting, Anxiety, Mydriasis – caused by dopamine.

Endorphin is the reward of labor.

Serotonin: comes when you get close contact: skin to skin, kiss, hugs, embracing, intimating acts, or the feeling of belonging and significance. Dogs can make the owner have this feeling. When doing good, kind, and helping others. An act of goodness: the doer, the receiver, and the watcher will have the feeling caused by this. Dopamine and Serotonin is the chemical that all psychic medication used to increase in patients. All medications for depression aim at increasing these.

Lastly, the chemical is oxytocin: sex, love, skin contact, and giving birth are high with this.

Scientists find that oxytocin may help autistic mice. they will do more research in the future to apply to the autistic child. They do not know that these happy chemicals are secreted when they treat well with each other with love, close contact, connection, supporting and trusting. Using smartwatches to know the emotion, thinking of people is the good suggestion by observing physical figures: heartbeat, blood pressure during the days, events, years and important Missions.

When people can sense the changes in the body with these chemicals- it called Gut Feelings: tighten the muscle, throbbing in head muscle, sweating or chill. It is there even we consciously know it or not as the conditioned responses with the environment

How about the fragile kid who is forming the immature brain in stress, best of all is calm stress down by

1. Unconditional love

2. Connection: people, animal, nature, parents

3. Unstressed environment: happy, warm, cheering; then make them have

4. Ability to deal with facts of life - the fact that some people may think is a big threat, problems, or danger

Simple breathing meditation helps children better than medication in ADHD and Autism. Father said: "the day autistic child happy he will less over-react than the stressful day."

Really good with meditation, it calms the mind and brings the mind to the body. Live in mindfulness by simple breath. Daniel Goleman the author of Emotional intelligence has told a story of applying simple breathing meditation in elementary school in chaos areas. It works. When you are in nervous, anxiety, people usually advise you to calm down and breath slowly, deeply.

How to start:

Observe the body when breathing in and out. Or stick a small object on the lower abdomen near then let the kid breath in and breath out with observing the moving of body This kind of breath bring the mind of kid back to present. The kid does not have to live with the fear or stress of the past or future. When the mind is at ease with the body, the good chemicals flush the brain and the body, then the whole repair the defect in the brain. Zen masters are the mind master.

Countless phenomena create an event but the organs of senses of people only catch a few varieties into the brain or mind. Then the neocortex interprets small part of data in the brain into sensual language: sound, image, senses, order, spaces, and movement to translate for the next generation, scientists called multiple intelligences. The sages and enlightened one is right when they said "they are smart because they do not know any things at all, then they start to accumulate facts for decisions, not accumulate distorted facts for stubborn assumptions. The more of thinking, doing, examining, and trying makes more connections inside the brain. Enough huge amount of connection in good quality makes the mind jump to a higher level of thinking: "Quantity of connection change enough create the change of quality in mind." Perhaps, it may take 10.000 hours as Malcolm Gladwell. Meditation is the exercise of the mind that creates enough connection creates the powerful brain that Tibetan monks can create the highest brain's brainwave "Gamma wave, this gamma wave only catch in seizure attack."

Enough connection the cognitive mind can understand the information in the subconscious mind that cannot express in words, sound, images and sensual feelings; they have sharpened the intuitive mind. Artists have the highest intuitive mind that they can do, write or paint the works that carry the message but hardly understood by most ordinary people. it is out of words, out of images, out of sound to describe the beauty or ugly of the artworks. No one can describe the beauty of the painting of Picasso worth $ 90 million for the blind men.

Meditation awakens the mind, meditation awakens the body, and meditation awakens the world. The family is the only place where the enemies sleep shares the same bed; they may sleep, eat, and enjoy stress. The fact is all will sleep with the stress hormone very tired, terrible sleep: because they do not find trust or safety from the partner. It is devastating to both wife and husband. But the baby bears it all: the infant with the fragile, sensible brain. The immature brain is forming under stress.

UNFORTUNATELY, THE LEVEL OF STRESS IN THE MIND IS UNLIMITED, BUT THE PREPARE OF THE PHYSICAL BODY IS LIMITED.

Then the autoimmune started ignorantly but incredible collectively.

When all are high, the organ may send the feedback signal to the brain to stop secreting hormones. The brain still wants to raise the level of preparation of the body to find safety in fight and flight, as the nation raises money to build weapon and army. The lower organs start to send the feedback to calm the mind and effects down to regulate blood pressure, blood glucose and remain Biological homeostasis. The hysterical mind does not want that, Immune system obeys the order of the brain to attack the normal cells. Autoimmune diseases started, wars started, stress started.

The pain inside out, stress inside out, live with some people may worsen than dying. All perceptions are relative. Some conditioned chose the negative side. Sorry, some of them choose suicide.

Worst of all: most victims are good people. Rarely prisoners commit suicide. They become the victims mainly because of their goodness, considering other, weakness and helplessness.

I am sorry!

I am sorry!

I am sorry!

We need to help them.

Just remember the moment of doing kindly to each other, kindness, respect, trust... described by the positive adjective or positive adjectively, all will going to sleep easily, happily, and peacefully. You do not teach healthy kids to learn the languages: English, Japanese, Chinese, and Vietnamese... but kids can make it become their instinct. Walking, thinking, studying countless skills: one-year-old kids, two-year-old kids, three-year-old kids never have to sit at the table to learn. But that time kids can learn more than anybody can imagine. Playing is learning, watching is learning, sleeping is learning, and doing is learning... Their most powerful tools are the weakness, beloved, cute, enthusiasm, pay attention, curiosity, asking, imagining, and learn, try, fail, think, learn, try, fail, think, learn, try, fail, think with joy, enthusiasm and never said a negative work. Seeing my friend with a college degree take five to ten year to learn English but fail in communicating with English, I realize that how potential our kids are if we let them freely as themselves. Just give them the needed basic ones, they will grow and develop incredibly. We need to accept to let them grow.

Thank for reading, I hope that we can be awakened by our beloved people.

Contents

Awaken parents – the conversation of the old 1

    I love you 4

    I am sorry 4

    Please forgive me 4

    Thank you! 4

    Thank you, these are some of the feedbacks: 7

    We will discuss in this book: 11

Part I: The cause and possible cure for cancer and chronic diseases from applying Papaya, baking soda, aspirin, sugar, Vietnamese Qi Gong breathing and traditional medicine. 1

    Self-checking the health and trigger points points in the body, the hands, the foot. 2

    Chapter 1: Cells with metabolic reactions are the basic structure of all tissues and organs 5

        Table 1: Catabolic reactions 5

        Table 2: The factors that impact the catabolic reactions in the body 5

        Table 3: The signs and the effects of hypotension. 9

    Chapter 2: Hypoglycemia and hypothermia 12

        Table 4: The signs and the effects of hypoglycemia 12

        Hypothermia 15

        Table 5: The signs and the effects of hypothermia 15

Chapter 3: Possible results of metabolic disorders proves that metabolic disorders are the real cause. 17

Chapter 4: Science of the Qi 22

Table 6: Balancing Qi 22

Chapter 5: Effect of deep breathing, Vietnamse Qi Gong exercise and smoking on the glycemia. 25

Table 7: Experiments of quick, strong and deep breathing in respiration therapy 28

Table 8: Experiments of slow, gentle and deep breathing in respiration therapy 30

Table 9: Vietnamese Qi Gong instructed by master Do Duc Ngoc 33

Clapping, massaging, pressing on pain areas when having heat and enough sugar in the blood. 37

Chater 6: Applying self-healing techniques, the natural healing for pain, hypertension, hypotension, fibromyalgia, cancer, ulcer, respiratory diseases, and metabolic disorders 38

The simple techniques that give the healing for most illnesses. It is so simple that most people can do it. And this can give us a new view of most illnesses 38

A. Ten minutes to remove trigger points cause pain in the back, neck, head and shoulder 40

B. 10 minutes to reduce irritation bowel, irritation on the stomach or pain in the liver. 41

C. 10 minutes to make warm the hand and feet and the whole body..41

D. 30 minutes to have a natural sleep for the people with insomnia...42

E. Control glucose in the blood, blood pressure, metabolism of the body...42

F. Remove trigger point and balance metabolic reactions simply in three steps 42

- The first step: eat and drink first 45

- The second step: lie down and place an object on the lower abdomen..45

- Third step: clapping on trigger point until having the sensation of roughness. 47

Chapter 7: The cold, flu A, cough, asthma, bronchitis, pneumonitis, and Covid-19...49

Herbal oils for health, cold, flu, sinusitis and systemic body..49

"Keto flu", the key for the flu and the most chronic illnesses. 51

Tips to help self treating COVID-19, cold, asthma, coughing, difficult breathing, COPD, chest pain, Shortness of breath, cough with sputum.......................................52

Herbal oils for health, cold, flu, sinusitis and systemic body: head, heart, hormones, circulations...................52

A. First step: eat and drink first to warm up the body ..53

B. Second step: boosting the blood circulation, warm up the body and cut the fever by one or some of these exercises. 53

C. Third step: Removing trigger points in the lungs 55

D. Fourth step: finding and removing the trigger points on the whole body. 56

Some of traditional alternative healing techniques that help for pain, fever and systemic illnesses: 56

E. FACTS: Covid-19 mortality rate, profoundly disturbing. It is not by the virus, but it may reveal the weakness of the modern medical system. 57

Source of the oxygen in in the lungs, all health problems should check the health of the lungs 61

For self treating fever, pain, cough, phlegm, difficult breathing and many other chronic diseases: finding and removing the trigger points. 61

Chapter 8: Changing lifestyle, adequate diet is the advice for most diseases 62

Table 10: Mechanism of alternative therapies that help to prevent and heal chronic illness 63

The illnesses and diseases can be benefit from these exercises: 64

Table 11: Top ten causes of death in high income/affluent countries – lifestyle diseases 65

For self treating fever, pain, cough, phlegm, difficult breathing and many other chronic diseases: finding and removing the trigger points. 67

Some of traditional alternative healing techniques that help for pain, fever and systemic illnesses: 68

References: 70

Part II: State of Mind: Stress and Happiness. 85

Chapter 9: What happens in the body when we are in a happy state? 85

Table 12: the symptoms of excessive dopamine 87

References: 92

Chapter 10: What is happening when we are under stress? 93

Table 13: Side effects of three stress chemicals 97

Table 14: bad effects of short-term stress on body, mind, and performance 100

Table 15: The effects of long-term stress 102

Table 16: The early warning signs of mental disorders are also the symptoms of stress 105

The fifteen most common causes of death in the United States 107

Table 17: The most symptoms of stress that we can find in many patients 108

Table 18: The symptoms of Cushing's syndrome, adrenal insufficiency, and congenital adrenal hyperplasia 112

Table 19: The symptoms of epilepsy, fibromyalgia, and depression 114

References: 118

Part III: The Potential of Brain: Intuitive Mind and Gut Feelings 121

Chapter 11: How people and experts talk about gut feelings? 121

Chapter 12: Review the structure of the human brain 125

References: 127

Chapter 13: Multiple Intelligence 129

References: 131

Chapter 14: Immeasurable phenomena in one single fact 132

References: 140

Chapter 15: Mirror neuron, sleep, and EEG 141

EEG Frequency bands 141

References: 144

Part IV: Hologram: Brain, Mind, Body, Physical Heath, and Ego 145

Chapter 16: New understanding of telepathy 145

Chapter 17: The universe is a gigantic and splendidly detailed hologram of interconnected phenomena 151

We are interdependence for our happiness 161

Yin and Yang theory 165

Table 20: Yin and Yang in all phenomena 167

The first is Socrates: 169

The second is Jim Rhon: 170

The third is Adolf Hitler. 171

The fourth is Michael Jackson. 173

The fifth is the kings, heroes, and warriors 173

The sixth is you. 174

The seventh is an imagined story. 174

Chapter 18: New philosophy of relation between brain, mind, body, physical health, ego 178

Mind, body, health, life, and environment. 182

Questions to ponder to help people gain wisdom and enlightenment 183

Chapter 19: Outliers: a new level of brain, mind, physical body, and health 186

Part V: Conditioned Responses 191

Chapter 20: All the things we have are the results of conditioned responses 191

Chapter 21: Beliefs, religions, taboos and conditioned responses 197

Table 21: food, animals, religions and conditioned responses 206

References: 213

Chapter 22: Brief history of humankind 215

Table 22: Some religions in the world 226

References: 231

Chapter 23: Obsessing with characters and concepts of living environment, we forget who we are 233

Table 23: relativities between human being, cell, atom, electron, earth, solar system and the Milky Way 240

International System of Units 243

References: 249

Chapter 24: Hysteria and conditioned responses 251

References: 258

Chapter 25: The relation between mental problems, environment, and conditioned responses 259

Definition and understanding of mental disorders 260

Debating ideas about the relation between autism, ADHD and depression 267

Part VI: Belief System, Obsessed Desires, and the Work of Potential Brain 271

Chapter 26: Coding the mind, the role of practicing in learning skills 271

Chapter 27: The brain with obsessed desires 280

Chapter 28: What influence the belief system of individuals? 289

The wrong opinions of a child may become the child's belief 289

The good opinions of a child may become the child's belief 292

Chapter 29: The work of the potential mind 297

    The need for more 298

    Table 24: The videos on youtube.com help people understand the needs of human beings. 309

References 313

Part VII: Real Hunger in Abundance Living and Countless Problems 315

    Chapter 30: The real hunger of modern people and its consequences 315

        Table 25: The four causes of human problems 316

        Table 26: Basic symptoms of autism accompanied by other medical conditions 326

        Think out of the boxes: 343

        References: 346

    Chapter 31: The real cause of mental problems and social problems in older kids 347

        References: 365

    Chapter 32: Still ignoring? Autoimmune diseases and suicides are inevitable 369

        Table 27: Relief uncomfortable and best-selling OTC drugs in Britain in 2015 379

        Table 28: The top best-selling groups of the over-the-counter and natural supplements in the United States in 2016 381

Table 29: The top ten medications by sales in America are 382

The power of the focusing the mind, the power of thinking 386

Table 30: Summarization of some autoimmune diseases 388

Table 31: Relation between signs of autoimmune disease and stress 390

"The tragedies do not happen to me; I do not care" ..391

References: 397

Part VIII: Game of Mind Masters 403

Chapter 33: God does not bless any human beings. 403

Table 32: The cost of human life in the human World War II 404

Chapter 34: The killing of Jews 405

Chapter 35: Some are cheated and coded 412

Chapter 36: Worst of the worst: concepts in the funeral rituals 416

Chapter 37: The karma we have created for ourselves 419

Chapter 38: God does not need their blood to wash the human sins. 422

Well-known assassination in history 422

Chapter 39: Our gods, our Holy spirits also died because of the ignorance of his people 424

Chapter 40: How are some coded? 434

Table 33: Their farewells of warriors 435

Chapter 41: How did Hitler seduce the mind of millions of people and soldiers? 437

References: 441

Part IX: A Stressed World with Rainbow of Stress 443

Chapter 42: Stress syndrome and the rainbow of stress..443

Chapter 43: The geographical of diseases in the world....448

Chapter 44: The stressed world 455

Table 34: Top 10 American children's health concerns, 2011 466

Table 35: Attributions of cause and recurrence in long-term breast cancer survivors, 2001 475

Chapter 45: Nature does not answer or revenge human beings 476

Chapter 46: The hidden correlation 478

References: 480

Part X: Paradoxes of Mind and the Science of Achievement 488

Chapter 47: Real learning 490

Table 36: The process of learning 491

Chapter 48: What do create human beings? 492

Chapter 49: Paradoxes of the mind 495

Psychology focus on paradoxes of the mind to overcome it 495

Chapter 50: Science of achievement: mastering the mind by goals, visions, virtues, and principles 521

References: 528

Part XII: The Art of Happiness: Emotional Management and Meditation 534

Chapter 51: Mastering the mind by mastering the emotion 534

Table 37: Differences between ordinary people and successful people 537

D. The fourth way to control emotion is by taking action. 548

References: 552

Chapter 52: The role of meditation to have a healthy, happy life 553

Picture 1: sitting postures of meditation 554

Part XIII: Teaching of the Old 570

Chapter 53: The teachings of Buddha 570

The four foundations of mindfulness are: 573

Chapter 60: Understand the teaching of the old, great men 582

Table 38: Discretionary spending 2015 of America 585

Chapter 54: Gods and religions have taught us. 587

Table 39: Core teaching of some religions 587

Chapter 55: The teaching of Lao Tzu, Aesop, and Socrates 591

The teaching of Aesop 609

The teaching of Socrates 610

Ho'oponopono techniques and the combination to calm the mind 610

Chapter 56: Teaching of Benjamin Franklin 611

Chapter 57: Educators taught about the miracle of mind, principles, and lifelong learning 614

Chapter 58: Teaching of Dalai Lama 621

Chapter 59: Teaching of educators about education 624

Below are the invaluable suggestions of educators. 634

Chapter 60: We are the creators of our lives and the creators of our children 655

Table 40: The relation between abilities, problems, and stress 662

Chapter 61: Time to create heaven on earth 665

Part XIV: Questions, answers, and some advice..................674

1. The ten effective ways to help children with problems 674

2. Love is the verb, right understanding is unconditional love, how to get the right understanding? 679

3. Problem-solving skills: are you learning the root or learning tops? New view..684

4. How do parents affect their children? 689

5. I AM SORRY VICTIMS, WE ARE WRONG. 699

I love you 699

I am sorry 699

Please forgive me 699

Thank you! 699

Contents 708

www.ingramcontent.com/pod-product-compliance
Lightning Source LLC
Chambersburg PA
CBHW020851180526
45163CB00007B/2473